The Baby Solution

The Baby Solution

Your Essential Resource
for Overcoming Infertility

DANIEL KENIGSBERG, M.D.

with Lauren Hartman

AVERY
a member of Penguin Group (USA) Inc.
New York

AVERY

Published by the Penguin Group
Penguin Group (USA) Inc., 375 Hudson Street, New York, New York 10014, USA •
Penguin Group (Canada), 90 Eglinton Avenue East, Suite 700, Toronto, Ontario M4P 2Y3, Canada
(a division of Pearson Penguin Canada Inc.) • Penguin Books Ltd, 80 Strand, London WC2R 0RL, England •
Penguin Ireland, 25 St Stephen's Green, Dublin 2, Ireland (a division of Penguin
Books Ltd) • Penguin Group (Australia), 250 Camberwell Road, Camberwell, Victoria 3124,
Australia (a division of Pearson Australia Group Pty Ltd) • Penguin Books India Pvt Ltd,
11 Community Centre, Panchsheel Park, New Delhi–110 017, India • Penguin Group (NZ),
Cnr Airborne and Rosedale Roads, Albany, Auckland 1310, New Zealand (a division of
Pearson New Zealand Ltd) • Penguin Books (South Africa) (Pty) Ltd,
24 Sturdee Avenue, Rosebank, Johannesburg 2196, South Africa

Penguin Books Ltd, Registered Offices:
80 Strand, London WC2R 0RL, England

Most Avery books are available at special quantity discounts for bulk
purchase for sales promotions, premiums, fund-raising, and educational needs.
Special books or book excerpts also can be created to fit specific needs.
For details, write Penguin Group (USA) Inc. Special Markets,
375 Hudson Street, New York, NY 10014.

Library of Congress Cataloging-in-Publication Data
Kenigsberg, Daniel.
The baby solution : your essential resource for overcoming infertility /
Daniel Kenigsberg, M.D., with Lauren Hartman.
    p.   cm
Includes bibliographical references
ISBN 1-58333-264-2
1. Infertility—Popular works.   2. Human reproductive technology—Popular works.
    1. Hartman, Lauren.   II. Title.
RC889.K49   2006   2006042965
        616.6'92—dc22

Printed in the United States of America
1   3   5   7   9   10   8   6   4   2

BOOK DESIGN BY TANYA MAIBORODA

While the authors have made every effort to provide accurate telephone numbers and Internet addresses at the time of publication, neither the publisher nor the authors assume any responsibility for errors, or for changes that occur after publication. Further, the publisher does not have any control over and does not assume any responsibility for author or third-party websites or their content.

Neither the publisher nor the authors are engaged in rendering professional advice or services to the individual reader. The ideas, procedures, and suggestions contained in this book are not intended as a substitute for consulting with your physician. All matters regarding your health require medical supervision. Neither the authors nor the publisher shall be liable or responsible for any loss or damage allegedly arising from any information or suggestion in this book.

To my inspiring teachers:

J. Victor Reyniak,
for introducing me to the field

John A. Rock,
for showing me the power of determination
and high standards

J. Donald Woodruff,
who taught pathology and gave me the
foundation for understanding disease

Tom Klein,
for his insistence on evidence-based,
practical, and pure medicine

D. Lynn Loriaux,
whose brilliance and energy challenged us to
think beyond conventional treatments

Gary Hodgen,
whose uncanny ability to see the future
revolutionized reproductive medicine

Contents

Acknowledgments

I WANT TO THANK THE FOLLOWING PEOPLE FOR THEIR assistance in creating this book:

Science writer Jamie Talan and my agent, Faith Hamlin, for getting me involved in this project

Dara Stewart and Lynn Napoli, M.D., for editorial support

Jan MacDougal for illustrations

For information on male reproduction: Bruce Gilbert, M.D., Ph.D., and Scott Press, M.D.

For information on emotional and psychological health: Harriette Rovner Ferguson, LCSW, and Aviva Zigelman, MSW

For information on genetics: David Hymen, M.D.

For information about multiple pregnancy and multifetal reduction: Victor Klein, M.D.; Mark Evans, M.D.; Patricia C. Mele, RN, MSN, CNNP; and Maureen A. Doolan Boyle, executive director, MOST (Mothers of Supertwins), Inc.

For information about complementary medicine: Jacques R. Depardieu, MS, LAc, Andrea Huggler, and Lenny Izzo

For information about donor eggs and embryos and gestational carriers: Vicky Loveland, RN, and Andrea Braverman, Ph.D.

For information about IVF/infertility nursing: Karen Roach, RN

For information about finances and insurance: Adele Demsker

For information about adoption: Jeanine Castagna, JD

To the many patients who agreed to share their experiences and insights

Last, to my partners, Steven Brenner, M.D., and Kathleen Droesch, M.D., and my family for their support during the long process of writing this book

Introduction

OVER THE COURSE OF MY CAREER, I'VE WITNESSED sweeping changes in the field of infertility care, from the earliest developments in the field more than twenty-five years ago, when treatments were barely effective, to the present, when we are on the horizon of limitless possibilities for couples struggling to have children.

Throughout this time, I have been most impressed by my patients' bravery and optimism. As a young doctor, I was always amazed that people would let me take care of them. It was then that I began to understand the tremendous leap of faith people take when they place their trust in their doctors. Now, after having cared for thousands of patients, I never cease to respect my patients' heroism during the course of a treatment regimen that can be emotionally, physically, and financially grueling. Women, especially, may have to endure repeated tests and procedures, sometimes even sur-geries, to have children. It takes a certain kind of toughness and determi-nation to get through that.

I value truth and honesty. In writing this book, I don't seek to make you, the reader, enthused about getting treatment, nor do I want you to be unnecessarily discouraged about the possible results. I want to inform you of the facts about infertility treatment so that you can apply what you learn here to your own life to make a decision about treatment that is best for you. Although most people with infertility can be successfully treated, some people will not get pregnant. At best, a couple has a 50 percent chance of getting pregnant each time they try with infertility treatment, even with the most sophisticated technology. If you are older—that is, thirty-seven or over—your chances may be lower. When you consult with your doctor, it's important for you to know what your chances are, given your age and medical circumstances. It is much better to know what the odds are at the outset of treatment than to wait until you have exhausted your emotional and financial resources and your time. Whatever decision you make—whether it is to forgo treatment, to adopt a child, or to try that third in vitro fertilization (IVF)—it should be a decision based on medical facts and your considered desires.

The more knowledge you have about infertility treatment, the more control you have over this inherently uncontrollable situation. In this book, you will find not only information about state-of-the art infertility care, but also tips to help you negotiate a field where the cost of treatment is high and the business concerns of clinics and doctors can sometimes override a patient's best interests. In addition to the latest in treatment, this book will tell you how to get the most out of your insurance coverage, how to keep your relationship intact during treatment, and how to choose a doctor or a clinic that will give you the best chance of success. You'll learn about alternative means of creating your family and what's on the horizon for the future, among many other topics. You will also hear from women and men who were generous enough to share information about their experiences with infertility treatment—both the disappointments and the joys—to help you get a realistic sense of what treatment will be like. Knowing what you will face before you begin, taking control over what you can, and letting go of what you cannot control will help you get through this extraordinarily difficult time.

Doctors may also suffer the ups and downs of infertility treatment as they try to help their patients. It is sometimes frustrating to see a patient who shouldn't give up quit infertility treatment when success is likely. It's also hard to see someone struggle with repeated failures when her prognosis isn't good, though it's important to understand that each patient has the right to do as she sees fit. Of course, being an infertility specialist can bring extraordinary rewards. Even after years of practice, it is still thrilling to tell a couple that they are pregnant, to have patients return to our program to show us their big bellies, and at last to see their babies and even their grown children.

I hope you will use this book as a guide, referring to it at each stage of treatment to help you make decisions with your doctor. As you put this book away, it is my hope that you will leave treatment with a sense of closure, knowing that you did all that you could to get the best advice and treatment possible and that you made an informed decision to take the path that was right for you.

1 | Confronting Infertility

GROWING UP, ALMOST EVERYONE THINKS OF HAVING a child as inevitable. We naturally assume that we are going to be parents someday, and so before becoming a need, parenthood is understood to be a right, almost as if our children are waiting for us when we choose to have them. Even when we discover this desire later in life, perhaps after having achieved what we wanted or been disappointed in the things we sought, or when we watch friends depart into family life, it's difficult to imagine that anything could disrupt the natural course toward motherhood or fatherhood.

Very often, the intention to parent begins when a couple stops using contraception, saying, "If it happens, it happens." But this is a kind of denial, one of the first in many that must be overcome when facing a problem with conception. People are rarely indifferent to whether or not they have children. What we should really be saying is, "I want this to happen. I expect it to happen." This is much closer to the truth. Once you accept that you are trying to have a child, you will start to become aware of whether or not you are really on your way. If it becomes apparent that you are not, you can get help early when the chances of being able to have a child are better than if you delay treatment.

FACING FEARS ABOUT INFERTILITY

By the time most people go to see an infertility specialist, they are frustrated and scared. Most are less frightened of the medical procedures they might endure than of what a diagnosis of infertility might do to their lives. The prospect of being infertile, of facing an unfamiliar world of medical tests and procedures, and of acute emotional and financial vulnerabilities, can start to unravel every thread in an otherwise planned and secure life. Exposing your intimate relationship to anyone, much less to medical doctors, can feel threatening. And depending on your insurance coverage, the cost of treatment can actually be financially threatening, often adding up to more than a couple—and certainly a prospective single parent—can easily afford.

Among the many losses that infertility treatment can bring is the loss of control over your time. In vitro fertilization (IVF) is an intensive medical procedure; it isn't like going to the dentist during office hours. You may have to go to your doctor's office every day for a certain number of days every month, very possibly causing you problems at work or at home. You may have to take medications at very specific times, perhaps medications that cause mood swings. Couples may come under considerable stress when a treatment they thought would take a matter of months doesn't happen quickly. The emotional, financial, physical, and spiritual challenges that infertility treatment can create in your life can feel overwhelming. It's no wonder that couples find it hard to raise the issue with each other.

When you don't conceive right away, regrets can surface, and these can be hard to deal with, too. If you have had an abortion in the past, you may wonder if it hurt your chances of getting pregnant. With rare exceptions, pregnancy termination is almost never a cause of infertility. If you are in your midthirties or in your forties, you may regret not having started to plan your family earlier. With most things in life—and especially with infertility—looking back is counterproductive. You are who you are today because of everything that you have done up to this point. Maybe there was a better time in your life to start trying to get pregnant, but if you did have children earlier, you would be an entirely different person now. You can't do much about the past, but you can be effective in the present, making the best decisions you can, based on the options you have before you.

Single women and lesbian couples may start trying to get pregnant with inseminations, never suspecting that they have infertility. Still, some women who initially believe that being a lesbian or being unmarried is incompatible with childrearing come to find out that it's not, and choose to parent later on in life. You already know that medical intervention is going to be a part of creating your family, and so you may be in a better position than heterosexuals or couples, at least from a psychological point of view, to undergo the often rigorous process of infertility care with determination and perhaps fewer expectations to reconsider.

In the end, it's important to remember that infertility is a medical condition. You didn't ask for or cause your infertility, just as people don't ask to have any other serious health problem. While you may be worried that you do have a health problem, the best way to approach any medical issue is to find out what the problem is and what your options are to treat it. Find the best medical care you can and put together a plan of action to tackle it. This book will show you how to do that.

> *At first you were a couple standing alone at the altar. Now you are standing alone with the next phase of life ahead of you, and you're having a problem getting there. That's a very hard thing to accept. Then, when you realize that you are going to accept it and go for help, that help is not some-*

thing that you can easily fit into your schedule. All of a sudden you have to give up part of your life and your work. —ANN

You have to have a strong marriage to go through fertility treatment. You're scared. You feel like you have no control over what's happening. You feel inadequate because you can't have a baby on your own. Everybody and his uncle is telling you, "Have a glass of wine. That's all you need." You understand way too much biology, about what happens inside your skin, and no one gets it. It's almost like a secret clan, women who experience fertility problems. I can tell you the rudest question in the world is, "So when are you going to have a baby?" —CYNTHIA

I had a child already and then I had multiple miscarriages. I was thirty-six or thirty-seven at the time I decided that I wanted another child, but I said to myself, there is no chance I'm ever doing IVF. I thought, "I'm not taking drugs. I have a healthy child. I'm perfectly happy with what I have. There's no way I'm doing that to my body." But as you get into the process, it becomes something that you just can't drop. You are determined. The next thing you know, you're taking all these drugs. —SARI

WHAT IS INFERTILITY?

Contrary to popular assumptions, infertility isn't just a woman's issue. Infertility affects men and women equally, and each partner in a couple may contribute to that individual couple's infertility. About 40 percent of the time, it's male infertility that's causing the problem, and 40 percent of the time it's female infertility. In another 10 percent of cases, combined problems cause infertility. Infertility can also be unexplained, accounting for the last 10 percent of cases. Unexplained doesn't mean untreatable. Couples with unexplained infertility—where both partners have normal results on all the requisite fertility tests and still don't conceive—do just as well as, and sometimes even better than, other couples in infertility treatment.

Despite both partners' potential to contribute to infertility, the medical definition centers on a woman's age for reasons we'll talk about in a moment.

The standard medical definition of infertility for couples in which the woman is under thirty-five is one year of attempted pregnancy without success. If you are under thirty-five, your doctor may advise you to keep trying for a year before seeking infertility care. If you're thirty-five to thirty-six, the diagnosis is the same, but the standard recommendation is that you see an infertility specialist, called a reproductive endocrinologist (RE), for initial testing after six months of trying to get pregnant without success.

If you're thirty-seven or older, see a reproductive endocrinologist soon. There's no time to waste. As you age, fertility declines significantly and rapidly. No matter what your age, you may want to see a doctor sooner rather than later when you know that you have a condition that could be related to your fertility. If you have endometriosis, talk to the doctor who diagnosed you, if you can. Find out whether your fallopian tubes are affected. Even women with significant amounts of endometriosis can be fertile, but it helps to know the extent of your endometriosis.

If your menstrual cycles are irregular—for example, they are very far apart and/or you are on birth control pills to regulate your cycles—an infertility workup can tell you whether you are ovulating. (See Chapter 3.) If you are trying to have a child and you have had two or more miscarriages, see a doctor for complete pregnancy-loss workup. (See Chapter 10.)

Women who experience infertility after having already had a child are said to have *secondary infertility.* Here again, if you are under thirty-five, your doctor will tell you to keep trying to get pregnant for a year before seeing an infertility specialist, but again, even with secondary infertility, see a reproductive endocrinologist early on if you have a condition such as endometriosis or if you have had two miscarriages or more.

What Causes Infertility?

If, like most people, you spent your young adulthood trying *not* to get pregnant, you may be taken aback when you learn just how inefficient human reproduction can be. Without infertility, the average couple has about a 20 percent chance of conceiving during each menstrual cycle. When you have a fertility problem, the chances of getting pregnant are lower.

Ovulation dysfunction is the most common cause of infertility in women. Failing to ovulate regularly or at all, a low supply of egg-producing follicles in your ovaries, and/or poor egg quality are the most common female fertility problems. Other major factors for women include:

- blocked or damaged fallopian tubes, which make it difficult for sperm to reach an egg for fertilization or for an embryo (a fertilized egg) to make its way to the uterus to implant and grow (see Chapter 2 to learn more about the reproduction process);
- endometriosis, a condition in which endometrial tissue (the tissue lining the uterus normally shed during menstruation) is found adhered to organs outside of the uterus; and
- uterine problems, including fibroids, polyps, and uterine structural problems.

Male factor infertility can include a low (or no) sperm count, and problems with the quality of sperm and/or with the ability of the sperm to reach and penetrate an egg. It's not uncommon for couples to have more than one fertility problem, such as when a woman has blocked tubes and her partner has a low sperm count. In Chapters 5 and 6, we will look closely at the causes of infertility for women and men.

If You Have Infertility, You Are Not Alone

Having infertility—or even thinking that you have infertility—can be lonely, especially when everyone else seems to have babies without trying, when you feel that you are running out of time and options, and when there are few supportive people in your life. But chances are, you do know someone who can understand what you're going through. About one out of every six couples in the United States has experienced infertility. According to the Centers for Disease Control (CDC), more people than ever are turning to assisted reproductive technology (ART) to have their babies. The increased use and success of ART has resulted in a dramatic rise in the number of babies born through ART, growing 94 percent from 20,921 babies conceived through ART in 1996 to a staggering 40,687 in 2001.[1]

Does this mean that we are more infertile now than in the past? Not necessarily. It may just be that our ability to treat infertility has helped to identify more people who could have used treatment in the past. Are there environmental factors affecting fertility? In some populations, there is a documented decline in fertility among men, a decline that suggests the possibility of an environmental influence, but what that influence is remains to be seen. It's likely that the increased use of ART is due to the increasing numbers of people delaying their first child until later in life.

AGE AND FERTILITY: WHAT YOU NEED TO KNOW

For women, thirty-seven is a turning point in infertility care, because it's at this age that fertility starts to decline quickly. You are significantly more fertile at thirty-seven than you are at thirty-eight. At thirty-eight, you are more fertile than at thirty-nine. Conversely, these yearly changes aren't as significant when you are younger. Not only do you become less fertile as you age, you are less likely to get pregnant with infertility treatment. But let's be clear, you are *less* likely to succeed. It's not at all impossible. Every body is truly different. Some older women who think they are infertile because of the diminished number and quality of their eggs get pregnant.

Even if you're not ovulating, you may not be in perimenopause, the transition into menopause that usually happens between the ages of forty and fifty. If you aren't in perimenopause, you may just need some help ovulating to get pregnant. If you are ovulating, there may be a problem with your coital technique, in which case intrauterine inseminations (IUI) may help you conceive. (See Chapter 8.) On the other hand, your fallopian tubes may be blocked. If your tubes are blocked, you are unlikely to get pregnant without infertility treatment. But how do you know? An infertility workup, which includes basic testing of your reproductive status, will help you to find out. (See Chapter 3.) Without at least some testing to find out what's wrong, you may be wasting valuable time trying to conceive when you have a barrier to conception that can be corrected.

I think it's appropriate for a physician to say, "Don't wait too long to start having a family. It may not be as easy as you think." I don't think I ever heard that. I don't think people know that it's harder every year and that scientifically it's been shown to be harder to conceive after a certain age. The decline in fertility from twenty-five to twenty-nine is less than the decline from thirty to thirty-four. —BETH

There are statistics and then there are people. I cried in the beginning. I said my daughter is calling to me. The nurses looked at me with that knowing look that said, "We'll see," because they've seen so many failures. It was so satisfying to walk in with my baby and perhaps change their outlook for the next person who walks in there at forty years old. Nothing is impossible. —KATHLEEN

Why Age Is a Factor for Women

From time to time we are reminded of the changes age brings. In my early fifties, I am not as strong or as fast as I used be. I don't see as well as I used to, and I'm subject to conditions like heart disease and some types of cancer that would be rare in a person half my age. Arguably, medicine has improved dramatically over the last century, and our diets may be better than in the past. But although we may look and feel better at forty or fifty than our parents did at the same age, men and women at midlife are still subject to the same bodily changes. This aging process is especially critical for women, who are born with all the eggs they will ever produce.

Immature eggs wait to be ovulated, typically one a month, from the onset of menstruation at adolescence until you reach your last period at menopause. It's not the number of eggs that you have that matters to fertility, it's their age. Not only are you born with all the eggs you will ever have, your eggs are stored in the first stage of division on what's called a *spindle*, a microtubule apparatus that also deteriorates with age. This is a vulnerable state in which to store chromosomes in a cell and a second reason why older eggs tend toward chromosomal and metabolic abnormalities that can result in no pregnancy, miscarriage, or a pregnancy with a chromosomal abnormality, such as Down syndrome.

You may already know that it can be harder to time intercourse for conception as you get older. As you get older, your cycles can shorten, bouncing around, for instance, from twenty-eight days one month to twenty-six days the next month, and then twenty-five days the next. As this shift occurs, you are actually ovulating earlier in your monthly cycle. If your cycles are shortening, it is important to monitor them and time your intercourse earlier in your cycle. You may have conceived your teenager on day fourteen or fifteen of your cycle, but your new child may have to be conceived on day nine or ten. Having relations more frequently in the second quarter of your cycle ups the odds of conceiving. In Chapter 2, you'll find tips on timing intercourse before ovulation for the best chance of conceiving.

If you are a woman in your late thirties or forties, try to maintain a sense of realistic optimism. Don't delay seeing a reproductive endocrinologist and *don't give up hope* until you have examined all of your options, allowing yourself to be the best judge of the choices that are right for you.

Why His Age Is Less Important

Assuming that a man has no medical conditions, such as hypertension (high blood pressure) or diabetes—which is growing by leaps and bounds in the United States—age may not be a factor in a man's ability to father a child until he reaches his midfifties. About that time, there is an increased risk of chromosomal abnormalities in his sperm. If you are pregnant and your partner is over the age of fifty-five, your doctor will likely recommend amniocentesis to screen for fetal abnormalities.

High blood pressure and certain high blood pressure medications, such as calcium channel blockers, can be associated with decreased sperm function. Diabetes can create vascular problems that lead to sexual dysfunction as well as nerve damage that can cause retrograde ejaculation, a condition wherein semen does not leave the body through the urethra on ejaculation but returns to the bladder.

As a man ages, his testosterone levels gradually decline. Age-related declines in testosterone can lead to a lessened feeling of well-being for men. Men with low testosterone levels are sometimes given testosterone therapy to address decreased energy. While lower testosterone shouldn't directly affect a man's fertility unless it affects his ability to perform sexually, testosterone replacement therapy dramatically lowers his sperm count, because it shuts off the hormones that promote sperm production. This happened to a patient of mine who had a child with his wife through egg donation. When he and his wife came back to do egg donation for a second child, we did a semen analysis and his sperm count was zero! It turns out that he was feeling sluggish and his doctor had put him on twice weekly injections of testosterone, which decimated his sperm count.

I'M DOING EVERYTHING RIGHT BUT I'M STILL NOT PREGNANT: WHAT NOW?

Maybe you have tried for months to get pregnant or maybe you have been having relations for years without contraception. If you think you should be pregnant but you're not, see a doctor. If you are under thirty-five, you may want to start by talking with your general ob-gyn for testing. But see a reproductive endocrinologist if you are thirty-seven or older; if the intervals between your periods are irregular or if you are not menstruating; if you had two or more miscarriages; if you were treated for cancer; or if you needed hormones to assist you through puberty. You should also see an RE if you have been diagnosed with pelvic inflammatory disease. Chapter 3 will give you an overview of all the basic tests you need—and tests you don't need—to find out if infertility is the issue. Once you know whether or not you have a problem, you can decide what course of action is best for you.

Before You Start Infertility Treatment: What to Know, What to Do

One of the best things you can do for yourself before considering infertility treatment is to find out what infertility care may be like for you and make a plan of action based on the results of initial diagnostic tests, your age, your insurance coverage and financial resources, the time you can devote to treatment, and the course of treatment that makes the most sense to you and your doctor. Jumping into treatment without a plan can mean a loss of valuable fertile time and money, as couples can sometimes spend months, even years, in the wrong course of treatment.

Make Sure Your Treatment Is Based on Your Complete Initial Evaluation

Without a complete workup, you can waste valuable fertile time in treatment by not knowing the cause of your infertility and trying to get pregnant based on a general approach to care rather than on your specific medical problem or problems.

Plan to Be in Treatment for Six to Twelve Months

Most women or couples should either have their treatment resolved within a year or should have moved on to the most sophisticated ART treatments, such as IVF and donor eggs. Once you plan to be in treatment for a year, you can then break up that year into three- to six-month blocks of time. You can look at your likely reproductive issue, try an appropriate technique for your diagnosis for three to six months, and if that doesn't work, go to the next step, which will include three to six months of another treatment.

Understand the Risks of Miscarriage and Ectopic Pregnancy

Whether or not you are receiving infertility care, there is about a 20 percent chance that your pregnancy will result in miscarriage. That number can exceed 50 percent in women over forty. Most of these miscarriages are unpreventable and happen because the pregnancy isn't developing. (For more information, see Chapter 10.)

Know the Risk of Multiple Pregnancy

Anyone who receives ovarian stimulation (fertility drugs used to stimulate ovulation of more than one egg each month) should know about the risk of multiple pregnancy. Parents pregnant with what are called *higher-order multiples* often face the prospect of terminating some of the pregnancies to try to improve outcomes for the remaining fetuses. I recommend that all people entering infertility care honestly examine their feelings about this subject and receive counseling on the issue before going ahead with treatment. (See Chapter 11.)

Write Down Your Treatment Goals

Is your desire to have a child who is genetically related to you or would you consider donor eggs, donor sperm, or adoption, if necessary? You can use your thoughts about what you want from treatment as a kind of touchstone or guide as you go through it. You may find that your goals change, or that you change during treatment. You can revise your goals. It's important to allow yourself flexibility. Try not to think of disappointments in treatment as failure. Remember that there are aspects of treatment you can control and others you cannot control. Try to focus on what you can control.

Consider Whether You Need an Exit Plan

If you are thirty-seven or older, and especially if you are in your early to midforties, it can be helpful to think about alternatives, such as using eggs from a donor early in your treatment. Sperm donation is an alternative for heterosexual couples in which the male partner has severe infertility or a genetic condition that is passed down through the male. Sometimes couples cannot afford the expense of in vitro fertilization (IVF) with intra-cytoplasmic sperm injection (ICSI), a technique in which a single sperm is injected into an egg to increase the chance of fertilization. Some consider donor insemination when they experience other complicating factors, such as when a man must undergo surgery to have his sperm retrieved. Adoption is also an option. You will find an overview of alternatives in Chapter 12. Be honest with yourself. If you have hesitations, respect them and consider that these alternatives may not be the right choice for you. If you are interested in them as possibilities, start your research early so that you don't reach an end point in treatment without a sense of what you will do next.

Check Your Finances

Before you do anything else to prepare financially, check your insurance to find out whether you have coverage for infertility care, and if so, what is covered. (See Chapter 15.) Take a hard look at your resources and decide what you will and will not spend in treatment, setting limits before you start.

I thought all I needed was one IVF. I figured we'd have twins on the first time, because my husband only wanted one and I wanted two. I thought I'd have one pregnancy and one maternity leave, and life would be grand. After all, medical technology is so amazing now, right? We did insemination for quite a while. I needed a myomectomy (fibroid removal) before IVF. The first IVF worked, but I had a miscarriage at seven weeks. And then we had four more in vitro rounds that didn't work. A lot of people just take IVF for granted, but it doesn't always work. You like to hope it does, because if you don't hope that it is going to go work then you wouldn't even bother to try.
　　　　　　　　　　　　　　　　　　　　　　　　　　—REBECCA

I think you really have to figure out how you are going to deal with disappointment. You think after the first time, after the second time, "I'm going to get pregnant." After the fifth time, I still said, "I'm going to get pregnant." I even used somebody else's embryos. I kept thinking, "I'm going to get pregnant. I'm going to get pregnant this time," and it never happened. —MEG

PREPARE YOUR BODY FOR INFERTILITY TREATMENT AND PREGNANCY

Before planning to get pregnant, take care of routine medical exams, especially those that are more complicated during pregnancy, and take precautions to protect the health of a potentially developing embryo or fetus.

• If you smoke, quit. Smoking is the primary lifestyle detriment to fertility. Women smokers have an earlier age of menopause than nonsmokers. Smoking not only damages the ovaries, but can also contribute to higher incidences of pregnancy loss and ectopic pregnancy. Babies whose mothers smoked have a higher incidence of low birth weight than women who did not smoke during pregnancy. Smoking can damage the blood supply to the penis, increasing the incidence of erectile dysfunction in men who smoke. Smoking may also be detrimental to the offspring of fathers who smoke.[2]

- Ask yourself if weight is an issue. If you have a body mass index (BMI) greater than 30, your chance of succeeding with fertility care is statistically lower than women who are not overweight. This is because you are more likely to be insulin resistant and to have problems with ovulation associated with insulin resistance. You may need higher doses of fertility medication to stimulate ovulation for IVF, and surgery can be more difficult. We also know that a woman with less than 17 percent body fat may not ovulate. This often happens to athletes, for example marathon runners. A woman who is anorexic can also stop ovulating and menstruating. It's easy to find out your BMI. Ask your doctor for a BMI chart or search the Internet for the many BMI charts available online.

- Update your Pap smear. You should have a Pap smear within the year you begin trying to conceive.

- Test for diabetes. If you do have diabetes, work to bring it under control.

- If you are over thirty-five, have your annual mammogram. You should have a baseline mammogram at thirty-five and a yearly screening after forty. If you get pregnant, it may be more than a year until you can have another mammogram, as you will want to avoid exposing your developing fetus to radiation. A diagnosis of breast cancer is traumatic and life changing. Although rare, a diagnosis of breast cancer during pregnancy is extraordinarily tragic, as pregnancy can exacerbate breast cancer.

- Do any anticipated dental work. Dental work is more complicated when you're pregnant. Your gums are different, and there are limits to the local anesthetics dentists can use to treat you when you are pregnant. It would be a shame to go through your infertility treatment, finally get pregnant, and then have complications with this aspect of your heath care, when you could have taken care of your dental work before conception.

- If you are trying to get pregnant, make sure your ob-gyn or reproductive endocrinologist provides you with routine screening tests, including a check of your blood type and count, your iron level, hepatitis C and B, HIV, and sexually transmitted diseases.

- Have a TORCH titer test. TORCH refers to the diseases toxoplasmosis, rubella (or German measles), cytomegalovirus, and herpes. These diseases are associated with increased risk of miscarriage, and, for some, harm to your infant.

- Have your thyroid tested. There is a correlation between an underactive thyroid and impaired mental development of a fetus. (See Chapter 3.)

- Get tested for genetically inherited disease. Ask your ob-gyn what tests you need given your age, racial and ethnic background, and family history.

- If you are a teacher, get tested for fifth disease, which is very common among young children. It won't hurt a healthy young child, but can cause serious problems in a developing fetus.

- Avoid hair dye and beauty salons. Walk into a beauty salon, what do you smell? No doubt you can recall the strong smell of . . . chemicals. You are indeed exposing yourself to particulate chemicals. While there is no evidence that people who work in beauty parlors have shorter lifetimes, it is my bias to advise patients to limit chemical exposure, including exposure from beauty products, whenever possible.

- Avoid sushi and deli meats. Sushi may contain parasites. Deli meats and soft cheeses contain a type of bacteria called *Listeria*, which has been linked to miscarriages. Avoid fish that contain mercury.

- Take prenatal vitamins, the most important of which is folic acid. All you need to prevent neural tube defects, such as spina bifida, is 400 micrograms at minimum and from 800 to 1,000 micrograms (about a milligram) of folic acid daily. In addition to supplements, you can find folic acid in leafy green vegetables. Many foods are fortified with folic acids, so check your labels.

- Increase your calcium to keep your bones strong during pregnancy, either by taking calcium supplements or eating dairy products, or both.

- If you don't get sunlight or eat a balanced diet, take vitamin D. It helps you absorb calcium. Milk and salmon are good sources of vitamin D.
- Exercise moderately. Exercise is never a bad idea, unless it causes changes in your menstrual cycle, as might be the case with high-stress athletes.

LEARNING TO INTEGRATE INFERTILITY TREATMENT INTO YOUR LIFE

It may seem like a tall order, but the more you can integrate infertility treatment into your routine, the easier it will be to get through treatment. Try not to focus all of your energy on your infertility care. This is very hard to do, because you are spending time, money, and energy trying to get pregnant. Still, realize that worry doesn't make infertility problems better. Find out what helps you relieve stress. For some it's working, socializing, and going about their normal routine. Others find that exercise or practices like yoga, meditation, or biofeedback help to relieve stress. Find out what works for you and try to get on with the business of living as best you can.

You can have children. Some people get pregnant without treatment, some get pregnant quickly with treatment, and some may undergo many attempts before finally getting pregnant. Even people who do not get pregnant with infertility care can have a family with new options such as donor eggs or donor sperm. Along your journey, there will be lots of new information, new insights, and perhaps even new thoughts about what you value as you plan your family. Whether or not you really have infertility, you will come through this difficult time knowing more about your body, your health, and what really matters to you. Try to find a good doctor, and remember that you are always in charge of the decisions you make and that those decisions can have an impact on you for years to come.

2 | Reproduction Quick and Easy

BEFORE YOU CAN FULLY UNDERSTAND THE WAY INFER-
tility treatment works, you must first have an understanding of how the
female reproductive system works. In this chapter, you will find the basic
information you need to better understand your treatment.

FEMALE REPRODUCTION

The female reproductive system begins with the ovaries. The two ovaries
are the organs that contain your eggs, which carry the genetic material you
will pass on to your children. The ovaries are inside your abdominal cavity. Each month, one ovary typically releases one egg during ovulation. In
order for a woman to become pregnant, the egg must be fertilized with

sperm and then transported to the uterus to implant. The fallopian tubes are needed to transport the released egg or the fertilized egg (called an *embryo*) from the ovary to the uterus. *Fertilization* (fusing of the sperm and egg) actually takes place in the fallopian tubes. There, the embryo will begin developing for three to five days. The fallopian tube will then transport the embryo to the uterus, where it will implant in a uterine wall and grow into a pregnancy. Typically, pregnancy lasts about thirty-eight weeks from the time of implantation to delivery. At delivery, the baby is expelled from the uterus through the cervix (the opening of the uterus) into the vagina, which is the birth canal, and then through the vaginal opening.

A woman is born with all the eggs she will ever produce. Even as a baby, millions of eggs (*oocytes*) wait in her ovaries in an early state of development. But most will die before having a chance to mature and ovulate. By the time she reaches puberty, she will have about 200,000 eggs in each ovary. From the time of her first menstruation at adolescence to her last at menopause, she will release between 400 and 500 eggs.

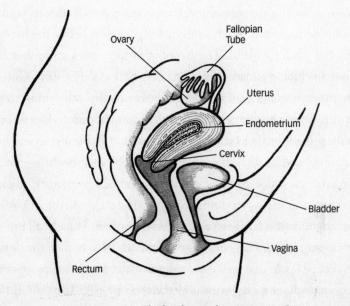

FIGURE I. *The female reproductive system*

When undergoing assisted reproduction, you'll hear a lot about follicles. Your *follicles* are essentially fluid-filled sacs in the ovaries that contain the eggs that will ripen and will be released through ovulation. Each month, many of these follicles begin development within the ovary, but usually only one will mature. This follicle is known as the "dominant" follicle. This follicle is also called the *preovulatory, primary,* or *lead follicle.*

Your menstrual cycle comprises two cycles that are tightly coordinated: the *ovarian cycle,* in which your brain and ovaries communicate to correctly time ovulation, and your *uterine cycle.* The uterine cycle prepares your uterus to receive and nurture a fertilized egg and, alternatively, to slough off the uterine lining and clean itself in the process known as menstruation. The average menstrual cycle lasts about twenty-eight days, although normal cycles can range from twenty-one to thirty-five days.

The Ovarian Cycle: Your Hormones and Ovulation

The hypothalamus, pituitary gland, and ovaries rule the ovarian cycle. The hypothalamus is an area at the base of your brain that controls major body functions, including appetite, thirst, temperature, sexual activity, your emotions, and the functions of your internal organs. Just below the hypothalamus sits the pituitary gland. The hypothalamus secretes a number of vital hormones, including gonadotropin-releasing hormone (GnRH). GnRH signals the pituitary gland, which sits right below the hypothalamus, to release follicle-stimulating hormone. Follicle-stimulating hormone does just that—it stimulates the follicles in your ovaries to mature. Typically, several follicles will be stimulated at the same time. As the follicles grow, they produce a form of estrogen called *estradiol* in anticipation of a pregnancy, thickening the lining of your uterus (endometrium) to create a hospitable environment in which to nurture a fertilized egg, called an *embryo.* Usually, all but one of the developing follicles degenerates each month. Remember, the dominant follicle is the follicle that will eventually ovulate. If you look at pictures of follicles, you will see an egg surrounded closely by cells. Later on, fluid suddenly surrounds the egg, as if the egg were a little island in a bay. It's the amount of the fluid, not the size of the egg, that grows. Follicles can grow from 1 to 2.5 centimeters before they ovulate.

Just before ovulation, estradiol levels peak and the dominant follicle pushes against the ovary, forming a tiny blister on the ovary's surface through which the ovulated egg is ready to burst. The great surge of estradiol from the ovaries stimulates the hypothalamus to signal the pituitary to lower the amount of FSH and start making *luteinizing hormone* (LH). It is the surge of LH that stimulates ovulation and final egg maturation. As the egg emerges from the ovary, it is literally picked up by the fimbriated (or finger-like) ends of the fallopian tube, which sweep over the egg and draw it into the fallopian tube.

Ovulation is traumatic. When the egg is expelled, it breaks through the ovary's surface like a volcanic eruption. There is a small amount of bleeding from the ovary. Soon the follicle fills with blood, forming an organized clot, and the cells that line the follicle transform into luteal cells, which are the ovarian cells that secrete progesterone. The ovulated follicle becomes a glandular structure known as the *corpus luteum,* literally "yellow body," which continues to emit estrogen but now also pumps out progesterone, which prepares the uterine lining for implantation of the embryo. The corpus luteum is yellow in part because it is laden with fats (lipids).

The ovary has its own blood supply. When luteinization (the transformation of the follicle to the corpus luteum) takes place, this blood supply enhances the secretion of progesterone. This is called the *luteal phase* of your cycle. If you get pregnant, the embryo will implant in the uterus, and the corpus luteum will continue making estrogen and progesterone to support the embryo until a placenta develops. (See Figure 2 on page 22.) If you don't get pregnant, the corpus luteum withers. This is followed by a decrease in hormone levels and menstruation as the endometrium is sloughed off on the first day of your next cycle.

It's not always easy to tell if you are ovulating, but there are signs that you may *not* be ovulating, including:

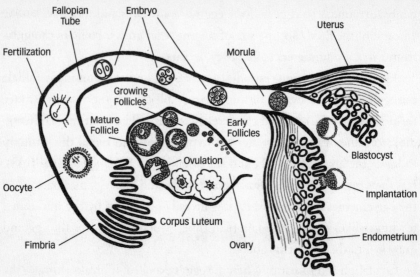

FIGURE 2. *Ovulation, fertilization, and implantation*

The egg develops in the ovary. It is then released at ovulation and picked up by the fimbria at the end of the fallopian tube. A sperm fertilizes the egg in the fallopian tube. As it travels down the fallopian tube toward the uterus, the fertilized egg becomes a developing embryo. Soon after entering the uterus at the blastocyst stage (the 5th or 6th day of embryonic development), the embryo attaches and implants into the wall of the uterus, beginning a pregnancy.

- You have irregular periods that seem to happen "out of the blue."
- You used to have PMS and now you don't. Signs of PMS include bloating, cramping, moodiness, food cravings, breast tenderness, and tingling. Signs of PMS are due to exposure to progesterone during the second half of your cycle. When progesterone is present, you are ovulating. If you have regular periods and even one symptom of PMS, you are most likely ovulating.

Cramps are a good sign. Menstrual cramps are caused by prostaglandin in the muscular walls of the uterus. Generally induced by progesterone, prostaglandin causes the uterine muscles to contract in order to expel the uterine lining during your period. Periods with ovulation are usually crampier than uterine bleeding not caused by ovulation, called *anovulatory* periods. Less pain may mean less chance of ovulating. In a nutshell, if you have relatively painful periods, regular cycles, and PMS, you are probably ovulating. Periods so painful that you miss work or school, though, may be a sign of endometriosis. (See Chapter 5.)

If your cycle is twenty-one days, you may be ovulating around day seven of your cycle. The concern with shorter cycles is whether you are going to build enough uterine lining to be receptive to implantation, having just shed it in menstruation. If your cycles are longer than thirty-five days, you may not be ovulating often enough during the year to be fertile. If you think this is true for you, talk to your doctor.

The Uterine Cycle: Your Uterus Prepares for Pregnancy

As your brain and ovaries prepare for the release of an egg at ovulation, your uterus prepares for the potential arrival of the fertilized egg, called the *embryo*, for implantation.

To understand the uterine cycle, it is helpful to remember that day one of your cycle is the first day of your period. The whole of your endometrial (uterine) lining sheds with blood during menstruation. Estradiol levels produced by the ovaries begin to rise, stimulating the rebuilding of your uterine lining in preparation for a new implantation. At about four to five days after the first day of your period, the glands of your uterine lining and the connective tissue between them, called the *stroma*, begin to grow. Blood vessels grow in the tissue. As these glands get longer, they extend almost from the base of the endometrium to its surface, which is the inner part of the uterus. This is called the *proliferative phase* of the uterine cycle.

Just after ovulation, the corpus luteum formed in the ovary drives the final stages of preparation for implantation, pulsing progesterone along with plenty of estradiol. A nutrient called *glycogen* is secreted into the uterus to aid implantation of the embryo. In the second half of the uterine cycle, called the *secretory phase*, the cells, once lengthened and filled with glycogen, become exhausted and flat, and the tissue, or stroma, is shed.

During the secretory phase, there are two things that can happen: you can get pregnant, in which case the corpus luteum continues making progesterone, or you don't get pregnant and the uterine lining is expelled, and a new cycle begins. After about seven to ten days of working, the corpus luteum can no longer function on its own. It needs a new source of stimulation to keep going. If you are pregnant, that source is the hormone human chorionic gonadotropin (hCG) produced by the placenta. The hormone hCG can be detected in your system about a week to ten days after fertilization.

MALE REPRODUCTION

A man's testicles, or testes, are the equivalent of a woman's ovaries. Just as the ovary produces both hormones and eggs, you can think of the testis as being a factory for testosterone and sperm. FSH and LH from the pituitary also in-

Not Just Chutes and Marbles: Your Reproductive System Is Active

A woman's reproductive organs are not passive structures awaiting entry of active sperm. Cervical mucus, or cervical fluid, admits and conducts sperm into the uterus toward the fallopian tubes where implantation takes place, and far from being merely a potential space, the uterus is made primarily of muscle tissue that can assist in implantation.

The uterus is influenced by progesterone. Progesterone relaxes the uterus and changes the waves inside the uterine cavity. In the first phase of your cycle, from the first day of your period until ovulation, the waves move from the top (the *fundus*) of the uterus to the bottom (the *cervix*). At menstruation, which begins the cycle, the uterine lining is shed through the cervix away from the body. But at ovulation, when progesterone appears, the waves reverse. Exactly then, when conception is possible, the uterus can move sperm up into its cavity toward the fallopian tube. A Japanese study looked very meticulously at the placement of embryos in the uterus at the time of in vitro fertilization (IVF). Consistently, the embryos implanted either where they were placed or higher. They almost never moved down.[1] And this accords perfectly with the direction of the waves in the uterine cavity after ovulation.

In the same way, the egg released from the ovary does not simply roll down the fallopian tube, but is assisted by *cilia,* microscopic hairlike projections that line the tube, and the muscular contractions of the tube itself, which becomes more muscular the closer it is to the uterus. Fluid produced by the fallopian tube nurtures the embryo and prevents it from sticking within the tube so it can progress to the uterine cavity, where it will implant and develop.

fluence the testes. Just as elevated FSH levels can signal ovarian failure in a woman, elevated FSH levels in a man may indicate testicular failure.

The testicles develop in the abdomen early in fetal life, gradually descending into the scrotum, outside the body, where the temperature is slightly lower. Sperm begin life inside the seminiferous tubules. These microscopic canals coiled inside the testes are lined with specialized Sertoli cells, which support the development of immature germ cells, called *spermatocytes*. Each spermatocyte has its own Sertoli cell to support it. Testosterone is made by the Leydig cells, which are grouped between the seminiferous tubules. Only a relatively small volume of Leydig cells are needed to supply a man with all the testosterone he will ever need.

The seminiferous tubules account for most of the mature testicle's volume. If stretched out to their full length, the seminiferous tubules would on average be about twenty feet long. While there is no relationship between the size of a man's testes and testosterone, there is a correlation between the size of a man's testicles and the content of the seminiferous tubules. A man with relatively small testes may have plenty of testosterone but very few sperm.

It takes about seventy-six days for an immature spermatocyte to become a mature sperm cell, but this process is continual. Men replenish their sperm daily, making millions of sperm in an attempt to ensure that one will penetrate and fuse with an egg. Not all sperm in a man's ejaculate are motile, that is, capable of swimming to the egg. The average ejaculate is between 2 and 5 milliliters (about $^2/_5$ of a teaspoon to a teaspoon), containing about 60 million sperm per milliliter. Only half of those may be motile. Even so, the average ejaculate contains from 60 to 150 million *moving* sperm. More volume to the ejaculate does not equate with more fertility.

Maturing each step of the way, sperm migrate from the seminiferous tubules to the tubules that travel to the epididymis, a coiled network of tubes that contain developing sperm. There, they are stored and continue to mature. Sperm must develop from immature round cells with no tail to mature spermatozoa with a head, a midpiece, and a tail. This takes approximately seventy-six days. By the time sperm leave the testes, they have their tails, but they continue to develop even through the vas deferens, the long tubes that transport semen to the urethra. The vas deferens exits the testicles and goes up behind the bladder, where it then empties into the

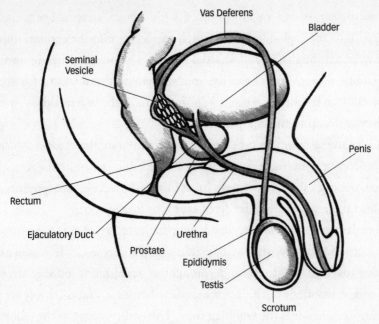

FIGURE 3. *The male reproductive system*

urethra in an area between the prostate and the bladder. The urethra carries the sperm out of the body through the penis.

Covering the head of the sperm is the *acrosomal cap*. This coating contains enzymes to help the sperm penetrate the *zona pellucida*, the egg's protective "shell." The chemical change that allows for penetration is called the *acrosome reaction*. As far as we know at present, the sperm's midpiece and tail simply provide the sperm cell with energy and ability to move.

Upon orgasm, contractions of the epididymis and the vas deferens force the sperm to the urethra, where the seminal vesicles add seminal fluid. Over 95 percent of the ejaculate comes from the seminal vesicles, which also contain the fructose that provides the semen with its protective alkalinity.

FERTILIZATION: WHEN EGG AND SPERM MEET

Contractions of the penis force the ejaculate out of a man's body into his partner's vagina, where, ideally, they are deposited near the cervix. At ovulation, the cervix and vagina are filled with cervical mucus. Sperm is deposited into the vagina, moves through the cervix into the cervical mucus and swims through the endometrial canals in the uterine lining up into the fallopian tube. Sperm can live in a woman's cervical mucus for about forty-eight to seventy-two hours. Contractions of the uterus aid the sperm as they swim up to the fallopian tube.

Once in the fallopian tube, sperm must penetrate the egg, break down the protective membrane surrounding the cell, and penetrate the zona pellucida, the egg's shell. One sperm must fuse with the egg, incorporating itself into the egg's nucleus, for fertilization to finally occur.

Implantation typically occurs during the secretory phase of the uterine cycle, around day twenty-one of a twenty-eight-day cycle. If you ovulate on day fourteen or fifteen, and you achieve fertilization on day sixteen, you might wonder where the embryo was before it found its way to the uterus. The answer is the fallopian tube. The embryo stays in the fallopian tube for three to five days and is almost at what is called the blastocyst stage (day five or six of growth) by the time it reaches the uterus. At the blastocyst stage, the embryo hatches out of its shell and attaches to the uterine wall to develop.

EARLY AND OFTEN: WHAT YOU MIGHT NOT KNOW ABOUT TIMING INTERCOURSE

Sperm can live in the female reproductive tract for up to forty-eight to seventy-two hours, but an egg has only twenty-four hours during which it can be fertilized after it is released from the ovary. If you have sex one day after ovulation, you've missed your monthly opportunity, but if you are three days early, you're in business. You want sperm to be present *before* the egg is released. Studies suggest that the best way to conceive is by having intercourse early and often *before* you ovulate.[2]

The middle of your menstrual cycle is the best time to conceive. To calculate the best days to time sex, divide your cycle into quarters. (You can find the length of your cycle by checking off the first day of your menstrual period on a calendar for a couple of months and counting the days in between.) If your cycle is twenty-eight days long, each quarter will be about seven days. So day eight would be the first day of the second quarter of your cycle and day fifteen will be the last day of that block. During a twenty-eight-day cycle, trying often from days eight through fifteen will maximize your chances of getting pregnant.

While the mechanisms of human reproduction are complex and fascinating to many, not everyone is interested in the fine points of conception. Still, knowing how your hormones affect your cycle and how conception occurs will help you to understand the rationale for fertility drugs—how and why they work—how to time sex for conception, and why your particular fertility issue may be preventing you from having a baby. Unfortunately, most of us were not sufficiently educated in human sexuality to be comfortable and conversant with the terms of reproduction, especially with the way in which our hormones affect us. But if you are undergoing infertility care, you will hear a lot more about FSH, LH, estradiol, and progesterone. More than likely, you will become more familiar than you ever were with the way your body works, and that can only be a good thing, giving you a real advantage when it comes to participating in your treatment plan and making sure that you are getting the best care possible.

3 | Get the Right Tests

AFTER A DIAGNOSIS OF INFERTILITY, PEOPLE OFTEN move from asking the question "Why me?" to "What's wrong with me?" In the age of in vitro fertilization (IVF) wherein it's possible to apply reproductive medical techniques to the broad symptom of infertility, you could very well undergo sophisticated infertility treatments without ever knowing what is wrong with you. Instead of trying simply to treat symptoms of a problem, *effective* medicine attempts to cure the underlying disorder. To treat your infertility effectively and efficiently, you and your doctor must isolate and treat the problems that may be keeping you from having a baby. Accordingly, your physician should do a number of initial tests.

THE ESSENTIAL INITIAL INFERTILITY WORKUP

The following tests should be part of you and your partner's initial evaluation:

- semen analysis
- transvaginal ultrasound
- day three FSH/estradiol test
- hysterosalpingogram (HSG)
- postcoital test
- luteal progesterone test
- thyroid-stimulating hormone (TSH) test
- prolactin test (in some cases)

Get Your Initial Testing Done Within One Month

You can do all of your initial screening tests within one month, and you should. Chances are that you have waited at least six months to a year to recognize that you have infertility, and certainly the medical definition of infertility generally requires you to do this. But now you may be facing a treatment process that takes time. Without IVF, you have only a 20 percent chance of getting pregnant each month with intercourse or insemination—those are nature's odds. And when your age is a factor, time becomes more critical. Why delay your chances of getting pregnant by delaying your initial workup? Do it soon, and you will be on your way to making decisions about your infertility care and getting the treatment you need to get pregnant.

Ideally, your reproductive endocrinologist should do your initial testing. But if you live in an area with few reproductive endocrinologists, these tests can be done by a good general ob-gyn. The essential thing is that you get them all done within one month.

During treatment I really did feel like a science project. This was something that was supposed to happen naturally, and it didn't happen naturally for me. I needed to go in for blood work and go in for the sonogram and show up three hours later for this other test, and don't forget to take this medication beforehand and that medication. I felt so micromanipulated that I was no longer in control. —SHARON

At first when they would tell me I had to take another test, I would cry hysterically, thinking, "Why me? Why do I have to go through this?" It takes you a long time to get to the point where you can say, "Thank God I can go for the tests. Thank God I can take these shots." At first you're very angry. —BARBARA

Be Prepared to Give Your Doctor Information about Your History

Your doctor will want to know about:

- *Your menstrual period.* When was your last menstrual period? When was the period before that? How often do your periods come? Has there been a change in your periods from a year ago? Five years ago? Ten years? Naturally, you may not have been charting your periods for ten years, but give your doctor a sense of any changes in your menstrual pattern. You can chart the length of time between your periods simply by marking the first day of each period on your calendar, if you haven't been doing this already.
- *Whether or not you'd been in a situation where you should have gotten pregnant but didn't.* This information could be very significant when you were previously partnered with someone known to be fertile—for example, if you had no children in your first marriage, but your ex-husband remarried and had children.
- *How often you have sexual relations.* It may seem odd, but it's not always easy to assess exactly how long you've been trying to get pregnant.

Sometimes people think they've been trying diligently for a year but in fact they may be partnered with someone who is out of town frequently or for large blocks of time. Have you been trying every month for over a year or six months? It's also possible for couples who have not been using contraceptives in a long-term partnership to start "trying" but to in fact have been exposing themselves to a possible pregnancy for much longer. Remember to factor in the total number of years you have been having sexual relations with your partner without contraceptives.

- *Your birth control history.* This is important, especially if you have used an IUD. IUDs are associated with pelvic infection, which can affect your fertility.
- *Your weight.* This is an issue when your cycles are irregular. If you are significantly overweight or underweight, you may have stopped ovulating.

Your doctor will do a pelvic exam and most likely a breast examination. You should be very concerned when a reproductive endocrinologist (RE) or ob-gyn treating you for infertility does not do a pelvic exam, even if you have already had a pelvic exam with another doctor. If this is the case, you are not getting a thorough evaluation.

Transvaginal Ultrasound

Also called: Vaginal sonogram

What it is: An ultrasound imaging technique done with a vaginal probe using sound waves to view images of the ovaries and uterus. These images are visible on a monitor. The vaginal probe used in ultrasound is called a *transducer*.

Why it's done: A transvaginal ultrasound is a potent and relatively accessible way to visualize the ovaries and uterus. The ovaries normally sit very

Tests You Need if You Are Seeing an RE for the First Time After Miscarriage

In Chapter 10, we will look closely at the possible causes of recurrent miscarriage. Although your initial workup will be different than if you first visited your RE without having had a pregnancy loss, many of the tests in your initial workup are described at length elsewhere in this chapter. Your workup should include:

- *A day three FSH/LH/estradiol test.* Higher LH levels are associated with an increased incidence of chromosomal mistakes, which can bring about miscarriage. Recurring miscarriage can also be a sign of perimenopause.
- *A hysterosalpingogram* to rule out uterine structural anomalies. (See page 40.) Other tests such as ultrasound, hysteroscopy, and possibly an MRI may be used to evaluate your uterus as well. A hysteroscopy is a narrow telescope introduced through your cervix to allow a surgeon to look directly into your uterus for problems.
- *A luteal progesterone test* or *endometrial biopsy.* Hormonal or endocrine problems may be the cause of miscarriage. These tests are described later in this chapter.

Other tests you may need after recurrent miscarriage:

- thyroid stimulating hormone (TSH) test
- prolactin test (page 50), because there is a small association between an elevated prolactin level and recurrent miscarriage
- fasting blood glucose (also known as fasting blood sugar) to rule out diabetes
- karyotype (an actual picture of your chromosomes) to look for chromosomal problems
- blood tests for blood clotting disorders, called thrombophilia testing

If you have had more than two miscarriages, be sure to read Chapter 10, where we will cover these tests in detail.

close to the vaginal walls, so a transducer pressed against the vaginal walls can transmit information about the location of the ovaries, the number of follicles in the ovaries, and anything that looks abnormal, such as ovarian cysts. A transvaginal sonogram can detect fibroids (*leiomyomas*) and can tell you whether your uterine lining is normal or abnormal. You can also see the relationship of the ovaries to the uterus. Normally, they sit near one another, but an ovary that looks plastered to the uterus is abnormal and may be a sign of *adhesions* (scar tissue adhered to an organ). Although a transvaginal ultrasound cannot visualize normal fallopian tubes well, if you do see fallopian tubes on a sonogram, it's usually because they're blocked and full of fluid. This is an early warning of tubal disease. Discomfort during the exam, which can happen when the doctor probes to the left and to the right, can reveal pelvic tenderness, which can be a sign of endometriosis, which is only visible on ultrasound when it causes cysts involving the ovary, known as *endometriomas*, or, theoretically, a sign of adhesions.

To prepare for the exam: There is no preparation for the exam other than emptying your bladder, which you can do right before the sonogram.

The procedure: You will lie on the table as you would for a pelvic exam. The doctor will insert a long, narrow probe called a *transducer* into your vagina to do the ultrasound. Transducers are invariably made of plastic and are not like cold, metal speculums. The probe is covered with a latex barrier, or, if you have a latex allergy, a covering that is not made of latex. The transducer will be lubricated with a gel to ensure continuous contact between the transducer, its covering and the vaginal walls, because any air pockets will disturb the sound waves. You may be able to see the monitor as the ultrasound is performed. Be sure to ask any questions you have about the procedure and its findings.

What will it feel like? It may feel a little strange, but few women complain that it is more uncomfortable than a pelvic exam. Unlike a pelvic exam, there is no cold, rigid speculum with which to contend, and no one is going to give you a rectal exam or press against your abdomen. It's important to note that this is not an examination in which an instrument will be inserted into your cervix, which causes cramping. The transducer enters your vagina only.

How long does it take? The exam should take about five minutes or less.

What does it cost? The standard cost is about $200. Check your insurance to see if diagnostic tests are covered. This advice extends to all procedures described here.

> *Despite a probe being inserted into the vagina, a transvaginal ultrasound is a very noninvasive procedure. It's a great window to the ovaries. But I think that because it's gynecologic, because you have to be undressed from the waist down, because you may have other people with you, whether it's a spouse or a partner, and the doctor, possibly a nurse, and maybe even an ultrasound technologist, you may feel like you are at a party with your legs up and everything off from the waist down.* —ANN

OVER-THE-COUNTER INFERTILITY TESTS?

You can walk into any drugstore today and buy a home pregnancy kit or an ovulation detector kit. You can get an HIV test without going through a third party, but why can't a man or a woman who merely wants to learn his or her reproductive status get a test over the counter? The answer in part lies with the medical community's fear that patients will rely less on their doctors. High levels of expertise and sensitivity are not required to interpret these tests. Considering the privacy desired by patients using these tests, they should be readily available without a prescription, and perhaps one day they will be.

The Day Three FSH/Estradiol Test

What it is: The day three FSH/estradiol test is a simple blood test done on day three of your cycle to suggest your ovarian reserve—simply put, the number of follicles and the quality of the eggs that you have left in your ovaries.

Why it's done: The day three FSH/estradiol test gives you information about the feedback between your ovaries and your pituitary gland. When your ovaries are functioning well, you should have relatively low FSH levels and low estradiol levels around day three of your menstrual cycle. If, on the other hand, the ovaries don't respond to FSH, the pituitary sends out more FSH to try to get the ovaries to work, in effect hammering on them to do their job to keep you ovulating as long as possible. High amounts of FSH or estradiol in your bloodstream on day three can mean that your ovarian reserve is diminished.

High estradiol and low FSH levels on day three can happen as you enter the perimenopausal transition. Your cycles shorten and in a sense overlap with earlier rises in FSH and earlier follicle development. Normally, your FSH level declines at the end of your last cycle, starting out very low at the beginning of the next cycle, eventually beginning to rise again. But as your menstrual cycles shorten, your FSH actually starts to rise in the previous cycle so that you begin developing new follicles even before your last cycle ends, making your cycle shorter. Your estradiol levels are high because the follicle is already secreting estradiol, which is starting to suppress your FSH. That is why a low FSH level on day three in the context of a high estradiol level is also good evidence that you have an ovary that is not functioning properly and, specifically, one that is in an advanced state of deterioration.

The day three FSH/estradiol test can be used to determine whether you are a candidate for IVF and how aggressive you might be with treatment.

What's normal, what's not? Your estradiol level should be below 75. As far as your FSH level is concerned:

- below 10 is very good;
- below 12 is acceptable;
- between 12 and 15 is worrisome;
- above 15 is problematic;
- above 20 is almost menopausal.

When it's done: Day three of your period. If you are going to err in scheduling the test, err on the side of day two. Your estradiol goes up naturally as your cycle progresses. If you take the test too late, you may have a high estradiol that is normal, for instance, on day five, but not on day three.

If you have a high FSH on one test, can you try again? Yes, you should generally do two tests in two different months to make sure your levels are accurate. However, even one abnormal test is usually meaningful.

Does age matter? Almost everyone knows someone past thirty-five with high FSH levels who still got pregnant. Your fertility doesn't come to a screeching halt as you age. It's just that the percentage of women who are still fertile in their late thirties and forties is much smaller than the percentage of women who are not fertile. You may have a relatively high level of FSH, but that doesn't mean you won't get pregnant. It may mean that you are less likely to get pregnant, which is why some clinics may screen out women with high FSH levels.

Recent research indicates that a high FSH level is not as dire for a young woman as it may be for an older woman. Even though a younger woman's FSH level may be high and even though she may have few eggs left, her eggs are statistically more likely to be chromosomally intact than those of an older woman. Still, amniocentesis should be recommended for young pregnant women with a history of FSH elevation. A thirty-one-year-old with a high FSH level might carry the same risks of having a child with Down syndrome as a woman in her late thirties.

Some young women who have had premature ovarian failure experience an odd phenomenon wherein they reverse themselves temporarily for about six months or so and then return to ovarian failure. There's also some capacity for younger women to recover from ovarian damage. For example, a young woman treated for cancer with chemotherapy may have ovarian failure and a very high FSH level but find that her cycles return a few years after chemotherapy. No one really knows why this is, but it may be due to the greater volume and resilience of the young ovary. This is also seen in young men treated for Hodgkin's disease. They may be completely *azoospermic* (that is, they have no sperm) and then five years later begin producing sperm again. The younger the person, the more common the phenomenon is.

To prepare: The test does not require fasting, but you must *not* be on medication that will affect ovulation, such as birth control pills, progesterone, Provera, or Lupron. It's meaningless to test while on these drugs. Prolactin can interfere with ovulation, and antianxiety or psychotropic drugs can raise your prolactin levels, which can in turn interfere with ovulation. (See "Other Tests Women May Need" on page 50, for more information about prolactin.) Make sure to tell your doctor if you are taking psychotropic medication. Thyroid medication will not affect your day three FSH/estradiol level.

What will it feel like? A typical blood draw.

Who should take the test: It's not unreasonable to suggest that every woman who is considering infertility care get this test, and some insurers require this test before they will cover treatment. Some insurance companies want everyone screened in order to deny coverage to people who are less likely to have therapeutic success.

The cost: Around $60.

Do different labs have different values? Today, most labs use ELISA assays. (ELISA stands for *enzyme-linked immunosorbent assay*.) Some specialty labs have their own methodologies, but the day three FSH/estradiol test is now fairly standardized.

Hysterosalpingogram (HSG)

What it is: An invasive X-ray with a contrast dye done in order to determine whether your fallopian tubes are blocked and if your uterus is structured normally. As intimidating as this test seems, it's very important to have it in order to fully evaluate your anatomy.

The procedure: Your doctor will schedule your appointment at a radiology facility. You will lie on the table in the same position as if you are having a pelvic exam. Some tables may have stirrups; others may be flat, in which case you will be asked to lie in a frog-leg position. A speculum will be gently inserted into your vagina. Your cervix will be visualized and grasped with an instrument, usually a *tenaculum*, which is a long-handled clamp. There are many types of tenacula, but the type most often used in gynecology is called a single-tooth tenaculum. Although the instrument is a bit scary-looking, the cervix has fewer nerve endings than your uterine wall, clitoris, or even the tip of your finger. Still, it may cause discomfort, and the amount of discomfort can vary from patient to patient. If you have had a tenaculum applied in the past and had discomfort, you might ask your doctor to numb your cervix.

After the tenaculum is placed, your cervix will be cleansed. A narrow *cannula* (flexible tube) will be inserted into your cervix through which the contrast dye will be slowly infused. As it is infused into your uterine cavity, the dye will spread out through your fallopian tubes. (See Figure 4 on page 44.) X-ray images will be taken of your uterine cavity and tubes. You may be asked to change positions slightly to take side views of your uterine cavity.

What will it feel like? The hysterosalpingogram has in some ways deserved its bad reputation among fertility patients. If done incorrectly, this test can be painful, but *in the vast majority of cases,* it can be done with a minimal amount of discomfort, causing hardly more discomfort than a Pap smear. Problems arise when the doctor performing the test is unaccustomed to performing procedures that are routine for ob-gyns. Some radiologists specialize in doing hysterosalpingograms and do a significant number of them as part of their practice, but not all radiologists are experienced. The most common problems are unfamiliarity with inserting a speculum and manipulating a cervix—again, the kind of things that ob-gyns do every day. Also, radiologists tend to use balloon catheters to obstruct the cervix and hold in the radiologic dye. The balloons cause undue cramping when inflated and can prevent the radiologist from seeing a complete picture of what's inside the uterus.

Importantly, only a minimal amount of contrast dye is needed to visualize the uterus and fallopian tubes. The uterus is very sensitive and very small in a woman who isn't pregnant. Only a tiny amount of dye, maybe 3 to 5 milliliters, is required to visualize the uterus and fallopian tubes. The dye must be infused slowly. The more slowly it is infused, the more likely you are to have a painless procedure. A common mistake is to inject too much, too fast.

Who should do the HSG: It's best if your RE does the procedure. Not only will your RE be conversant with the procedure, causing you minimal pain, you will be able to get your results immediately and put those results in the context of your individual fertility plan. If you find out that you have a problem, you can ask your doctor right then and there, "What are we going to do about this?' and begin to develop a strategy. Otherwise, you will have to wait several days or a week until the results come back to your RE. If your doctor does schedule you with a radiologist, ask who will do it and whether or not that person does these procedures all the time. You most definitely want to schedule with someone who has done a significant number of these procedures.

When it's done: Early in your cycle, after your period.

To prepare for the test: You are going to have some degree of uterine cramping, either from manipulation of your cervix or from expansion of your uterine cavity during the exam. I recommend a painkilling agent, such as ibuprofen (up to 800 milligrams), an hour or two before the procedure. You should also be pretreated with an antibiotic, especially if you have blocked fallopian tubes, a history of infection, or if you have a known infection at the time of your HSG, because it's possible for the dye to push bacteria further up your reproductive tract. Taking an antibiotic before the procedure can treat the infection should the HSG stir up an old infection or cause a new one.

You may be asked to have a blood count before the hysterosalpingogram to make sure that your white blood count is normal, again, to rule out an existing infection. Also, a pregnancy test should be rechecked.

Tell your doctor if you are allergic to shellfish. Some people are allergic to the contrast dye, which contains iodine. These same people tend to be allergic to seafood, particularly shellfish. There are special dyes that can be used in such cases.

After the test: You're going to have some discharge, because some of the contrast dye, which is clear, is going to come back through your vagina and may be mixed with blood, because of irritation to the uterine lining. Having an HSG will be a little bit like going home with your period again for a day or two. You may have some residual cramping while your uterus is contracting and expelling the dye. But you shouldn't be so uncomfortable that you can't drive yourself home. Of course, you may prefer to have someone drive you home and lend support after the test. This is a good time for husbands or partners to be present and supportive. If your infertility doctor is doing the test, your partner can listen as the results are shared.

Watch for signs of infection. If you develop a fever or if you have pelvic pain the day after your HSG, call your doctor right away. You could have an infection, which should be treated immediately.

If your doctor finds an abnormality: If you doctor finds something unusual about your uterus, you may have a diagnostic *hysteroscopy.* This is a procedure in which a narrow telescope is introduced in the cervix so that your doctor can visualize your uterus clearly. However, if your fallopian tubes are blocked, you and your physician may talk about whether or not it is appropriate to have a laparoscopy to directly visualize and possibly unblock your tubes or to do IVF and bypass the problem of blocked tubes. (See Chapter 5 for more about tubal problems and Chapter 9 for information on IVF.) Laparoscopy involves the insertion of a telescope into the abdominal cavity, allowing the physician to view and operate therein. Laparoscopy and hysteroscopy are often done in the same setting. (See Figure 7 on page 130.) Again, one of the benefits of having your RE do the hysterosalpingogram is that these discussions can take place right after the procedure before you go home.

Will you have to repeat the test? Most women will have the test only once, but if your tubes are blocked and you do have surgery, you could have another hysterosalpingogram three months later to make certain they are still open.

Will a hysterosalpingogram improve your chance of getting pregnant? Occasionally, hysterosalpingograms are therapeutic. There are reports of women having a higher incidence of pregnancy within three months of an HSG. Some women have had pregnancies after a hysterosalpingogram, returned to infertility care to have their second child, and gotten pregnant the same way after another hysterosalpingogram. If you are a young woman with a relatively short period of infertility and your initial workup is normal, then you might consider waiting two or three months after a normal HSG to see if the procedure does the trick by itself. But if you are in your midthirties or older, when time is of the essence, you don't want to take a wait-and-see attitude.

When might you defer your HSG? If you are young (under thirty-five), do not ovulate, and are just starting on a fertility drug called clomiphene

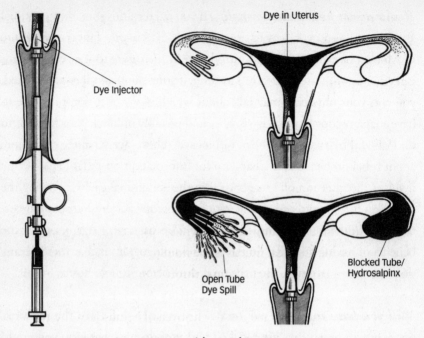

Dye in Uterus

Dye Injector

Open Tube
Dye Spill

Blocked Tube/
Hydrosalpinx

FIGURE 4. *A hysterosalpingogram.*
Contrast dye is injected into the cervix, uterus, and fallopian tubes.

citrate, which you might know as Clomid or Serophene, your doctor may say, "Well, you've only had one sexual partner. You've never had abdominal surgery, never had an IUD, and do not have very regular periods. We are going to try to see if clomiphene makes your ovulation more regular. Therefore, why don't we just assume your tubes are open, and if you aren't pregnant after three ovulations, then we'll check them." This is reasonable. Otherwise, always make sure that you know whether your tubes are open. Remember that your infertility treatment should not be a voyage of discovery, but rather the execution of a logical plan. Testing is part of that plan.

I didn't have any problems with the HSG. I had mild cramping. I've heard some people say that they had severe cramping, and they would never do it again. But mine went very smoothly. —JENNIFER

The people I know who said it was horrible also said that no one told them what it was going to be like. It's scary when all of the sudden you get these cramps, especially when you're in fertility treatment and you don't know what's going on inside. The anxiety makes it more painful. This is what people who have had children say about childbirth. Those who are realistically prepared for it don't seem to be as overwhelmed by the pain of labor and delivery, because it hurts, you know it's going to hurt. —REBECCA

The Postcoital Test (PCT)

What it is: A simple examination in which your cervical mucus is tested after intercourse. Cervical mucus is the fluid that plays a key role in transporting sperm from the vaginal canal through the cervix to the uterus.

Why it's done: The postcoital test is controversial because health professionals worry about its cost-effectiveness. Yet it is one of the cheapest fertility tests in your doctor's array of diagnostic techniques. The test is done to investigate the quality of your cervical mucus, its hospitability to your partner's sperm, and how your partner's sperm functions in your cervical mucus. The test can tell you whether you are having sexual relations for conception appropriately and whether your cervical mucus and your partner's sperm are compatible. Sometimes couples with normal semen analyses and good cervical mucus have no findings of semen in the mucus on a postcoital test. This could indicate an ejaculatory problem or perhaps a problem with your sexual technique. Semen should be ejaculated into the deeper half of the vagina.

In addition to telling you about the relationship between your cervical mucus and your partner's sperm, the postcoital test can be a good indication for intrauterine insemination. Inseminations can help when a man has a poor semen analysis. I think there is a good case for three to six months of intrauterine inseminations for a couple with a bad postcoital test. However, while many reproductive endocrinologists start couples out with inseminations even if the man's sperm is normal and the woman's cervical mucus is fine, there is no evidence that insemination will help a couple with a good semen analysis and a good postcoital test.

The procedure: Many couples believe and are told they have to have relations and get to the doctor's office within an hour for a postcoital test. Logistically, this can be a real nightmare, and there's really no need for this amount of rush. People can have relations twenty-four hours before the test or a half an hour before. It makes no difference. To complete the test, the woman can come to her doctor within twenty-four hours after having had intercourse. You will lie on the examination table in your doctor's office, just as you would for a Pap smear. You will have a speculum examination and your doctor will use a syringe to collect your cervical mucus, which will then be examined under a microscope.

Good results are: There should be moving sperm in your cervical mucus. Sperm should be seen to be swimming forward.

Bad results are: Sperm that shake in place may be victims of sperm antibodies. (See "Initial Infertility Tests for Men" on page 55.) Sperm that swim in small tight circles may have abnormal motility. Many white blood cells present in the cervical mucus may indicate inhospitable mucus or infection.

To prepare: If you need a lubricant when you have sexual intercourse, choose a non-spermicidal one.

When to take the test: The test should be done just before ovulation because of the ever-changing nature of cervical mucus. In many women, there are only a few days per cycle when the cervical mucus is receptive, that is, abundant, clear, and stretchy, and this happens just before or during ovulation. If vaginal intercourse occurs within twenty-four hours of this period of time, moving sperm should be visible within the cervical mucus when placed on a microscopic slide.

How long will it take? About five minutes.

Will you have to repeat the test? You should only have to do a postcoital test once, if it's normal. You may want to have the test done again, if you had an abnormal postcoital test or if you began taking clomiphene citrate (a fertility drug) and are now coming off clomiphene. Clomiphene citrate can disrupt your cervical mucus.

The cost: Between $50 and $100.

The Luteal Progesterone Test

Also called: Serum progesterone or plasma progesterone test

What it is: A blood test to measure the amount of progesterone secreted by the ovaries. The ovaries secrete progesterone in the second half of your cycle in order to prepare the endometrium (uterine lining) for implantation and maintenance of an early pregnancy. A low level of progesterone in the second half of your cycle can indicate ovarian dysfunction, suggesting a luteal-phase defect in which there is either inadequate progesterone or the uterine lining does not sufficiently respond to progesterone. Very low levels of progesterone indicate that you haven't ovulated. When the uterine lining is not properly prepared for implantation, infertility or miscarriage can result. Women with high FSH levels are more likely to be among those with low progesterone levels and may benefit from supplemental progesterone to create a better uterine environment to increase the likelihood of implantation.

When it's done: Ideally, your doctor should check your progesterone level about five to seven days after ovulation—for example, between days twenty-one and twenty-three in a twenty-eight-day cycle.

- If you are timing your test with a urine LH kit, take the blood test a week after the LH kit turns positive.

- If you were timing the test after an insemination, take the test five to six days after insemination.
- If you are timing after a postcoital test, take the blood test a week after the postcoital test.

Good results are: Your level should be 10 nanograms or more. A level of 3 or above confirms that you are ovulating, but numbers below 10 are low for midluteal progesterone. Your doctor can repeat the test two to three days later to confirm or disprove your number, but a repeated low number suggests inadequate progesterone.

If your progesterone level is low: Your doctor might suggest ultrasound or an endometrial biopsy to further evaluate your endometrium. (See "Endometrial Biopsy: A Closer Look" on page 51.) Your doctor will also probably suggest that you take supplemental progesterone. You can take progesterone as a vaginal suppository—a micronized progesterone capsule taken vaginally. (Micronized progesterone capsules taken orally are not as active and therefore not recommended in this situation.) You can also use Crinone, a vaginal progesterone gel. Progesterone can also be given in oil injections, but this deep intramuscular shot is barely tolerable for many women, particularly because it must be given daily and may be required for several months. Although most people do prefer suppositories, some women favor injections, especially if they find the suppositories irritating. A longer-acting progesterone called 17-alpha hydroxyprogesterone caproate (Delalutin or Prodrox) can be injected twice a week, although it is not readily available to consumers. Interestingly, this drug was proven effective at prolonging pregnancies during the 1970s, but fell out of favor because of complications from other hormonal treatments in pregnancy, such as diethylstilbestrol (DES). (See page 97.) It was rediscovered recently at large multicenter trials and again proven to be beneficial for the same purpose.[1]

Knowing when to give progesterone can be a little tricky. For instance, if your doctor thinks that you are ovulating on day fourteen and starts you on progesterone on day fifteen, but you are really ovulating on day sixteen, your uterine lining will be made too advanced for an embryo to implant. It's best for your physician to use a window of time that's at least three to four days after assumed ovulation and start you on progesterone at that point, giving you a good amount of extra progesterone just when your own levels are starting to achieve their peak.

If you get pregnant, you will want to continue progesterone until your placenta can take over producing progesterone during the first nine weeks of pregnancy (or seven weeks after conception). Progesterone supplementation can prevent you from getting your period, so you may not know you're pregnant unless you take a pregnancy test. Many practitioners will suggest that you continue to use supplemental progesterone throughout the first trimester of pregnancy (the first twelve weeks).

What is a luteal-phase defect? A luteal-phase defect means that either your ovaries are not secreting sufficient progesterone in the second half of your cycle or your endometrial lining is not responding to progesterone, making it difficult for an embryo to implant in your uterine lining and grow. To diagnose luteal-phase defect, you will need this test, an endometrial biopsy, and possibly an ultrasound.

Thyroid-Stimulating Hormone (TSH) Test

Thyroid problems are not a major cause of infertility, but it's crucial for any woman who is considering pregnancy to have a thyroid test, because there is a very strong correlation between an underactive thyroid (hypothyroidism) and the impaired mental development of a fetus. Fortunately, thyroid problems are virtually always correctable. The gain of identifying and treating a thyroid problem before pregnancy to protect the health of your child is immeasurable. In Chapter 5, we will talk about a common fertility problem called polycystic ovarian syndrome (PCOS). Hypothyroidism can give you a PCOS-like syndrome. For more information and a discussion of PCOS, see that chapter.

OTHER TESTS WOMEN MAY NEED

Depending on your situation, your doctor may order some of these other tests.

Prolactin Test

This is a simple blood test. Prolactin is a pituitary hormone that stimulates lactation, or milk production. Lactating at times other than after having had a baby could be a sign of an elevated prolactin level, which can interfere with your ovulation. If you have regular cycles and no breast discharge, the odds that you have a prolactin problem are small. Otherwise, your doctor will most likely order a prolactin blood test. High prolactin levels are often caused by what are known as pituitary adenomas, or microadenomas. These little pituitary tumors, less than one centimeter in diameter, are slow-growing tumors that invariably shrink upon treatment with a dopamine agonist, most commonly bromocriptine. When first discovered, there was a rush to treat these tumors surgically, but they are no longer treated surgically and are little cause for alarm. Stress and irritation of your nipples by your clothing or bra can also raise your prolactin level, as can serotonin medications, such as medications used to treat depression. Tell your doctor if you are on any serotonin drugs. You and your doctor should discuss the best way to approach your care without jeopardizing your psychological well-being.

Adrenal Androgens Test

If you are not ovulating and you have characteristics of polycystic ovarian syndrome (see Chapter 5), your doctor may recommend a blood test for excessive levels of adrenal androgens, male hormones normally manufactured by the adrenal gland. Adrenal overactivity can cause an overabundance of substances that can interfere with normal ovulation and/or create side effects characteristic of masculinity, such as *hirsutism* (excessive hair growth). The most abundant adrenal androgen is DHEAS (dehydro-epiandrosterone sulfate).

Endometrial Biopsy: A Closer Look

In some cases your doctor may want to evaluate your uterine lining more closely. Your doctor might want to do this if there is some concern about your luteal phase or, for example, if you have a good luteal progesterone level, but your endometrium (uterine lining) looks thin on ultrasound. An endometrial biopsy is an excellent way to evaluate the effect of progesterone on your uterine lining. The characteristics of the uterine lining change almost from day to day. In a normal cycle, a pathologist can precisely determine what day of your cycle you are on by looking at a sample of your lining under a microscope, using a process known as endometrial dating. If your lining is more than two days behind where it should be in its development during your cycle, you may have a luteal phase defect. For example, if you have a biopsy on day twenty-seven, your uterine lining should look like it is on day twenty-seven, but if it is looks like it is on day twenty-two instead, you are five days behind. This means the development of your uterine lining is out of phase.

What it is: A biopsy of your uterine lining to determine whether it is developing properly during your cycle.

To prepare: To minimize cramping, take 800 milligrams of ibuprofen an hour before the procedure.

The procedure: You will be asked to lie in the same position as you would for a pelvic exam. Your cervix will be cleansed, and a very narrow strawlike instrument called a *Pipelle* will be passed through your cervix. Occasionally, a *tenaculum* (a long-handled clamp) will be used to steady the cervix. In some women, the uterus must be dilated before the Pipelle can be

Can an Endometrial Biopsy Improve Your Chances of Pregnancy?

A study in Israel published in the June 2003 issue of *Fertility & Sterility* suggests that endometrial biopsy may improve the chances of getting pregnant, if done soon before an IVF cycle.[2]

In the study, women who had failed with IVF were offered four endometrial biopsies. Those women who participated in the experiment had dramatically higher pregnancy rates than those who didn't have endometrial biopsies. The reason for this may be that damage to the uterus promotes growth factors in the healing process and that these growth factors contribute to a better uterine environment in the short term.

In our clinic on Long Island, we've offered this procedure to patients who want it, doing an endometrial biopsy one week before ovarian stimulation for IVF. Among those who accepted the procedure, half got pregnant with their next IVF cycle. While a 50-percent success rate is what we might normally expect with IVF, we don't expect it in people who have previously failed with IVF after a number of cycles. We offered endometrial biopsies to another 16 patients who were having frozen embryo transfer IVF. (See Chapter 9.) We did endometrial biopsies for these women a week after starting them on estrogen. Sixty percent got pregnant with their next IVF cycle. Normally, we would have expected a success rate of 30 percent for women using frozen embryos. It turns out that endometrial biopsy may indeed be beneficial for some patients and that the benefits may be specific to an embryo implanted through IVF. While physicians and researchers have focused on developing the best embryo for implantation in IVF, these results suggest that there is much to be learned about the optimal uterine environment for implantation.

passed through the cervix into the uterus. Once the instrument is inside your uterus, the doctor will pull back on a small stylet inside the instrument, creating a little suction, which will draw a sample of your uterine lining into the tube for evaluation. As the Pipelle is withdrawn, it is rotated to collect more tissue.

What it feels like: You may feel some pain when your cervix is grasped, and a sharp pain or bad cramping when the Pipelle is inserted or the tissue sample is taken. Some doctors inject anesthesia into the cervix to numb it, but that may also cause discomfort. If you have had a tenaculum applied before and found it particularly difficult, you might ask your doctor about a local anesthetic. However, most women will not need an anesthetic.

After the procedure: You will have a little bleeding and cramping, so you may want to bring a sanitary pad along with you to wear home. Make sure to call your doctor immediately, if you develop a fever or have pain after the procedure. This could be a sign of infection.

Cost: If not covered by insurance, this procedure will cost between $200 and $500.

> *If I had a question or I didn't understand something, I would pick up the phone and call my doctor's office, and I know a lot of people don't do that. People don't realize that it makes the process so much easier. If I was in any kind of pain, I would call them up and they were very, very good at giving me what I needed.* —JILL

TESTS YOU AND YOUR PARTNER DON'T NEED

There are certain tests described in the infertility literature that actually provide doctors with little or no additional information with which to guide diagnostic or treatment decisions. If your doctor orders one of the following tests, ask for the reason. These tests should only be ordered under very unique circumstances.

The Hamster Egg Penetration Test

The hamster egg penetration test is a labor-intensive, expensive procedure that in my opinion ought to be frowned upon. Briefly, the test involves taking an egg from a hamster and removing the zona pellucida (the covering of the egg) to allow penetration of the egg by a sperm of a different species; in this case, the human species. The zona pellucida is what confers species specificity. Once it is removed, one species can fertilize the egg of another. It was thought that if a man's sperm was able to penetrate a hamster egg, then he was fertile, and if not, he was infertile. The problem is that when IVF came along, it was apparent that many men who were not able to penetrate a hamster egg were very capable of fertilizing their partners' eggs. With so many false positives, the test became rather useless rather quickly. If your doctor orders this test, question it, and consider whether you should pay for something that is unnecessary.

The Clomiphene Challenge Test

Simply, a clomiphene challenge test involves giving a woman a day three FSH/estradiol test, putting her on clomiphene citrate (an inexpensive fertility drug), and measuring her FSH/estradiol levels again. The most valuable part of the test is the day three FSH/estradiol test. I have seen many patients who failed the clomiphene challenge test who conceived on the same cycle. Thus, the test, in my opinion, is a kind of glorification of the tests you are already being given. It doesn't add any new information.

Inhibin B/AMH (Anti-Mullerian Hormone) Test

Inhibin B and AMH are substances produced by cells surrounding your follicles. The health of these cells is somewhat related to the health of the follicle and the egg. Testing for inhibin B or AMH can be an alternative test to a day three FSH/estradiol test. There are no studies to show that these newer tests are superior to FSH/estradiol, but they are certainly more expensive. These tests may be shown to have some future utility beyond the day three /FSH estradiol test.

Cervical Mucus Tests that Are Not Postcoital Tests

In the past, doctors looked at cervical mucus in a number of ways, including matching the mucus of a number of women and adding sperm to look at the reaction of sperm in the mucus. These tests are no longer contemporary.

INITIAL INFERTILITY TESTS FOR MEN

Before you begin treatment, your doctor will ask you questions to ascertain any potential fertility problems. The most pertinent infertility questions for men are:

- *Have you been involved in any previous pregnancies?* Fathering a child or having been involved in a pregnancy in the past is the best test of your ability to father a child now.
- *Have you had surgery in infancy or childhood related to a hernia or undescended testes?* Hernias and undescended testes—especially undescended testes—are often a fetal expression of a testicular problem. The production of testosterone by the testes itself is one of the major catalysts to the normal descent of the testes. If there is a testosterone deficiency, the testes may not descend, and if the testicle does not descend, it will not function well. Although the vast majority of men with hernias are fertile, there is a relationship between hernias and infertility. Although a rare complication, the *vas deferens* (the tube that transports sperm) can be damaged in a hernia operation. This is especially harmful to fertility when it happens in childhood.

- *Do you have trouble maintaining an erection or having sexual relations?* You may need to address impotence or lack of interest as part of your infertility care plan.
- *Do you have any illnesses?* Some medications for hypertension (high blood pressure) impair sperm function. Diabetes can cause impotence or retrograde ejaculation, a condition in which semen enters the bladder upon ejaculation. Prostate and bladder surgery also carry the potential risk of nerve damage, as this is an extremely difficult area on which to operate. Some medications used to treat inflammatory bowel diseases, including Crohn's disease and ulcerative colitis, can impair sperm quality. Sulfasalazine is known to impair sperm quality, and there is evidence that long-term treatment with Azathioprine and 6-Mercaptopurine can do the same. Some people being treated for autoimmune disease might be given cyclophosphamide (Cytoxan), which can be toxic to sperm and eggs. Some treatments for gout, for example, colchicine, affect sperm quality. If you are taking any of these medications, or your doctor advises you to take any of these medicines, consider the possibility of banking (freezing and storing) sperm or considering other medications, if feasible. Be sure to tell your RE or ob-gyn about *any* medical conditions that you have to make certain there isn't something in your history that is having an effect on your fertility.

The Semen Analysis

What it is: A semen analysis is the single most important fertility test for men. It's a simple test that will not only tell you about your sperm count, it will also analyze other components of your semen that directly relate to your fertility. If you have an abnormal semen analysis, you will be referred to a urologist for further testing. If your semen analysis is normal and your answers to the key infertility questions for men (above) don't indicate a potential cause of infertility, you probably won't need a physical examination.

The semen analysis has a number of components. Those most important to your fertility are:

- *Liquefaction.* Semen goes through phases after ejaculation. At first, it is relatively liquid; it then congeals and liquefies again. Normal semen should go through this process.
- *The appearance of your semen.* Semen should have a milky appearance. Yellowish semen may indicate infection.
- *The volume of your semen* is the amount of liquid produced. This should be between 2 and 5 milliliters. Low volume doesn't indicate poor sperm quality, but it may indicate a need for intrauterine insemination (IUI) to help deliver sperm into the cervix.
- *Morphology.* Morphology refers to the size and shape of your sperm. Sperm have heads, necks, and tails. If you place very strict criteria on what normalcy is for sperm in terms of head and neck size and shape, and tail shape and dimension, you will find that only 14 percent of most men's sperm are normal and the other 86 percent are not. Use of this standard is called strict morphology, or Kruger morphology. When your morphology is lower than 14 percent using strict criteria, your doctor might worry that you have a varicocele (a varicose vein in the testes). Some varicoceles can be felt on examination. Sonography (ultrasound) may also be used to further detect a varicocele.

  Insurance companies contracting with large laboratories will most likely use another standard for morphology called the WHO (World Health Organization) criteria. According to the WHO criteria, more than 60 percent of sperm should have normal shape.
- *Your sperm count.* Also called concentration or density, the count refers to the number of sperm per milliliter of semen. In most labs, 20 million or above per milliliter is considered adequate.
- *Motility or movement of your sperm.* This is the percentage of sperm moving forward in a straight line. You want to see at least 40 to 50 percent of the sperm moving forward.
- *The pH (acidity or alkalinity) of your semen* may be a concern, if there is a possibility of retrograde ejaculation in which semen is ejaculated into the bladder. This is a condition associated with diabetes.

Other factors, such as fructose levels and consistency, are not as relevant to evaluating fertility as the factors above.

To prepare: You will be asked to abstain from ejaculation for at least forty-eight hours. The reason for this is that, at least in theory, frequent ejaculation may artificially lower your sperm count. But in actuality a man with a normal sperm count will continue to have a normal sperm count, even if he ejaculates once daily. Laboratories like to standardize the conditions of testing as much as possible, yet it's difficult to standardize something with as broad a normal range as a semen analysis, which can be normal anywhere from 20 million to 200 million. A borderline semen analysis may require you to repeat the test under these ideal conditions.

The procedure: You can prepare your semen sample at home or in a private room in your doctor's office by masturbating into a sterile cup. If done at your doctor's office, the cup should be immediately handed to a lab technician. It should not be allowed to sit at room temperature. Sperm motility is very sensitive to temperature changes. If your specimen is allowed to sit outside of an incubator or a warming device set approximately at body temperature (98.6°F), you may have normal concentration, but your motility (the ability of sperm to move forward) will be abnormal. Sperm should be transported to the lab within an hour of ejaculation. If you are bringing your specimen to the lab from home, be sure to carry it in a pocket or other warm place.

Once you provide your specimen, its volume will be measured and a portion of the semen will be taken to look at its morphology (size and shape) and a portion will be taken to assess the count and motility. This may be done either by looking under a microscope or by the use of an automated technique called CASA, or computer-assisted semen analysis. Either technique is fine, although CASA allows for more consistency between laboratories.

Will you have to repeat the test? If your analysis is completely normal, you may have to provide semen only once. On the other hand, you may have to provide a number of semen samples, depending on your fertility issues as a couple, for example, if you begin doing intrauterine inseminations.

When will you know your results? Motility and count, results of primary importance, should be known within a day. Sperm morphology results may take a week, as this evaluation requires a bit more labor and expertise. Still, knowing your motility and sperm count can immediately give you a very good sense of your overall sperm quality.

Making sense of the numbers: Some patients only want to know whether or not their semen analysis is normal. Others want to know what their numbers are. If you ask for a copy of your semen analysis, be sure to ask your doctor to help you put the numbers in context. It's important to realize that once you get above a certain threshold, you are fertile, and that's that. A sperm concentration of 35 million, for example, is not necessarily inferior to a sperm concentration of 70 million, and motility of 65 percent is not necessarily better than motility of 55 percent. Likewise, a sperm concentration of 175 million doesn't make fertility certain.

When your semen analysis shows that sperm is absent or low: Most reproductive endocrinologists are trained to perform male examination, but will generally refer men to a colleague in urology when a problem is suspected. In Chapter 6, we will look more closely at diagnosis and treatment for men, delving into topics related to male infertility at length.

Cost: A basic semen analysis, which includes concentration and motility, should cost about $100, but once you get into specialized morphologies, the price can double because of the extra work involved in doing them.

Tests for Infection

If you have a semen analysis that is suggestive of a lot of immature sperm cells, find out whether these are really immature sperm cells or white blood cells, which can appear very similar and can indicate an underlying infection. This will require a special test to distinguish the two. Either peroxidase /orthotoluidine or immunocytochemistry with a CD45 marker for white blood cells will be used.

Test for Antisperm Antibodies

You've read about the postcoital test to look at the quality of a woman's cervical mucus and its hospitality to her partner's sperm. If the results of your postcoital tests are poor, or if you have had a vasectomy, your doctor may test for antisperm antibodies, usually with what's called an *immunobead-binding assay*.

An antibody is a protein made by the immune system that recognizes and fights foreign invaders. Sometimes men make antibodies to their own sperm. Normally, a man's bloodstream will never see his sperm because of the blood-testes barrier that separates them. But when that barrier is broken, as can happen during a vasectomy, and sperm escapes into the bloodstream, the blood sees the sperm in a way that it never has before. The immune system can treat these sperm as foreign bodies and attack them. When this happens, there can be damage to the sperm that affects the sperm's movement and ability to bind with an egg.

HEADING TOWARD PREGNANCY

Once you have completed your initial testing, you are ready to make sense out of the results of these tests and to obtain an accurate diagnosis. If you choose to go forward with infertility care, your next task will be to find a good doctor who is educated in reproductive endocrinology and to get organized to get the best care. In Chapters 5 and 6, you will find questions and answers about the most common fertility problems to help you discern what your problem might be and get the best care from your doctor.

4. | Get a Good Doctor

OPEN THE YELLOW PAGES OR GO ONLINE AND YOU will see an array of ads for infertility specialists and clinics, but how do you know if any provide quality contemporary care? The truth is, you don't. In order to find good care, you are going to have to do some investigation, including gathering referrals, asking questions of the doctors or clinics you're considering, and learning how to evaluate a doctor's or clinic's practice and success rates. The quality of the care you receive depends on your doctor's skill and experience. It's well worth the trouble to find the right doctor or clinic because the decisions you make about your infertility care will have a significant impact on your physical and emotional well-being for some time to come.

WHEN YOU CAN SEE YOUR REGULAR OB-GYN

While there are distinct advantages to starting infertility care with a reproductive endocrinologist (RE), who is an ob-gyn with a dedicated subspecialty in reproductive care and infertility treatment, there are some instances when you may want to start care with your ob-gyn, particularly if you are under thirty-seven, your insurance does not cover RE visits, or there is no RE in your area.

If you are under thirty-seven, some of the things you can do with your regular ob-gyn include:

- Semen analysis to evaluate the quality and quantity of your partner's sperm.
- Day three FSH/estradiol test to determine how many egg-producing follicles you have left, how well they are functioning, and whether they will respond to stimulation. (See Chapter 3.)
- Hysterosalpingogram, an X-ray study performed with a clear dye that is visible on an X-ray and allows your doctor to see whether your fallopian tubes are open and whether your uterus is shaped normally. (See Chapter 3.)
- Treatment with the fertility drug clomiphene citrate for three to six months. (But see Chapter 7 for more details on this advice.)
- Intrauterine inseminations.

As with any practitioner treating fertility, a general ob-gyn treating infertility should have office hours seven days a week. If you are having IUIs, for example, and you ovulate on a day your doctor's office is closed, you won't conceive through insemination on that cycle.

Your ob-gyn should have a reasonable and logical plan to treat you based on your test results. Always ask your doctor why he or she recommends a particular test and on what basis your treatment plans are being made. You should also be able to do other tests relevant to your general health and ovulatory function, such as a thyroid test, glucose tolerance test, and blood count, with your general ob-gyn or family-practice doctor.

> *I think people are wasting time using regular gynecologists, especially when they are older. You're losing a year or two, key years. No matter how much your primary-care doctor or gynecologist loves you and wants you to be pregnant, that love and that hope is not going to work. You need scientific evaluation, and I don't think that people know that.* —BETH

WHEN TO SEE A REPRODUCTIVE ENDOCRINOLOGIST

There are times when it's best to start infertility treatment by seeing a reproductive endocrinologist, such as when:

- your partner is diagnosed with a low sperm count;
- you have blocked fallopian tubes;
- your period is not regular or you are not having a period;
- you have had two or more miscarriages;
- you were treated for cancer;
- you needed hormones to get through puberty;
- you have been diagnosed with pelvic inflammatory disease;
- you have done three to six months of clomiphene citrate without success;
- you have done three to six months of IUI without success;
- you are thirty-five to thirty-seven or older and you have not had a complete diagnostic workup within two months of visiting your regular ob-gyn about infertility concerns.

Some couples may want to work with their ob-gyn and an RE, although this is usually not the best practice, because it requires a high level of coordination between both doctors' offices. However, this can be a viable option for a couple living in a remote area with little access to a reproductive endocrinologist.

Reproductive endocrinologists (RE) are ob-gyns with additional training in reproductive endocrinology and infertility. Reproductive endocrinologists should be board certified (or board eligible) and have completed a fellowship approved by the American Board of Obstetrics and Gynecology (ABOG). To date, there are fewer than 800 fellowship-trained reproductive endocrinologists in the United States.[1]

The Society for Reproductive Endocrinology and Infertility (SREI) is a membership organization that admits only those physicians who are certified reproductive endocrinologists. Associate membership is available to those who are eligible for certification. Membership requires seven years of formal specialty and subspecialty training after medical school and certification. You can visit SREI's Web site at http://www.socrei.org.

FINDING A DOCTOR

Choosing a doctor for any medical problem can often pose a conflict between selecting a personable doctor to whom you relate and seeing someone whose manner may be more detached but whose approach is methodical. Sometimes you may find both assets in the same doctor, but you shouldn't choose a doctor simply because he or she is a great person. Your goal is treatment success. Before you look for a doctor, make sure you seek referrals based on that doctor's knowledge, reputation, and skill. Finding the right doctor can be daunting, but here are simple tips to start.

Gather Referrals

The best way to begin searching for referrals is to ask people you know. Perhaps you know someone who has been successfully treated or someone who has a friend who had a good experience.

If you have a good relationship with your ob-gyn, and he or she has a range of patients who have had infertility treatment, she or he can refer you to an RE. Referrals from other doctors can be a bit tricky. It's natural for physicians to form friendships with one another, particularly when they are in the same specialty. Your doctor may be recommending a friend who may indeed be a great doctor. But as a consumer you have the right to ask why your doctor recommends one doctor over another. Questions asked in a nonconfrontational manner will not be viewed as offensive.

RESOLVE, Inc., is a national consumer organization that provides education, advocacy, and support to men and women facing an infertility crisis. Visit the Web site at www.resolve.org or call 888-623-0744 to access the organization's physician referral service. A physician must meet objective criteria for training and practice in order to be included on the list.

Online chat groups can be a good source of information. Ask what other people's experiences have been at the clinic or office you are contemplating. But balance the information you hear with facts. If someone recommends or warns against a particular practice, find out why from an

objective source. Be aware that an excellent clinic may have a few dissatis-
fied patients and that those who participate in online chat groups may still
be receiving treatment while those who have had children, and who are
satisfied with the services they received, may have stopped visiting.

Ask About Your Doctor's Qualifications:
What You Want to See

Choosing a reproductive endocrinologist involves a considerate assessment of her or his professional expertise and experience, the type of services offered, and your comfort level with the doctor and staff, as well as
other factors. When choosing a doctor, look for the following:

- board certification
- undergraduate and medical degrees and residencies taken at reputable American educational institutions
- fellowship completed
- a teaching appointment at a good educational program is also reassuring

Publishing is one indication that a physician is current in his or her field. But some physicians are so inundated with patient caseloads that they seldom find the time to publish. Others work in settings where publication is encouraged or rewarded. If your doctor has published, you can go online to look at abstracts of medical articles by doing a search for "PubMed," or typing in http://www.ncbi.nlm.nih.gov/entrez/query.fcgi. PubMed is service of the National Library of Medicine. It includes over 15 million citations for biomedical articles. Try typing your doctor's name into the database to see if he or she has published articles. Often, you can read summaries of those articles online.

Ask Questions Over the Phone

Here are some initial questions you can ask to get a sense of whether to make a first appointment:

- How much of the doctor's practice is devoted to treating infertility? The answer should be more than 90 percent.
- Does the doctor have a fellowship in reproductive endocrinology? The answer should be yes.
- Is the doctor board certified or board eligible? *Yes* is what you want to hear.
- Is your doctor's office open seven days a week? Again, *yes* should be the answer.
- Does the doctor accept your insurance?
- Does the office have an insurance counselor on staff to help you get the most out of your insurance?

- Where does the doctor have hospital privileges?
- Will you be able to see the same doctor consistently? Will a nurse or doctor return your phone calls promptly?
- What professional memberships does the doctor hold? Membership in the Society for Reproductive Endocrinology (SREI) suggests that your doctor has met the criteria discussed above.

Does your doctor have access to the services you may need? We will talk about choosing a clinic later in this chapter. There you will find further discussion of the services clinics may have available.

Working with your doctor is a team effort. You should be confident that your doctor will explain treatment plans and their rationale. Some patients are uncomfortable questioning their doctors, but remember that you have a right to information and to be an equal player on your medical team.

I had to sit down and talk to the doctor, and if I couldn't talk to him, I wasn't staying. I wouldn't have been able to spend three years of my life in that office. So if a doctor puts you off, if something makes you feel uncomfortable, such as feeling the doctor was condescending, which is a big complaint, go elsewhere. You're going to share many intimate issues with this doctor, so you have to be comfortable. Understand what it is that you need, and find someone to match your needs. If I had one of those really mushy, moon-eyed people who held my hand through everything, I probably wouldn't go back, because that doesn't work for me. But some people need that. —PAM

My doctor was direct. He didn't play any games and he didn't tell me everything was rosy, like, "I'm definitely going to get you pregnant. You're fine." This is what my first doctor did. If the doctor is positive that you're going to get pregnant, question that. —LAYLA

Worshipping the "Fertility Gods"

Is there such a person as "the best doctor in the world"? Given the widespread dissemination of medical knowledge and techniques, are there individual human beings endowed with unusual powers to deliver medical care? When a patient of mine has twins, did I "give her twins" or did I merely perform the medicine correctly? Because infertility care centers on reproduction, the basis of new life, there is a tendency for magical thinking and egotism to creep into fertility doctors' practices.

"Fertility gods" are not necessarily unethical or bad doctors, but they may have a tendency to put their own interests ahead of their patients'. How can you tell if your doctor is one of the so-called fertility gods? Are you comfortable with your doctor? Does your doctor listen and consider your needs? Do you hear phrases like, "I gave her a baby," or "You owe it to yourself to get care with me"? Does your doctor refer to herself or himself as a pioneer? Do you see an excess of promotional literature in the office? Does your doctor refer to your embryos as "babies"? (This should never happen.) Trust your instincts. If you feel that your concerns are not being met or that your decisions are being unduly colored by your doctor's influence, you might consider whether the doctor you are seeing is a god or a monster.

CHOOSING A FERTILITY CLINIC

There are several considerations to bear in mind when choosing a fertility clinic, one of which is the composition of the program or staff. The American Society for Reproductive Medicine (ASRM) publishes and reviews minimum standards for fertility clinics performing ART. Among criteria, the guidelines recommend that a clinic staff include:

- a licensed physician who directs the program, which should have a medical director, a practice director, and laboratory director, although one physician may fill more than one of these positions;
- an RE who has completed an ABOG-approved fellowship;
- an RE with experience in infertility surgery;
- an ultrasonographer with specialized training in gynecologic sonography (ultrasound);
- a professional who is familiar with male reproduction and who has competence in semenology;
- an embryology lab director with experience organizing and maintaining a clinical embryology laboratory. As of 2006, lab directors should hold HCLD (High Complexity Laboratory Director) certification or ABB-ELD (American Board of Bioanalysis Embryology Laboratory Director) certification or should seek such certification;
- an available mental health professional with experience in reproductive issues;
- a specialist in gamete (egg and sperm) and embryo cryopreservation (freezing), if the services are offered by the clinic;
- a specialist in oocyte (egg) micro-operative techniques, such as ICSI.

ASRM also recommends that

- each physician directing egg retrievals should have done at least twenty follicular aspirations under direct supervision and should continue to do a minimum of twenty egg retrievals or transfers a year;
- each staff embryologist (including the embryology laboratory director or supervisor) should perform at least sixty ART (assisted reproductive technology) procedures a year.[2]

First, make sure you are choosing a reputable doctor or fertility center. Ask about results, but remember that everybody is different. You want their results on people from your age group and with your specific fertility issue.

Never go into a doctor's office without a list of questions. That's your forum. That's your time to ask questions, because it will be difficult to get them on the phone later. If you ask at the time, you get an answer. Be sure to ask whether the doctor will answer questions via e-mail. —CINDY

Ask Questions of Clinics: What You Want to Know

- Is the lab accredited? The most common accrediting body is the College of American Pathologists (CAP), because CAP is affiliated with the American Society for Reproductive Medicine (ASRM) for the purposes of accreditation. CAP was the first organization to offer accreditation. Labs may also be accredited by the Joint Commission on Accreditation of Health Care Organizations or by state departments of health.
- Is the clinic a member of the Society for Assisted Reproductive Technology (SART)? SART requires member clinics to meet specific standards.
- Does the program report statistics to the Centers for Disease Control and Prevention (CDC)?
- Does the clinic follow and meet ASRM guidelines?
- Are all the REs board certified? Some doctors may be between training and certification, in which case they are called "board eligible." This is certainly acceptable.
- Is there an IVF program at the clinic? Clinics without IVF programs may push procedures short of IVF for too long, while a program structured to perform IVF primarily may move to this procedure before trying other alternatives.
- Are donor sperm and egg services offered?
- How much cryopreservation (embryo freezing) does the clinic do? This will become important to understanding a clinic's success rates (see page 74).
- Does the program have an age limit? Many clinics do not like to treat women over forty-two. When it comes to donor egg cycles, fifty is a common, if arbitrary, cutoff age. If you are over forty, be sure to ask about age limits.

- Can the program treat your particular infertility diagnosis? How many other patients with your diagnosis have been treated?
- How many embryos are typically transferred during a cycle? More embryos transferred could increase your chances of pregnancy but also increase the risk of multiple pregnancy. (See Chapter 11.)
- What is the cost of an IVF cycle? What services are not included in the cost?
- Most IVF programs have a global fee that covers the IVF cycle, the office visits, ultrasounds, and all of the blood tests, as well as egg retrieval and embryo transfer. But additional procedures may not be covered. Find out about additional costs for:
  - ICSI (see Chapter 9), which will be important if your partner has a very low sperm count;
  - assisted hatching (see Chapter 9);
  - cryopreservation (embryo freezing) (see Chapter 9 and below);
  - fertility drugs;
  - the pre-IVF workup and other tests such as screening for HIV, rubella, and thyroid problems, as well as blood-count tests;
  - any tests of your uterus that you may need;
  - testing after the IVF cycle is completed to verify pregnancy, such as pregnancy tests, hormone-level tests, ultrasounds, and office visits;
  - immunotherapy; also ask about the clinic's position on intravenous immunoglobulin (IVIG), the most common form of immunotherapy and a very controversial issue in fertility treatment. It can be extremely expensive and is normally *not* covered by the global fee. Although few clinics use immunotherapy, it is something to ask about when assessing potential costs. It can also be associated with a number of extremely expensive and dubious tests. Inquire about the costs of all testing.

A physical plant disaster can destroy frozen embryos. The liquid nitrogen canisters that keep embryos frozen should be checked and replenished on a regular basis. Also, electricity that keeps the incubators running can fail, for example, in a blackout. You can ask the clinic what method they use for checking the tanks holding the embryos and whether or not the clinic has a UPS (uninterrupted power supply) backup generator. During a power outage, this type of generator can make a very smooth transition back to electricity. Ask what the exit plan is for the embryos in case of fire. Long-term storage facilities can be used to hold embryos in the rare event that a clinic has to close its doors. Importantly, you must rely on the reputation of the clinic you have chosen.

Get the Facts: Read Clinic Statistics

The Fertility Clinic Success Rate and Certification Act of 1992 mandates all American IVF clinics to report their success rates. The Centers for Disease Control (CDC) is charged with the administration of this law. Like all data, this data is subject to manipulation. Although they are supposed to report statistics on all their patients, some clinics are selective about who they include in their reporting. However flawed, this is the most complete overview of IVF clinics in the country. The information is available at the CDC Web site at http://www.cdc.gov/ART/index.htm.

Because fertility treatment involves a number of processes and not a single treatment, reports are based on cycles started by each clinic. A cycle begins when a woman begins taking fertility drugs. If the woman produces eggs, those eggs will be retrieved and united with sperm in the laboratory. The embryo will be transferred to her uterus (or in some cases, fallopian tube), and if successful, she will become pregnant, and if the pregnancy is successful, she will deliver an infant.

Naturally, your goal is to have a baby. The statistic you may be most interested in is the *live birth rate for your age group.* Your age is a crucial factor in determining your potential for pregnancy and delivery of a live infant with younger women (under thirty-five to thirty-seven) having a higher chance of success typically than women thirty-seven and older. The only statistic that modifies the live birth rate is the cryopreservation rate, or the rate at which embryos are frozen, a statistic that we will talk about momentarily.

The *live birth rate per egg retrieval* is the most important statistic for judging the quality of an IVF clinic, because up until the point of egg retrieval and fertilization, nothing has been done in vitro. In other words, IVF has not been performed.

Of course, you don't just want a baby, you want a healthy baby. Some IVF labs may raise their pregnancy rates by transferring more than two embryos to women who are likely to do well with IVF, increasing the likelihood of pregnancy but increasing the chance of multifetal pregnancies, not only putting mother and fetuses at risk for severe complications, but possibly exposing women to the necessity of multifetal reduction, in which some fetuses may have to be terminated with the hopes of improving the lives of the others. Some clinics raise their pregnancy rates by transferring more than two blastocyst embryos to the mother. (A blastocyst is an embryo grown to day five or six. We also talk about this detail in Chapter 9.) Transferring more than two blastocysts can put you at risk for having more than two fetuses and having to make a decision about reducing your pregnancy. When transferring at the blastocyst stage, the replacement of more than two embryos is strongly discouraged. If you don't want to have more than one child, if you don't want to be put in a position of having to make a decision about pregnancy termination, be very careful about the number of embryos you have transferred. When reviewing information about a clinic, look at the *average number of embryos transferred* as well as the *clinic's multiple birth rates* to get a sense of whether or not the clinic tends to transfer high numbers of embryos. Lowering the risk of multiple pregnancies by transferring fewer embryos also lowers the clinic's overall pregnancy rate. That's why it's very important not to look solely at the pregnancy rate but consider other factors as well.

Find Out About Embryo Freezing (Cryopreservation): Why You Need to Know

The most important statistic is one that is not reported, one that I call the "total pregnancy rate." This refers to the chance of pregnancy and delivery, not just from the transfer of a fresh embryo, but from additional frozen embryos as well. Embryos derived from a cycle can be frozen and used later after the fresh transfer. If you can try to get pregnant by using your fresh eggs and frozen embryos later on, not only will you increase the possibility of getting pregnant, but you can do so with less intervention because you will not have to go through the stimulation and aspiration process each time to create these additional embryos. By increasing the possibility of live births per cycle, the clinic also increases its overall success rate. For instance, let's say Clinic A has a 50 percent fresh live birth rate and a 10 percent cryopreservation rate and the rate of live births from cryopreservation is 30 percent. Out of 100 patients in Clinic A, fifty women give birth after a fresh cycle, and two more have children from frozen cycles. Fifty-two births result. But let's say Clinic B has a 45 percent fresh live birth rate, a 50 percent cryopreservation rate, and a 30 percent birth rate from cryopreservation. In Clinic B, forty-five women have children from a fresh cycle, and fifteen women have children from a frozen cycle. This now means than the clinic has an additional fifteen live births, bringing the total number of lives births to sixty.

If you had looked only at the live birth rate for fresh eggs you would think that Clinic A was superior to Clinic B, when in the long run Clinic B had the most births.

The "total pregnancy rate" is difficult to track annually because the frozen cycles can continue into the year following the fresh cycle, especially if the frozen cycle involves a second or third attempt at pregnancy

U.S. NATIONAL AVERAGES ARE HIGH

The average rate for live deliveries in American fertility clinics is between 30 and 40 percent per cycle, about 50 percent higher than in Western European countries.

from a single IVF stimulation and retrieval. Although the total pregnancy rate isn't to be found in the statistics, you can get a feel for it by looking at the clinic's combined fresh and frozen pregnancy rate, keeping in mind that it is very important to look at the proportion of frozen embryos compared to the fresh transfers for your age group. For more information about IVF and frozen embryo transfers, see Chapter 9.

Consider Other Features a Clinic May Have

You may ask, is the size of the clinic important? Clinics with more patients have, on the average, tended to do better than those with fewer, but there are exceptions. You also have to ask yourself why a clinic has such a high volume. Could it be that they have so much repeat business because their pregnancy rates are low? Some practices have a lot of patients because of their good reputations. Some have low volumes because of their remote location.

Like all other considerations, the size of a practice is an important feature, but one that must be weighed against other features and facts. In Chapter 9, we talk about ICSI, a procedure in which a single sperm is injected into an egg. This can be useful to couples with male factor infertility or borderline male infertility, but has extra costs associated with it. Most clinics are able to individualize their procedures for couples, but in some extraordinarily large programs they perform ICSI on all cases. This is not only overkill but also overcharging for services that aren't necessary. You can rest assured that this would not be done, if there were no extra charge for ICSI.

Understand the Number Crunching:
How Clinics Can Inflate Their Success Rates

As you now know, fertility clinics are very competitive, especially when insurance doesn't cover many provided services. Although clinics are required to verify that their data on reported cases is accurate, there is no mechanism in place to assure that all cases are reported. A clinic can do 2,000 cases but choose to report only 1,000 and not be discovered. This, of course, can lead to clinics appearing to be more successful than they actually are. Unfortunately, there is almost no way for patients to tell if they are in a program that is underreporting. However, if you are told that you are in a "special program" in which you will receive IVF only if your stimulation phase goes well, it is possible that your cycle may not be reported, because reported cycles must be entered at the time of the cycle start.

YOU HAVE CHOSEN YOUR DOCTOR: ARE YOU GETTING THE BEST CARE?

You have gathered referrals, researched statistics, and asked all the right questions of your clinic or doctor before making your selection. Now you want to know if you made the right choice. Naturally, your doctor's experience and expertise matter, but you want to be a proactive consumer, fully involved in understanding and monitoring your care. Ask yourself:

- Does your doctor's advice make sense? Infertility care is a structured, logical, process. Decisions are made based on your diagnosis and what occurs in treatment.
- What is your infertility diagnosis? Ten percent of couples have truly unexplained infertility, but do you know if you really fall into this category?
- Is the strategy for treatment to determine the cause of your infertility and address it accordingly or is it just to send "bombs away," overloading your system with fertility drugs? Always ask for explanations.

About every three months, doctor and patient should reassess treatment. For example, a doctor might try three months of clomiphene or three months of IUI before moving to another phase of treatment. At each stage, assess where you are and the progress you have made. Do you have a plan? Does it make sense?

Try the "doomsday scenario." Sometimes doctors must be cold dispensers of facts, and sometimes we can be coaches or cheerleaders. Not everybody has the same chance of conceiving a pregnancy. People with favorable characteristics like youth and good ovarian function will almost certainly succeed (although even among people in this group, there are no guarantees). So, if you're thirty-one and you're making a lot of eggs and embryos, and your doctor tells you in times of discouragement that you have a 90 percent chance of succeeding, your doctor is probably right. But if you are in your late thirties or in your forties and things are not going as well, and you know that there are problems, and your medical team is acting as though everything is just great, you are probably not getting realistic information. Ask your doctor what your alternatives are, if you don't succeed. This doomsday scenario can tell you about your doctor's attitude and professional practice. Be wary if your doctor promises pregnancy or guarantees an outcome.

Getting a Second Opinion

No doctor should discourage a patient from seeking a second opinion. If your doctor does, find another doctor. On the other hand, your doctor should not give you unsolicited advice about who should provide that opinion. A second opinion should always come from an unrelated institution, which should not accept you as a patient, because to do so would be unethical.

Changing Doctors?

As time passes, you may begin to feel frustrated with treatment, especially if you have been with a program for while. At some point, you may ask yourself if you made the right decision. Infertility care is very complex. More often than not, worries about quality care are not justified. Your fertility problems may be such that you may do no better with another physician. However, it's fair to bring up your concerns with your doctor, especially if you have been with a program for a while, say, six or nine months. Talk to your doctor. Assess your doctor's response. Are your concerns being dismissed? If this is the case, you might consider another practice. But if the care is logical and organized and everything that should be done is being done, it may be that there are physiological issues in question—or even just bad statistical luck. Here too, you want a realistic assessment of your chance of having a child so that you can make informed decisions about your future.

WHAT YOU SHOULD KNOW ABOUT OTHERS INVOLVED IN YOUR CARE

A chain is only as strong as its weakest link, and complex infertility cases may require a multidisciplinary approach. The qualifications and communication between all of those involved in your care is crucial. The following individuals may be key members of your infertility team.

The Infertility Urologist

If you're having difficulty getting pregnant the old-fashioned way, your partner may see a urologist at some point in treatment. Your urologist should be board certified. Some urologists who specialize in male infertility are fellowship trained. This means that after completing a residency in urology, an infertility urologist will undergo one to two years of additional training in male infertility. However, some of the most noteworthy urologists do not have a fellowship and were instead "grandfathered" in to this criterion by virtue of their experience and achievements. When looking for a urologist, consider:

- recommendations from your reproductive endocrinologist
- publication in peer-reviewed medical journals

The Embryologist

The embryologist is the person who views and selects the embryos for transfer, among many other duties. Although embryologists work behind the scenes, their role in maintaining the function of the IVF lab is a vital one.

Most embryologists slowly master all of the components of IVF through an apprenticeship. Though they are usually not medical doctors, they are crucial links in the chain of care. Some have credentials after their name, and some don't, but for practical purposes there may be no difference in the skill level of either practitioner.

The head embryologist designs and sets forth all of the procedures for the lab, which includes every step of the lab process from selection of culture media (the media around the embryos in the dish) to dish preparation, to setting incubators, to making certain all the components of the lab are running well, to all of the lab's policy procedures and paperwork.

Importantly, the head embryologist chooses the embryos for transfer. Like an art critic, the embryologist uses visual criteria for selection of the best embryos. While there may someday be a test of the culture media to choose the most viable embryos, it is still done by sight, and the head embryologist must have a very good eye.

Ultimately, your doctor is responsible for your case and its outcome, but the doctor and the embryologist work closely together. You have a right to ask a clinic:

- Who is the embryologist?
- How long has the embryologist been practicing?
- How long has the embryologist worked with you?

Patients often want to talk to the embryologist about the embryos. In my dream IVF lab, I would have an embryologist available to patients for one-to-one consultation on an ongoing basis. Our head embryologist in my practice is unusually outgoing, and we are able to offer educational meetings in an informal group setting for questions and answers. Although having an embryologist available for consultation is ideal, the reality is the people who work in the IVF lab are on a tight schedule and most embryologists are not available for phone or live consultation for good reason. For example, when an embryologist is supposed to inseminate eggs at a precise hour, that person must be on time and cannot be held up on a phone call or by a conversation in the hallway. Most patients who are concerned about the timing of their own procedures understand how punctual and efficient embryologists must be and have no problem allowing for questions in a group setting. Ask by what means your clinic educates patients about the embryology questions.

Once you have had initial testing and chosen a doctor or a clinic, the next step is to make sure you have the right diagnosis of your individual problem, so that you don't end up spending more time and money than necessary. In Chapter 5, you will find information about common infertility issues for women. In Chapter 6, you will find a discussion of medical problems that can affect male fertility. Most people do find out why they are having trouble having a baby. The sooner you and your doctor discover the problem, the sooner you will be on your way to getting the right treatment.

5 | Get the Right Treatment: For Women

In Chapter 3, you read about preliminary tests that your doctor can use to investigate the potential causes of your infertility. In this chapter, we will go further, looking at additional tests you may need not only to diagnose the cause of your infertility but to treat it as well.

There is a 90 percent chance that the cause of your infertility can be determined. In vitro fertilization (IVF) is an option for many with infertility and ultimately may be the right treatment for you. But undergoing IVF without finding and treating the root cause of your infertility is both inefficient and impractical, potentially exposing you to treatment that is unduly invasive when there are many problems that can be fixed with relatively inexpensive and minimal therapies.

This chapter is designed to help you identify your potential diagnosis. Bear in mind that it is only intended to help you better understand a medical condition that may underlie your infertility and is not meant as medical advice. Always consult your doctor. If you are seeing your doctor because of recurring miscarriages, turn to Chapter 10. There you will find in-depth information on testing and treatment for recurrent pregnancy loss.

POLYCYSTIC OVARIAN SYNDROME (PCOS): THE MOST COMMON FORM OF OVARIAN DYSFUNCTION

Polycystic ovarian syndrome (PCOS) is one of the most common forms of ovarian dysfunction, affecting up to 10 percent of women of reproductive age. You may also hear this condition termed polycystic ovarian disease, or Stein-Leventhal syndrome, after the two gynecologists who first identified it. Polycystic ovarian syndrome is a complex hormonal disorder in which your normal cycle is disrupted. You can develop PCOS at any time of your reproductive life from adolescence to the onset of menopause, but because PCOS has health consequences that reach beyond infertility, detection is important.

Women with PCOS have enlarged ovaries in which there is an accumulation of cysts developed from unreleased follicles in arrested development. These follicles can be seen on an ultrasound in a characteristic "string of pearls" formation. With PCOS, the follicles stop growing in the secondary phase of development when the cells proliferate and divide. Fluid accumulates in the follicular cells and surrounds part of the egg. Looking under a microscope, you would see a fluid-filled structure in the ovary—the ovarian follicle, which is a cyst, since the very definition of a cyst is a fluid-filled sac. With PCOS, the follicles neither regress nor continue past this point, and over time hundreds of these follicles halted in their development accumulate in the ovary, giving it its polycystic appearance. As different generations of follicles grow but fail to ovulate, they continue to pump out hormones. Rather than rising and falling as they would normally, they secrete continuously, disrupting your cycle so that ovulation doesn't happen. The more follicles that accumulate, the more hormones you are pumping out, keeping you on a cycle of anovulation, or lack of ovulation. High levels of androgen (male hormone, including testosterone) levels and irregular or absent periods are defining features of this syndrome. If you have PCOS, you may never ovulate or ovulate only rarely.

While disorders with symptoms similar to PCOS originate with your adrenal glands or pituitary (the master gland in your brain that controls many body functions), true PCOS is a disorder of the ovary, the "seat of the soul" of ovulation. Because the ovary drives your cycle, anything that affects your ovary affects your cycle. Too much estrogen, too much androgen, or inappropriate feedback from the ovary to the brain can interrupt your normal cycle and keep you from ovulating.

Some of the key factors that can disturb your cycle in PCOS include:

- *Overproduction of androgens.* Along with estrogen, the normal ovary produces androgens (male hormones), most of which become converted to estrogen by the enzyme aromatase. With PCOS, you have less relative aromatase activity because there is excess raw material, called substrate, leading to the production of more androgen than usual, causing the male-type characteristics that can be so troubling to women with PCOS: excess hair growth, acne, and in severe cases, thinning of the hair in a male pattern. While most women have testosterone levels that range between 20 to 80 nanograms, women with PCOS will generally have levels between 50 to 120 nanograms, the upper range or just above the upper limit of normal. But the amount of androgen in your system is not the only factor that affects you. Two women can put out exactly the same amount of testosterone, but one may have more cellular receptors to testosterone than the other, enabling her to receive more of the androgen hormone's message. Receptors are proteins on or inside a cell that await a matching hormone and can combine with it just as a lock allows a key to turn it. The hormone then affects the metabolism of that cell. If you are of Southern Italian heritage, for example, you may have more receptors for androgens than someone who is Scandinavian, so your response to androgen is going to look different. You may have more hair growth.

- *Excess estrogen production.* While you are putting out an abundance of male hormones, your ovaries are also making lots of estrogen every day. Your hormone levels don't ebb and flow, as they would if you were cycling. Excess estrogen is both a cause and an effect of PCOS. When you don't cycle regularly, your body isn't making progesterone in the second half of your cycle. Progesterone causes you to shed your uterine lining during menstruation. Instead, too much estrogen unopposed by progesterone can cause you to overgrow your uterine lining. This condition, called hyperplasia, predisposes you to endometrial cancer (cancer of the uterine lining).

- *High levels of luteinizing hormone (LH)* affect about two-thirds of women with PCOS. Chronic high levels of LH prevent the low to high hormonal fluctuation that is necessary for normal follicular development and ovulation. There is a relationship between high LH levels and miscarriage as well as increased levels of androgen.

- *Excess weight.* Body fat (adipose tissue) contains the enzyme aromatase, which causes the conversion of androgens to estrogens. Excess body fat can result in an overabundance of estrogen. Again, too much estrogen causes inappropriate signaling to the pituitary and disrupts the normal ebb and flow of FSH and LH secretion necessary for follicular development and ovulation. To exacerbate the problem, PCOS makes it difficult to lose weight. If you are not losing weight or you are gaining weight, you can become increasingly resistant to insulin. Insulin resistance can be a very important factor in PCOS.

- *Resistance to insulin.* Insulin stimulates ovarian androgen production, causing inappropriate feedback from your ovaries to your pituitary, disrupting your cycle, and causing hirsutism and acne. The hormone insulin carries glucose (sugar) into your cells to be used as energy in your body. As your cells become resistant to insulin, the levels of sugar in your blood increase, causing glucose intolerance that can lead to many of the problems related to diabetes, including obesity and risk for heart disease; stroke; kidney, eye, and foot problems; and other complications. Insulin resistance predisposes you to type 2 diabetes. This is different from insulin-dependent diabetes, where one is deprived of, rather than resistant to, insulin. Women who are insulin-dependent tend to ovulate when given insulin, just as women who are insulin-resistant will ovulate when given metformin or other insulin sensitizers.

Because you are not ovulating frequently or at all when you have PCOS, it's hard to get pregnant without intervention. Because your LH (luteinizing hormone) levels are higher than normal, your risk of miscarriage is increased, too. Women with PCOS are more likely to develop diabetes during pregnancy (called gestational diabetes) and to have larger babies, requiring cesarean delivery (C-section).

Do You Have PCOS?

When you're trying to have a baby, you are likely to be paying a lot of attention to your cycles, but there may have been other times when you were not as concerned about the regularity of your period. You may realize that you have PCOS only after you notice you are having trouble getting pregnant. On the other hand, you may have noticed irregularity early in your adolescence. Many women with PCOS start birth control pills in their teenage years to regulate their periods and to decrease hair growth and acne. There are noticeable signs of PCOS, including:

• Absent, infrequent, or irregular periods, or irregular periods punctuated by extremely heavy flow. Many women with PCOS have never had a regular period. A long history of irregular cycles and no PMS suggests the possibility of PCOS;

- Hair growth on your body that is excessive and differs from what is usual for your family or ethnic background;
- Excessive acne—more than you are used to or more than other family members;
- Obesity and a tendency to have difficulty losing weight no matter how much you restrict your caloric intake (though women can certainly have PCOS without obesity);
- Darkening of the pigment in skin folds (called acanthosis nigricans). This symptom and skin tags (below) affect a small proportion of people with PCOS;
- Skin tags, which look like little fragments of velvety hanging skin;

- Abnormal cholesterols levels: low levels of the good cholesterol (HDL) and high levels of bad cholesterol (LDL), which can be due to PCOS, obesity, or both conditions.

Most of the time, doctors begin to suspect PCOS based on your medical history, menstrual history including your premenstrual symptoms, and a history of any other symptoms, such as those listed above. Importantly, your doctor will suspect PCOS, if the "string of pearls" formation of visible cysts on your ovaries can be seen on your ultrasound. Your doctor will ask you:

- When was your last menstrual period?
- How often do you get your period?
- When you get your period or just before you get your period, do you notice any other kinds of symptoms, such as bloating, sore breasts, cramps, cravings, mood changes?

Is PCOS Genetic?

There may be a genetic link to PCOS. Your risk for PCOS increases if someone in your family has it. There is also a genetic link between PCO-like syndromes, such as those caused by increased adrenal production or other inherited steroid abnormalities. (See "PCO-like Syndromes." on page 88.) If a family member has a PCO-like syndrome, you are more at risk for developing that syndrome but not true PCOS. Lastly, some adrenal problems associated with PCOS are more common in Ashkenazi Jews and Eskimos.

Testing for PCOS

If you and your doctor suspect PCOS, you should have:

- An ultrasound, which should be done at your first visit.
- A day three FSH/LH/estradiol test. (See Chapter 3.) For PCOS, the

ratio of LH to FSH is important. A ratio of LH to FSH greater than two to one is abnormal. It's advisable to add LH to a day three FSH/estradiol test for patients who have cycles that are not perfectly regular or have suspicious findings for PCOS on a sonogram.

- Prolactin test. A high prolactin level can indicate hyperprolactinemia, a PCO-like syndrome.
- Thyroid-stimulating hormone (TSH) test for thyroid disorders. Hypothryoidism can give you a PCO-like syndrome as well. This test is sensitive for both "hypo" (low) thyroid and "hyper" (high) thyroid.
- Testing for testosterone is key for PCOS, because the vast majority of people with PCOS will have above-average testosterone levels.
- Testing for DHEAS, a weak androgen, and 17-hydroxyprogesterone can suggest adrenal issues that cause PCO-like syndromes.
- Fasting blood glucose and insulin, to test for diabetes. Although most people who have PCOS will be treated with a medication called metformin, and most show normal blood fasting sugars and insulin, getting tested for diabetes matters, because people with PCOS are at risk. It's important to have a record of your baseline should you develop diabetes in the future.

Treating PCOS

There is medication that will reverse PCOS for prolonged periods of time if taken continuously. Metformin is an insulin sensitizer that can help women with PCOS ovulate. As pointed out previously, 50 percent of women taking metformin ovulate. Even women who are not insulin resistant ovulate when taking metformin, perhaps because insulin resistance in this syndrome may be localized at the ovary and not measurable in the bloodstream, making some degree of insulin resistance undetectable by currently available tests. It may also be that we ultimately need to redefine insulin resistance as it relates to PCOS, substituting the concept of metformin-responsiveness instead.

For over a decade, doctors have treated women with PCOS with clomiphene citrate, the most common fertility drug, before treating with metformin. There is no doubt that combining metformin with clomiphene citrate works better than clomiphene citrate alone, because metformin enhances the action of clomiphene. But at the time of this writing, it seems that the tendency to treat initially with clomiphene is being reversed, that the first line of treatment may be metformin, followed by clomiphene citrate if metformin alone fails. There are good reasons for this. Unlike with clomiphene citrate, there is a lower incidence of miscarriage with metformin. You can also avoid the monthly visits to your RE that are necessary when you're on clomiphene citrate, having a new ultrasound, a new set of drugs, and possibly new blood tests at each pregnancy attempt. If you are on metformin and respond to it within about three months, you can keep attempting to get pregnant without having to go back to your doctor to try to induce ovulation again or for frequent monitoring. For some women, clomiphene robs their cervical mucus of its clear, voluminous abundance at ovulation, increasing the need for intrauterine insemination (IUI). With metformin, your need for inseminations is no less or greater than any other woman's need for IUI.

Weight loss is another benefit. Many women who are on metformin find it easier to lose weight, which means lowered insulin resistance, because being overweight makes you more insulin resistant. When you lose weight, you tend to feel better about your body. Feeling better about how you look can inspire you to keep exercising and dieting, important tools in lowering insulin resistance.

Metformin is a pill typically taken two or three times a day. The jury is still out on whether you may need to take the drug throughout your life, but this recommendation is foreseeable in the future. If clomiphene is added, you will generally take this oral medication for five days during the month.

Gastrointestinal problems are the most common side effects of metformin. For those who do have bowel disturbances, they usually subside soon after taking metformin, although for some, they are significant enough to be intolerable. In my practice, I usually introduce metformin gradually, building up to a full dose. You will know within two to three months whether you are responding to metformin and starting to ovulate.

Taking Care of Yourself for Life

Having PCOS means being vigilant about your health, recognizing symptoms of other PCOS-related conditions before they progress. Here are some things you can do to stay healthy and prevent problems:

- When you are not ovulating, a chronic excess level of estrogen can cause an overgrowth of the uterine lining. Birth control pills, taken when you are not trying to get pregnant, can help prevent your uterine lining from thickening, which predisposes you to endometrial hyperplasia and uterine cancer. As well, birth control pills can help keep your cycles regular and reduce hair growth and acne.
- Have your uterine lining (endometrium) checked with the most noninvasive method, transvaginal ultrasound. If you have a reassuring vaginal ultrasound, you may not need an endometrial biopsy, a more invasive means of evaluating your uterine lining. On the other hand, if your ultrasound indicates that your uterine lining is over 5 millimeters, you may need a biopsy to further investigate your endometrium. Even if the biopsy is negative, you should still have an ultrasound the following year. If that is negative, you may not need a biopsy again. Overgrowth of the endometrium can be treated with a high-dose progestin pill, such as Provera or Megace.
- Although you may not be diabetic now, remember that women with PCOS have a higher risk of being insulin resistant during pregnancy or later in life. If you have PCOS, have your fasting blood sugar checked annually. If you do develop diabetes, treatment with diet changes and possibly medication is in order. Exercise, always important, is especially important in patients with PCOS in order to optimize lipid levels and fat/muscle ratio.

DIMINISHED OVARIAN RESERVE

At the opposite end of the spectrum from PCOS is diminished ovarian reserve. With PCOS, the ovaries are full of follicles and working overtime, but with diminished ovarian reserve, both the number of eggs in the ovaries and the amount of hormones being put out are reduced. Although diminished ovarian reserve normally occurs with aging, loss of full ovarian function before the age of forty is considered premature. Partial loss is referred to as decreased ovarian reserve, perimenopause, or just as high FSH. Total loss of ovarian function before forty is called premature ovarian failure. In the vast majority of cases, the causes of diminished ovarian reserve are unexplained, yet there are genetic and environmental factors that can accelerate it. Risk factors include:

- previous ovarian surgery
- previous chemotherapy or radiotherapy
- systemic autoimmune disease, such as systemic lupus erythematosus

The age at which you go through menopause is, to some extent, determined by your family history. But having female relatives who went through menopause at a normal to late age (average is fifty-one) or who had children past forty is no insurance that you will not suffer from early diminished ovarian reserve.

Because it generally worsens over time and is associated with less success in virtually all infertility therapies short of the use of donor eggs, diminished ovarian reserve once diagnosed requires immediate attention.

TUBAL PROBLEMS: BLOCKED OR DAMAGED FALLOPIAN TUBES

Far from being passive conduits through which an egg or embryo travels to the uterus, the fallopian tubes are vital muscular and glandular organs that facilitate the joining of sperm and egg. The fimbria, the fingerlike projections that extend from the fanned ends of the fallopian tube, sweep over the ovary to actively draw in a newly released egg. After fertilization, the fertilized egg, or embryo, stays in the fallopian tube for about three to five days until it begins to make its way to the uterus. The fallopian tube provides the fluid that nurtures the early embryo, prevents it from adhering to the tube, and facilitates transport to the uterus. (Scientists have modeled a media in which to support embryos growing in the IVF laboratory after this fallopian fluid.) Finally, the fallopian tube actually moves the egg along to the uterus through contractions and the beating of tiny hairlike projections called cilia, which line the tube's interior.

When fallopian tubes are damaged, due to blockage, scarring, or destruction of the internal lining, conception without assistance can be difficult or impossible. Damaged tubes can also cause a potentially life-threatening condition called ectopic pregnancy, in which an embryo begins to develop outside the uterus, most often in a fallopian tube. (See Chapter 10.)

How Your Tubes Can Be Damaged

Generally speaking, there are a few ways your tubes can be damaged. We will discuss the ways tubes can be blocked or damaged, but first let's discuss how damaged tubes can affect your fertility.

Usually, fallopian tubes are blocked at one end or the other, and are rarely blocked in the middle. Blockage at the end of the tube, toward the uterus, in the portion of the tube known as the isthmus, is called proximal tubal obstruction. Proximal obstruction can be seen on a hysterosalpingogram (HSG—see page 40) and may be caused by inflammation, infection, plugs of mucus or tissue in the tubes, or by spasm of the wall of the tube. In many cases of proximal tubal obstruction, the cause is unknown and there is no predisposing factor. Proximal obstruction is much less common than blockage at the farthest end of the tube near the ovaries, called distal tubal obstruction.

The innate delicacy of the fimbria may be the reason for the greater likelihood of obstruction affecting the farthest end of the fallopian tube. The late stage of distal obstruction is called *hydrosalpinx*, a condition usually caused by infection. At this stage, the fingerlike ends of the fimbria become stuck together and shut. Unable to drain, fluid becomes trapped, and the fallopian tube swells to a "sausage" shape characteristic of hydrosalpinx. In addition, the fluid from the hydrosalpinx is toxic and can discharge into the uterine cavity, creating an environment hostile to embryo development. Therefore, having a hydrosalpinx profoundly reduces your chances of getting pregnant both with and without IVF. This is why a tube damaged to this extent should be removed or closed off near the uterus— that is, at the proximal end—before attempting pregnancy or pregnancy with IVF. Although hydrosalpinx is a dramatic destruction of the fallopian tube, you may have no symptoms. You may not know you have this condition until you discover you are infertile.

If one of your tubes is damaged, it's very likely that the other is, too. However, there are times when differences between tubes are pronounced, such as when damage occurs from irritation or appendicitis. (See page 96.) The following are some common causes of tubal damage.

Spasm

Spasm is not a true blockage but can look and function as an obstruction because it, at least temporarily, obstructs the connection between the uterus and tubes. This is a phenomenon limited to the proximal fallopian tube. One can't actually witness a fallopian spasm, and the cause is unknown. A physician may conclude that a tube is blocked due to spasm after seeing a proximal obstruction during a first inspection of the fallopian tube and then seeing the same tube open at a second investigation, for example, during a laparoscopy (see page 99). The reverse can also happen: a doctor may see a formerly open tube in a closed state at laparoscopy. Rarely, during a hysterosalpingogram, a doctor may give an injection of glucagon, a hormone that acts as a muscle relaxant, in order to try to relieve a tube blocked by spasm. In this case, the doctor may be able to see the spasm open up. The problem in these situations is always the unanswerable question of whether the tube is *usually* open or *usually* closed.

Pelvic Inflammatory Disease

Pelvic inflammatory disease (PID) is an infection of the uterus, fallopian tubes, and ovaries, most often caused by untreated chlamydia or gonorrhea, ascending infections that can be transmitted through sexual intercourse. Bacteria are introduced into the vagina through sex with an infected partner and travel through the cervix, the uterus, and fallopian tubes and out into the *peritoneal cavity* (the space in the abdomen that contains the liver, stomach, and intestines), causing inflammation. Over a period of time, inflammation can cause scar tissue, which can completely destroy your reproductive organs and increase your risk of ectopic pregnancy. Early symptoms of PID include pelvic pain and fever, but PID can also be silent, causing no symptoms.

Appendicitis

Appendicitis can cause damage. Lots of bacteria live in the appendix, the colon, and in the cecum, which is a part of the large intestine that leads to the appendix. If the appendix becomes infected and subsequently bursts, bacteria can spread over your reproductive system, damaging your reproductive organs. However, it's possible for the right tube, the tube nearest the appendix, to be affected and for the left to be unharmed.

Inflammation or Infection from Surgery

Lower abdominal or pelvic surgery can expose you to risk of infection and inflammation. An organ may also be accidentally scraped, pushed, or compressed during surgery, leading to inflammation that can occur without infection. In the past, surgical gloves were covered with a sterile talcum powder that also had the potential to irritate organs, cause inflammation, and increase the likelihood of causing adhesions and scarring. Today, surgical gloves are no longer coated with talcum.

IUDs (Intrauterine Devices)

IUDs are contraceptive devices that were much more common in the 1970s than today because of the infamous recall of the Dalkon Shield IUD, which was linked to pelvic inflammatory disease. Yet it may not have been the IUD portion of the device that was at fault, but rather the multifilament string on the IUD that allowed bacteria to travel into the uterus and up into the fallopian tubes, causing infection. After the Dalkon Shield debacle in which numerous lawsuits were brought against the company that manufactured it, IUD use declined dramatically. Contemporary IUDs are not like the Dalkon Shield. Although PID risk is possible, it has not been shown with contemporary IUDs. Still, because there is some question as to whether there is a risk with IUD use, it's reasonable to suggest that this method be reserved for monogamous women who are fairly certain that they have completed their families, but who are not yet ready for tubal ligation.

Diethylstilbestrol (DES)

Diethylstilbestrol (DES) is a synthetic estrogen that was prescribed to prevent miscarriage until 1971, when the FDA issued a bulletin advising against its use because of its link to a rare form of vaginal cancer in the daughters of women who took DES. Although not all DES daughters have reproductive abnormalities, exposed women are at increased risk for clear-cell adenocarcinoma of the vagina and cervix, pregnancy complications, and infertility. Women exposed to DES tend to have smaller uteruses and longer fallopian tubes. DES daughters have an increased risk of ectopic pregnancy, but the cause of this higher risk is unclear. It is most likely associated with a developmental abnormality of the fallopian tubes.

Endometriosis

Endometriosis can cause inflammation, yet it is a sterile process, not an infection. For reasons that aren't understood, endometriosis is less likely to affect the fallopian tubes than other organs. It's not unusual to find healthy fallopian tubes even in the midst of severe endometriosis. However, endometriosis can cause scarring around the ovaries that can prevent even functional fallopian tubes from doing their job of picking up and transporting an ovulated egg.

Peritubal Adhesions

Sometimes fallopian tubes are open but not functional because their location or mobility is limited by scar tissue around them known as peritubal adhesions. This is also the result of an inflammatory process such as one of those mentioned above. Peritubal adhesions are more amenable to surgical correction than other forms of tubal damage because peritubal adhesions are less destructive to the inner lining of the fallopian tube.

Salpingitis Isthmica Nodosa (SIN)

Salpingitis isthmica nodosa (SIN) is a severe abnormality of the tube at the isthmus, the portion of the tube near the uterus. Salpingitis means tubal inflammation, and nodosa means nodular in appearance. If you were to actually feel the part of the tube that extends into the uterus, it would feel nodular. On hysterosalpingogram, you can see invaginations (pockets), causing a honeycomb pattern along the tube. Tubes damaged to this extent don't function. SIN is considered irreparable, and in vitro fertilization (IVF) is used to bypass the affected tube.

Diagnosing and Treating Blocked Fallopian Tubes

When your tubes are blocked, you may face a choice between a procedure to open the tubes, called *tubal catheterization*, and forgoing such a procedure, moving directly to in vitro fertilization (IVF). Whether one option or the other is best depends on the extent of the damage to your tubes and your age, among other important factors.

Proximal Obstruction

If you have proximal obstruction, your options include a procedure called tubal catheterization (also called *tubal cannulation*) that can be done with two other procedures: laparoscopy using a hysteroscope (a narrow telescope with a fiber-optic light that enables your doctor to look directly into your uterus) or radiographically during a hysterosalpingogram (HSG). Whether done using a hysteroscope or during a hysterosalpingogram, this procedure involves the use of a small catheter inside of which there is a fine coated guidewire. The catheter with the guidewire is inserted through your cervix and your uterus in an attempt to push open the blockage.

Diagnosing and treating proximal obstruction with laparoscopy. Laparoscopy is a minimally invasive procedure that is the best way for a surgeon to see your entire reproductive system, to fully inspect your uterus, ovaries, and fallopian tubes, and to detect the extent of tubal damage and additional problems, including endometriosis and scarring (cobweblike adhesions). This is an outpatient surgery done under general anesthesia. A .5- to 1-centimeter incision will be made just under your navel, and about 2 to 3 liters of harmless carbon dioxide gas will be slowly pumped into your peritoneal cavity to expand it, allowing the surgeon to visualize your entire reproductive system.

A fiber-optic telescope called a *laparoscope* will be inserted through the incision in your navel. Another probe may be inserted through a second incision so that the surgeon can move organs in order to see whether there is scar tissue or endometriosis.

If upon laparoscopy everything looks normal and your tubes are only blocked proximally, your surgeon may attempt to open the fallopian tubes using a hysteroscope, a tiny telescopic device that is inserted through your vagina and cervix to look into your uterus. Although most illustrations of the uterus show the uterus as an open, pear-shaped organ, the walls of the uterus actually rest together when you are not pregnant. This is why the surgeon must expand your uterine cavity to see within. During a hysteroscopy, a catheter fed through an operating channel in the hysteroscope can be used to push open the blockage.

After surgery you may feel nausea from the anesthesia and bloating from the gas used to expand the abdominal cavity. It's not unusual to have shoulder pain and some bleeding like your period. You should be back to your usual activities within two or three days.

Later in this chapter, we will talk about the difficulties of finding a surgeon experienced in doing laparoscopy. Ideally, your laparoscopy should be used to diagnose as well as treat tubal damage, if possible. Not every surgeon is trained to use a hysteroscope during laparoscopy. If your surgeon feels unable to remove the blockage hysteroscopically, a hysterosalpingogram (HSG—see page 40) can be scheduled to try to unblock the tube radiographically. This can be a good option when you know that you do not have distal blockage.

Before scheduling a laparoscopy, you and your doctor should have a serious discussion about the likely findings of your surgery. What will your doctor do, based on those findings? Should a blocked tube be opened, if possible? Or should the tube or tubes be removed? Understanding the risks and benefits of any surgery is part of informed consent.

Never hesitate to schedule a discussion with your doctor. Ask for explanations. The amount of explanation your doctor gives you and the extent of investigation into your individual case is indicative of whether or not your doctor has sufficient interest and expertise to handle your concerns effectively. Remember that you are in control of the decisions you make about your body. You have a right to know the details of your diagnosis and treatment.

Personally, I recommend that patients have a laparoscopy before unblocking a proximal obstruction so that any other problems, such as a blockage at the end of the tube, can be seen and addressed. Not only can your doctor see additional problems during laparoscopy, the problems can be treated at the same time. If, for example, at laparoscopy you find out that you have damage at the end of the tube (the distal portion) as well as proximal damage, you know that the tube is damaged in two places. A tube damaged in two places cannot effectively be repaired. It should be left alone, or even removed, and IVF should be considered.

If you have distal damage, with or without proximal damage, you may wonder how a surgeon will know if the distal damage is bad. The surgeon will assess this by looking at the fimbriae, the fingerlike projections at the end of the tube. As you recall, they are very delicate. They are the part of the tube most susceptible to damage. Normally, they are soft and vascular. Their fingerlike projections should be separated, not stuck together. If you introduced a fluid through the tube directed toward the fimbria, you would see the fimbria flow and open up. The fimbriae should be able to pivot around the ovaries for about 360 degrees. If the tubal disease is bad enough that the ends of the tube are stuck together and obstructed, surgery will yield only a 20 percent chance of success. This means that with severe tubal disease, you have a one in five chance in your lifetime of getting pregnant after tubal surgery alone. Undergoing a procedure that isn't going to give you a great chance of success doesn't make sense in the world of IVF, which allows many women with no or damaged fallopian tubes to get pregnant and with which you have a 50 percent chance of success.

You are more likely to salvage your tube through surgery when your tube is only partially blocked. When not removing the tube, the goal of surgery is to normalize the anatomy of the tube and the surrounding organs as much as possible. If there is scar tissue around the tube, your surgeon will remove it. If the tube is open, but the opening is smaller than it ought to be, the surgeon will try to open it a little more, stretching it or making an incision so that it will be more functional. If the fimbriae look slightly abnormal, the surgeon will try to normalize them and make sure that nothing interferes with their ability to get close to the ovary to receive an ovulating egg. Unless damage and scarring are so bad that surgical treatment is risky or unlikely to help, it is absolutely incumbent upon a surgeon doing a laparoscopy to remove mild to moderate scar tissue. It is irresponsible and inappropriate for someone not to repair mild to moderate adhesions simply because in vitro fertilization (IVF) is an option. In some cases, for the wrong reasons, it does happen that some surgeons will stop an operation earlier than would be optimal, neglecting to remove scar tissue. You should have confidence that your doctor is dedicated to giving his or her best effort to treat you before allowing that doctor to operate on you.

Treating proximal obstruction during an HSG. A radiologist or a reproductive endocrinologist can also perform tubal catheterization for proximal obstruction during a hysterosalpingogram. This procedure is known as selective salpingography. Just as with a hysterosalpingogram, this procedure will be scheduled at a radiology facility. You will be awake during the procedure, although you may be given some sedation. You will be in a position similar to the one you must lie in during a Pap smear. Your cervix will be exposed and cleansed. A narrow, hollow tube called a catheter will be inserted into your cervix and guided toward the corner of your uterus. A radiocontrast dye will be injected to outline your upper cervix and uterus while an X-ray is taken. This allows the radiologist to see your uterus and fallopian tubes. If the dye stops in your fallopian tubes rather than flushing through the fimbria, indicating a blockage, the radiologist will then try to unblock your tubes. A fine, coated guidewire is fed through a catheter inserted into your cervix. The guidewire is used to probe the fallopian tube, potentially poking the blocked tube open. A contrast dye is injected a second time to confirm that your tubes are open.

Treating hydrosalpinx: alternatives to removal

A hydrosalpinx can be irreparable and can interfere with IVF pregnancy, if left open to the uterus.[1] Even if your other tube were to be miraculously unaffected by the disease process that caused the hydrosalpinx, an untreated hydrosalpinx still reduces your chances of getting pregnant with or without IVF, because the hydrosalpinx can interfere with the fertility of the opposite tube and make the uterine environment toxic.

Yet, a hydrosalpinx doesn't always have to be removed for IVF. An alternative is to close it off near the uterus in a procedure called *tubal occlusion* (also called proximal tubal salpingectomy). The surgeon will separate the connection between the fallopian tube and the uterus so that the fallopian tube doesn't drain into the uterine cavity. Studies have shown that, as far as IVF is concerned, there is no difference between these two alternatives. In my practice, if I can easily remove the hydrosalpinx in its entirety, I will. But sometimes the hydrosalpinx is stuck to other vital organs, such as the intestines. Of course, no surgeon wants to risk causing damage to other organs by trying to remove an adhered hydrosalpinx. Here again, the tube can be separated from the uterus and left in.

Very rarely, a hydrosalpinx left in can twist. This is called torsion and can happen when the tube is free from other organs but separated from the uterus for the purposes of IVF. A tube that is stuck to other organs is not likely to twist. When torsion occurs with a hydrosalpinx, the hydrosalpinx should be removed.

Be sure to meet with your surgeon before your procedure to discuss the possible findings at laparoscopy and the likely course of action your surgeon will take to treat them. You do not want to come out of surgery with a procedure that wasn't done as well as it could be. (For more information on how to talk to your doctor, take a look at the section "Before You Have Surgery: Choosing the Most Qualified Surgeon," on page 130.)

Treating Peritubal Adhesions: Scar Tissue Around Your Fallopian Tubes

Scar tissue (called *adhesions* or *extrinsic tubal disease*) can hurt your fertility in a number of ways. Although the ovary sits on a stalk, it's basically free and most of its surface should be accessible to the fimbriated end of the fallopian tube, which must be able to pivot over the surface of the ovary to pick up the egg as it emerges from its ruptured follicle. If the surface of the ovary is inaccessible, either because scar tissue has plastered the ovary to the pelvic wall, for example, or restricted the fallopian tube's movement, you may ovulate, but your egg won't be picked up by the fallopian tube. Fertilization must take place in the fallopian tube, and the fertilized egg must arrive at the uterus through the fallopian tube three to five days later.

Scar tissue can be removed surgically during laparoscopy with what's called tuboplasty. Tuboplasty is a very general term that describes any surgical intervention to normalize a fallopian tube. You may also hear operations to remove adhesions called lysis, in this case lysis of peritubal adhesions.

Lysis means "to cut." You may also hear the term *salpingolysis,* which means "to cut the adhesions from around the tube." Your fallopian tube won't be cut. In fact, the object is to remove the adhesions without doing damage to the tube.

With as little trauma as possible, the surgeon will try to remove scar tissue without cutting the tube or the ovary or any other structure to which the scar tissue is adhered. The surgeon will also take care to expose you to minimal bleeding, because in the surgical field, blood is a potentially inflammatory substance that can cause further scarring or adhesions.

Most often, these operations are done through a variety of techniques in conjunction with laparoscopy, which we'll discuss below. Sometimes surgeons prefer or advertise the use of a surgical tool that sounds very sophisticated, such as a harmonic scalpel or laser. Whether the surgeon is using a blade or another tool, remember that what matters is not the tool, but the delicacy with which the surgeon uses that instrument.

If you have scar tissue around your tubes and ovaries, but no internal damage to the tube creating blockage, your chances of surgical success are better than if you had blockage, precisely because your surgeon is not operating on the tube so much as on the adhesions around the tube.

In such a case, the success rate is approximately 50 percent within twelve months of surgery. Or to put it another way, you have a one in two chance of getting pregnant within the first year after your operation. These odds are about as good as the odds for one cycle of IVF. If you do have a successful pregnancy after removal of your adhesions, you can most likely have another successful pregnancy without further surgery, if you plan to get pregnant again.

There is a caveat here. Sometimes, removal of scar tissue improves the tubes, if they heal with less scar tissue. But in some cases, removal only makes matters worse, causing increased scar tissue. This may be in part due to individual genetics and the way we heal. One person can have surgery with relatively light scarring, while another will have thicker scarring. The same surgeon can do the same operation on two different people, each of whom will heal differently. Here again, if you had your scar tissue repaired and you don't get pregnant within six to twelve months, you may want to consider IVF.

A less destructive procedure may make you a candidate for reversal of tubal ligation, called *tubal anastomosis*. Through microsurgery (under magnification), the blocked part of the tube is removed and the fresh ends of the fallopian tube are put back together. Although there are some unusually technically adept laparoscopic centers where tubal anastomosis is done laparoscopically, it's usually accomplished through a laparotomy, a major operation with a hospital and a recovery time between two and four weeks. Otherwise, if the procedure can be done laparoscopically, you can go home the same day and recover in two to three days. After a tubal anastomosis, you can usually try to get pregnant within the next month.

Success rates for tubal anastomosis can be as high as 80 percent in people who have had reversible tubal ligations, who are good candidates for surgery, and who are relatively young—generally thirty-five and younger. There is about a 10 percent chance of an ectopic pregnancy after a tubal anastomosis.

Facing Choices: Surgery or IVF?

As we've pointed out, you may find yourself having to make a decision between a procedure to unblock or remove a damaged tube or in vitro fertilization (IVF), the latter being the most common artificial reproductive procedure. (See Chapter 9 to learn more about IVF.) Women undergoing IVF are given ovarian stimulation to produce eggs, which are then united with their partners' sperm in the laboratory to form embryos. The embryos are then placed inside the uterus to implant and grow. You don't use your fallopian tubes to get pregnant because your embryos are placed directly into your uterus. Unless you have a hydrosalpinx, IVF allows you to forgo procedures to fix a damaged tube.

Whether you choose to have a procedure to open your tubes and/or remove scar tissue or to go straight to IVF depends on a number of factors. The severity of the damage to your tubes dictates whether a tube can be salvaged. For instance, a tube that is only blocked at the proximal end can most likely be opened. Still, if you have proximal damage only, you can choose to go directly to IVF, because there is no harm in leaving in a proximally obstructed tube. It won't interfere with IVF, because it's not open near the uterus, and fluid will not drain into the uterine cavity as with a hydrosalpinx. If your tubal disease is bad enough that the ends of the tube are stuck together and obstructed, surgery only brings about a one in five chance of getting pregnant in the first year of surgery and thereafter. If your tube is damaged in more than one place or you have severe damage such as a hydrosalpinx, your tube is irreparable. If you only have peritubal adhesions, and you are young, the chances of getting pregnant after a successful removal of the adhesions is about 50 percent within twelve months of surgery, odds that are competitive with IVF. If this is your situation, you might remove the adhesions and see if you get pregnant spontaneously.

Your age can affect your choice. The younger you are, the more time you have to find out if an operation works. If you get pregnant within six to twelve months, the procedure worked. If you don't get pregnant within a year's time after surgery, the procedure was unsuccessful. (Usually, you can start trying to get pregnant within one month of your procedure. You don't have to wait for a healing period. Even with laparotomy you can start trying within the month.) If you are younger, for example, under thirty-five, you may be able to try tubal catheterization and then do IVF later, if the tubal procedure didn't work. If you are thirty-seven or older, you face a kind of double-edged sword. You don't have the luxury of time to wait and see if tubal catheterization works. At the same time, you are less likely to be successful with IVF, because of the age of your eggs. Older eggs tend toward chromosomal and metabolic abnormalities that can increase risk of having no pregnancy or of having a miscarriage. While IVF may not be ideal for someone in her late thirties and early forties, it's certainly faster than waiting six months to a year to find out if a tubal procedure worked or not and then moving on to IVF. When you consider that your fertility declines significantly each year after thirty-seven and that the chances of IVF success diminish accordingly, starting with IVF may be your best alternative.

Another consideration is whether an experienced surgeon is available. Your surgeon or radiologist's skill is another factor to keep in mind when deciding what to do. A tubal catheterization is usually done through laparoscopy, or it can be done during a hysterosalpingogram by an interventional radiologist experienced with tubal procedures. All laparoscopies are done microsurgically, because the laparoscope magnifies the fallopian tube. The surgeon is able to see the fallopian tube many times larger than it is in actuality. Any procedure to reattach a tube, such as reversal of a tubal ligation, is usually done with a laparotomy, surgery performed through an incision in the abdomen. This means major surgery with all its attendant risks and a much lengthier recovery time than laparoscopy. Both laparoscopy and laparotomy demand the skills of a surgeon who is expert in microsurgery. Experience is key. Yet tubal surgery is a dying art. Fewer and fewer reproductive endocrinologists are versed in treating blocked tubes with procedures other than IVF. Before getting any type of tubal surgery, be sure to find out if your doctor is truly qualified to perform your surgery. (Be sure to read the section "Before You Have Surgery: Choosing the Most Qualified Surgeon," on page 130, to help you better assess your options.)

As if you didn't have enough to contend with, insurance is also a factor. Very often, IVF isn't covered by insurance, whereas procedures to correct reversible tubal damage are covered (with the exception of a reversal of a tubal ligation). Of course, if you do have universal coverage for IVF, you have another reason to consider it as a first choice. As you can surmise, lack of coverage for IVF and fewer surgeons experienced in doing laparoscopies can put a woman who is in need of tubal surgery in a perilous position. Again, take a look at "Before You Have Surgery" for an in-depth look at the issues affecting your choices.

The Choice Between Tubal Reversal and IVF

If you are young, tubal anastomosis may be your first choice, especially if you want to have more than one child, because once your tubes are open that is a possibility. If you are past thirty-five and have had a tubal ligation, you may very well be facing a common dilemma. As you age, your chances of success with IVF diminish. Nonetheless, you will know fairly soon after IVF whether it is likely to work for you. For example, a woman who is thirty-eight may respond well to ovarian stimulation, produce a lot of eggs, and make good-looking embryos. But it's just as possible that a different woman of the same age may not stimulate well, and she and her partner may not make embryos that look as though they have potential to succeed. Both IVF and tubal anastomosis are often specifically excluded from insurance plans. So what should you do?

There is no one right answer, but you could do the following:

- If you have had a tubal ligation, you know that you were fertile at some point. If you are at an older age, such as at least thirty-seven, when you have less of a chance of succeeding at IVF, you might just go ahead and reverse your tubal ligation, if it is reversible. If you don't get pregnant, you might go on to try IVF the following year. The downside is that your fertility diminishes each year after thirty-seven, and you may be less likely to do well at IVF as you age.
- Try IVF first. If it doesn't work, you can try tubal reversal in the future.
- Pursue both options simultaneously. If you are of a mind to do everything you can to get pregnant, or you wanted to try having more than one child, you could do IVF and reverse your sterilization around the same period of time. You might get pregnant through IVF and/or spontaneously later on after a tubal reversal. There is nothing about having a reversal of sterilization that enhances your chance of IVF, but in this scenario you might be able to battle time more effectively.

Bearing in mind that you may not have coverage for either procedure, both are probably comparable in cost. The surgical fee for a tubal reversal may initially seem lower than IVF, but you will have to factor in costs of general anesthesia, the operating room, recovery room, and if your surgery is done with laparoscopy, the one-time use of equipment for that procedure.

Ectopic Pregnancy Risk after Tubal Surgery

In general, the risk of ectopic pregnancy (see Chapter 10) after tubal surgery is about 10 percent. Your doctor can diagnose ectopic pregnancy through the use of very sensitive pregnancy tests and ultrasound.

Sorting the Surgeries: A Quick Guide

If the names and definitions of the various procedures discussed in this chapter are intimidating, take heart. They can be confusing at first, but you will become familiar with the procedures that are relevant to your care. Here is a quick breakdown of the most common surgical and radiological procedures:

- *Hysterosalpingogram (HSG).* An X-ray of your fallopian tubes done by inserting a narrow tube (called a catheter or cannula) through your cervix and flushing a contrast dye through the fallopian tubes. A tubal catheterization (see below) can be performed during a hysterosalpingogram to attempt to unblock fallopian tubes.
- *Hysteroscope.* A thin telescopic instrument, about the diameter of a pencil, with a small light attached. Inserted through your vagina and cervix into your uterus, the hysteroscope is used to examine your uterine cavity. Surgical instruments can be inserted into the hysteroscope to treat abnormalities. If used alone without laparoscopy, you will not have an incision. However, a hysteroscopy can be combined with laparoscopy to treat abnormalities.
- *Laparoscopy.* A surgical procedure in which a tiny telescope is inserted into one or more small incisions in your abdomen. Treatment for abnormalities such as endometriosis and adhesions can be done during a laparoscopy. Laparoscopy can also be combined with hysteroscopy. Instruments can be inserted through the hysteroscope to unblock fallopian tubes or remove polyps and fibroids.
- *Laparotomy.* This is major surgery in which an incision is made into your abdomen. Some procedures, such as the removal of fibroids (myomectomy) and reversal of tubal ligation (tubal anastomosis), must be done at laparotomy.
- *Salpingectomy.* Removal of a fallopian tube.
- *Salpingostomy.* Opening up a blocked fallopian tube.

- *Fimbrioplasty.* Removing adhesions (scar tissue) from the fimbriated (or fingerlike) ends of fallopian tubes.
- *Tubal anastomosis (also called tubal reanastomosis).* A way of reversing a tubal ligation by cutting out (excising or resecting) the damaged area of a tube and reconnecting the tube, usually involving a laparotomy (surgery through the abdomen).
- *Tubal catheterization.* A procedure used with hysteroscopy or hysterosalpingogram to unblock fallopian tubes.

UTERINE PROBLEMS

In this section, we will talk about diagnosis and treatment of three major uterine problems: fibroids, polyps, and Asherman's syndrome.

Fibroids

Fibroids, also called *leiomyomas* or *myomas,* are benign smooth muscle tumors found in the uterus. It's not uncommon to have multiple myomas. They occur in up to 25 percent of women and are usually harmless but can cause symptoms, such as heavy uterine bleeding. When found incidentally, such as during a routine physical examination or on a sonogram, the usual advice to someone anticipating pregnancy is to go ahead and try to get pregnant and see what happens. Although there is a somewhat higher incidence of miscarriage or premature delivery with fibroids, the vast majority of pregnancies have good outcomes, and therefore myomas are not usually treated preventively. When they press against the bowel or bladder, they can cause urinary frequency or bowel pressure. Fibroids are treated when they cause symptoms, grow rapidly, or affect your fertility.

Fibroids can impair your fertility—and we'll talk about that in a moment—but determination of whether they are the primary cause of infertility depends on the exclusion of other more potentially significant factors. That's why even if you know you have fibroids, you want to make sure that your fallopian tubes are open, that you have a good semen analysis from your partner, and assurance that you are ovulating. When all of your other tests are fine, but you continue to have difficulty conceiving, or you have recurrent pregnancy loss, you and your doctor may suspect fibroids as a contributing factor in your infertility.

How Fibroids Can Affect Both Your Fertility and Pregnancy

Fibroids can complicate a pregnancy in a number of ways. They can increase risk of miscarriage. If you don't have a miscarriage, there is still a risk of degeneration of the fibroid during pregnancy, causing pain because fibroids are comprised of muscle tissue, and muscle death is physically painful, although it can be managed with analgesics. Most fibroids will grow with a pregnancy. As the uterus gets bigger, the fibroid gets bigger, increasing its potential to rob the developing fetus of its blood supply. There is also the risk of premature labor or premature rupture of your membranes, and depending on the location of the fibroid, obstructed labor. A cervical fibroid can obstruct vaginal delivery, requiring a C-section. Still, fibroids often don't complicate a pregnancy. Whether your fibroids affect your fertility depends on their size and location. Whether to treat them is sometimes a bit of a judgment call. Some women don't have their fibroids removed before trying to get pregnant, and doctors may rightly tell women with no other fertility issues to go ahead and try to get pregnant despite a small fibroid, that is, a fibroid under 5 centimeters in diameter, with the caveat that the risk of complications isn't as low as it might be if she didn't have that fibroid. This is reasonable advice for women who are trying to get pregnant for the first time, because most women with fibroids can still get pregnant.

You'll hear fibroids referred to according to three different locations:

- *subserosal fibroids*: fibroids beneath the outer surface of the uterus
- *intramural fibroids*: fibroids within the uterine wall
- *submucosal fibroids*: fibroids that protrude into the uterine cavity
- *pedunculated fibroids*: fibroids that develop on a stalk

These distinctions are in some ways most useful when talking about a small fibroid, but a fibroid can actually have two or three of these characteristics. (See Figure 5 on page 122 to get a better understanding of what fibroids look like.) A fibroid can be big enough to be beneath the surface of the uterine wall and protrude into your uterus. Fibroids that distort your uterine cavity can impair your fertility regardless of their size. That's why a smaller fibroid, a fibroid under 5 centimeters, can be more clinically significant than a larger fibroid, when the small fibroid distorts the uterine cavity and the larger one does not. Additionally, once a fibroid gets to be larger than 3 or 4 centimeters in diameter, it can compromise blood flow to the uterus, impeding implantation of the embryo.

Importantly, fibroids can also decrease the likelihood of success with IVF. According to the literature on IVF, women with fibroids have a significantly lower pregnancy rate with IVF than women without fibroids. Even women with fibroids of 3 centimeters do worse, and one study found that women with fibroids as small as 2.5 centimeters in diameter did worse.[2] This may be because the fibroid interrupts implantation or negatively affects uterine blood flow. When your doctor suspects that fibroids are significantly related to your infertility, you may want to consider having them removed.

We did insemination for quite a while before we went through the first surgery. I needed the myomectomy before doing IVF. The first one actually worked, but then I had a miscarriage at seven weeks. And then we had four more in vitro rounds that didn't work. You really don't appreciate what a miracle it is until you go through something like this. A lot of people just take it for granted, but it doesn't always work. You like to hope it does, because if you don't hope that it is going to work then you wouldn't even begin to try. I really thought I would be home with my babies the following year. But I had to have another hysteroscopy and another mass removed. I'm lumpy, that's one of my problems. It was tough, and it got harder and harder as more and more acquaintances and friends got pregnant.

—CYNTHIA

Diagnosing Fibroids

Your doctor can detect fibroids through a pelvic examination and ultrasound, a readily available tool for determining the size and number of fibroids. A sonohysterogram (also called a saline sonogram) is similar to a hysterosalpingogram (HSG) (see Chapter 3) except that a saline solution is injected into the uterus used instead of a contrast dye. This is an excellent way to view fibroids that affect the uterine cavity.

If I am planning a surgery and I think fibroids are affecting a woman's uterine cavity, I will do a preoperative hysterosalpingogram or a saline sonohysterogram. An advantage of the HSG is that your doctor can see the relationship of your fibroid to your fallopian tubes. This is important because if the fibroid is very close to the fallopian tube, there is a danger of cutting the fallopian tube during surgery. The HSG gives your doctor a kind of road map to follow, depending on your unique situation. An MRI (magnetic resonance imaging) is the best way for your doctor to get a complete overview of your entire uterus and identify the location of every fibroid. It can also rule out a more uncommon condition called *adenomyosis,* which is not amenable to surgery.

Adenomyosis is a condition where glands normally found in the uterine lining occur within the uterine wall. It is like having endometriosis within the wall of the uterus. Sometimes, the areas within the uterine wall form a mass (or tumor) that resembles a fibroid. But unlike a fibroid, these areas are not encapsulated and cannot be easily removed. This condition is more common in women who have had previous pregnancies, even if they were only first-trimester terminations. How adenomyosis affects fertility is not clearly defined. However, it is important to rule out adenomyosis before having a myomectomy, because operating on adenomyosis is a futile exercise without proven benefit. Occasionally adenomyosis can also occur within a fibroid (called adenomyoma). This is less of a concern because the myoma and the adenomyosis within it can be removed.

Treating Fibroids

If you are in infertility care, myomectomy, or the removal of fibroids, is the best option for treatment. There are two types of myomectomies: procedures that are done abdominally and procedures done through your cervix.

Removing Fibroids with a Hysteroscope.

Myomectomies done through the cervix are called hysteroscopic (or transcervical) myomectomies. They are done with a hysteroscope, a tiny telescope that can be inserted through the vagina and the cervix to visualize the interior of the uterus and treat identified problems. (See Figure 7 on page 130.) When a fibroid protrudes into the uterine cavity, it may be removed through a hysteroscopic procedure. Whether or not a fibroid can be removed hysteroscopically depends on how much of the fibroid extends into your uterus. If most of the fibroid—that is, most of its diameter—is seen inside the uterus, it is more likely that your doctor can treat it hysteroscopically. Submucosal fibroids are the most likely to be treated in this way. Sometimes, a physician will treat a fibroid that protrudes only partially into the uterine cavity, wait a few months for the remaining portion to extrude (poke out) into the uterus, and then remove the newly emerged portion. In my own practice, I have never had to do more than three hysteroscopies to remove such a fibroid.

The advantage of hysteroscopy is that no surgical incisions are made as they are with laparoscopy or, to a much greater extent, with laparotomy. Laparoscopic myomectomies are possible, but they require extraordinary laparoscopic surgical technique. Moreover, doctors are concerned about doing laparoscopic myomectomies for women who want to have children. The feeling is that a surgeon can better reconstruct the uterus after myomectomy using his or her own hands as opposed to laparoscopic surgical tools. This means that if your fibroids cannot be removed using a hysteroscope, laparotomy will most likely be necessary.

There are two types of hysteroscopies: diagnostic hysteroscopies done in an office setting, and operative hysteroscopies, which are performed under general anesthesia and often combined with laparoscopy or other procedures. Before having an operative hysteroscopy, your cervix will be dilated to accommodate the hysteroscope, which in the case of an operative hysteroscopy is generally 5 millimeters and larger. A distension medium, a saline solution or other clear liquid, will be slowly infused into your uterus in order to hold the uterine walls apart so that surgeon can see within the uterus. The hysteroscope will then be introduced into the uterus through the cervix. The uterine cavity can be inspected and surgery can be performed to remove the fibroid.

If you have an operative hysteroscopy performed in a hospital or surgery center, you will likely be asked to fast for six hours before surgery and will require someone to drive you home when you wake up. Recovery time for a hysteroscopy alone is usually quick. You should be able to go back to work in the next day or two. Because your uterus has been distended, you may have cramping. Because of the instrumentation of your cervix, you may also have some bleeding similar to a period.

Diagnostic hysteroscopies are done with hysteroscopes under 5 millimeters, requiring minimal cervical dilation. Anesthesia may not be necessary, and often the procedure takes a matter of minutes. Carbon dioxide may be used instead of a distention medium to expand your uterus. Because your uterus has been stretched, you're likely to feel cramping after the procedure and to have some bleeding, but you should feel well enough to drive yourself home.

Removing Fibroids with Laparotomy. Myomas removed through the abdomen are generally done with laparotomy. A laparotomy is an in-hospital surgical procedure, usually requiring two to five days of hospitalization and up to four to six weeks wherein you can do only limited work so that you can heal. However, most people are back to work between two to four weeks after surgery.

NEW TREATMENTS FOR FIBROIDS

There are two important recent developments in the treatment of uterine fibroids: uterine artery embolization and magnetic resonance guided focused ultrasound surgery (MRgFUS). Uterine artery embolization (UAE), performed by interventional radiologists, involves threading catheters into blood vessels to cut off the blood supply to fibroids, which usually causes the fibroid to shrink. However, this procedure is not recommended for people who wish to preserve their fertility, because there is concern about damage to the uterine walls beyond the fibroid itself, and there have been reported cases of decreased ovarian function after embolization.

Less invasive is magnetic resonance guided focused ultrasound surgery (MRgFUS). With this technique, high-frequency ultrasound beams are directed at fibroids under MRI guidance. This promises to be both the most precise treatment of certain fibroids while at the same time being the least invasive method. It is very likely that, unlike UAE, MRgFUS will be approved for women planning pregnancy, because all indications are that it is far less destructive than UAE or surgical myomectomy.

If you have a laparotomy, you will have a 4- to 10-inch transverse incision above your pubic hairline, called a Pfannenstiel incision, which will be a temporary weak spot in your abdomen and the site of postoperative pain.

During the procedure, your surgeon will typically remove the fibroids. The surgeon will make an incision into the uterine wall, identify the fibroid, which is often encapsulated by a tissue plane that distinguishes the fibroid from the normal uterine wall, and then remove the fibroid in its capsule. Once the fibroid is removed, your surgeon will then repair the cavity left in the uterine wall by sewing the cavity together in multiple layers. It's important that the surgeon make a judicious search to identify all of the fibroids, because it's easy to miss a fibroid if one isn't looking for it. This is why if I have any doubt about the location of each and every fibroid, I ask my patients to have an MRI. An MRI is a great way to view the uterus from multiple angles to make sure that every fibroid is identified and none will be missed during surgery.

Before Surgery for Fibroids: If you are anemic or you have a fibroid that is so big that shrinking it will make your operation significantly less invasive, your doctor may suggest that you take a GnRH-analog (synthetic versions of gonadotropin-releasing hormone), such as Lupron, to temporarily shrink your fibroid in order to make it more operable. If the fibroid is located near a vital structure, such as a ureter (ureters are the tubes that transport urine from the kidneys to the bladder), or is very low in the cervix, a GnRH-analog may also be used to shrink the fibroid to make the surgery easier and less risky to that structure.

GnRH-analogs suppress FSH and LH production, putting you in a hypoestrogenic (low estrogen) state, like menopause. Since most fibroids are estrogen dependent, when deprived of estrogen they shrink. Temporarily, you may experience hot flashes, vaginal dryness, short-term memory loss and/or insomnia, but these symptoms will subside once the drug is stopped.

You may be wondering if GnRH-analogs can permanently shrink fibroids, making surgery unnecessary. Unfortunately, GnRH-analogs cannot do that. After the medication is stopped, the fibroids will grow back within three months unless a woman is very close to menopause, when fibroids stop growing.

After Surgery for Fibroids: After the surgery, you will have some pain, which can be treated with pain medication. You shouldn't do any heavy lifting or any activity that causes tension in the abdominal wall, such as sit-ups, for about six weeks after surgery.

Possible Complications of Myomectomy: Occasionally, a fibroid can be so close to the ureters or the cervix that it can be too technically difficult to remove. This may be all right if you have, say, five fibroids, and four of them are removed. But it would be very disconcerting if you have one fibroid and your surgeon discovered that it was too difficult to remove during your operation. That's why your surgeon should make every effort to locate all of your fibroids and have a plan before you are in the operating room.

Myomectomies are fairly arduous procedures. You may lose some blood during the operation. Depending on the blood supply to the fibroid and its location, there is a risk of requiring a transfusion. Ask your doctor about banking your own blood for the operation in case you need a transfusion.

Importantly, there is a potential risk of damage to the structures near the uterus—not only the ureters, but the intestine, bladder, and blood vessels. Diminished ovarian blood flow, resulting in an ovary that may function less well, and scar tissue formation (adhesions) are other risks of surgery. Unfortunately, myomectomy can also lead to postoperative adhesions (scar tissue) that can damage tubal-ovarian relationships and contribute to infertility.

While not a complication of surgery per se, fibroid surgery may require that you have a cesarean delivery rather than a vaginal delivery. The usual rule of thumb is that if the uterine cavity is entered during the fibroid removal, cesarean delivery is recommended.

Getting Pregnant after Fibroid Surgery: A couple may start trying to conceive within the month following surgery or may have to wait up to twelve weeks after surgery in cases where a woman has had a very deep or extensive incision and needs a longer time to heal.

Is Your Surgeon Experienced Enough to Do Your Myomectomy?

Some doctors have more experience doing myomectomies than others. Ask your doctor:

- *How many myomectomies have you done?* While there is no specific number of myomectomies your surgeon should have done to be qualified, you want to know that your surgeon has substantial experience and has confidence in his or her ability to perform the surgery well. Listen to your surgeon's reaction to your question. If your surgeon suggests that you might want to see someone else, you probably should.

- *Have you ever had to do a hysterectomy during a myomectomy?* It's not alarming if your surgeon has had to do one or two hysterectomies in the course of a myomectomy, but the number should not be much higher.
- *Have you ever had problems with residual fibroids after you've done a myomectomy?* While this is a problem that even an experienced surgeon might have encountered, the way your surgeon answers this question is revealing.

You can also assess your doctor's interest in your case by asking yourself:

- *Has my doctor investigated my case before surgery?* A doctor who does an ultrasound and refers you to an MRI prior to surgery is likely to be more intent on identifying and removing all of your fibroids.
- *Has my doctor discussed all the facts of my operation with me, identifying the most likely findings during surgery and options for treating those findings?*
- *Has my doctor made me aware of all of the risks and benefits of my surgery?*

Polyps

A polyp is a mass (tumor) of glandular tissue in the uterine lining (endometrium). (See Figure 5 on page 122.) Almost always benign, polyps can develop when the uterine lining doesn't shed completely and instead becomes "polyploid." Irregular bleeding, spotting at midcycle, or heavier menstrual flow than you are accustomed to can be a sign of polyps. If left untreated, polyps can interfere with implantation of an embryo and should be removed. Rarely are they malignant in women under thirty-five. If you are over thirty-five, they should be removed and evaluated, even if you are not trying to get pregnant.

Along the course of your initial diagnosis, there are a number of ways to detect polyps. Sometimes polyps are fairly obvious on an ultrasound, which you should have at your initial workup. But you may still have

HYSTERECTOMY: IS YOUR SURGEON QUALIFIED TO TREAT FIBROIDS WITHOUT IT?

For too many gynecologists, the treatment for fibroids is hysterectomy (the removal of the uterus). While it should be an infrequent complication, there is a very small risk that a surgeon performing a myomectomy will be unable to reconstruct the uterus, and will have to remove it entirely. There's a lot of variability in ob-gyn training when it comes to myomectomy. While every ob-gyn should be comfortable doing a hysterectomy, not every ob-gyn—or RE for that matter—is trained in doing myomectomies, although reproductive endocrinologists are oriented toward saving, rather than removing, the uterus.

It may happen that a woman is told that she needs a hysterectomy solely because the doctor doesn't feel comfortable treating with myomectomy. This is tragic if someone has not completed her desired childbearing. It is imperative to find out the extent of your doctor's experience doing these operations and to get a second opinion before accepting surgery and especially before following your doctor's recommendation for hysterectomy.

polyps, even if your regular sonogram is normal, because ultrasound is not the most accurate way to diagnose polyps.

As you may recall, a hysterosalpingogram (HSG) involves infusion of a small amount of dye into your uterine cavity to outline your uterus and fallopian tubes. Providing your HSG is not done with an instrument with a balloon tip that expands inside your uterus, a hysterosalpingogram can also be used for diagnosis. A balloon-tipped instrument will obscure the contents of your uterus, making it impossible for your doctor to see a polyp.

The best way to visualize the architecture of the uterine walls and diagnose polyps is through a saline sonohysterogram (SSH), also called a saline sonogram. Essentially, a saline sonogram is similar to an HSG except that a saline solution is used instead of a contrast dye, there is no X-ray exposure during this procedure, and it can be done in your doctor's office. An SSH is typically ordered when there are questions about your hysterosalpingogram or if there were uterine abnormalities on your regular sonogram.

Hysteroscopy is another excellent way of diagnosing uterine polyps, although it is less comfortable than a saline sonohysterogram and demands that your doctor be skilled in using a hysteroscope, which is not an easy instrument to use. The advantage to a hysteroscopy is that your polyps can be immediately removed with instruments put through the hysteroscope. Whether your doctor will use a hysteroscope or a saline sonogram to further diagnose suspicious findings is a matter of your doctor's style of practice.

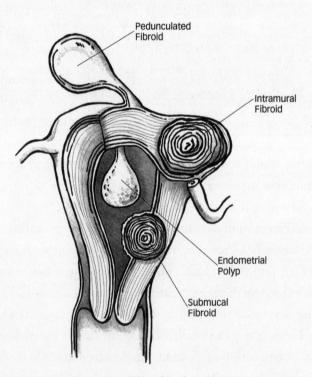

FIGURE 5. *A uterus with fibroids and a polyp.*
When they distort the inside of the uterus, these structures can interfere with implantation.

Removing Polyps

Treatment for polyps involves either a hysteroscopy or a D&C (dilatation & curettage), an outpatient procedure in which the cervix is dilated and the lining of the uterus is gently scraped. Your doctor may use a combination of both procedures.

Having a D&C. "Dilatation" means dilating, or opening, the cervix. "Curettage" means scraping a surface. D&Cs are intended to gently remove the uterine contents. Some women know D&C as a pregnancy termination procedure, but it certainly does have other uses—for example, the removal of polyps.

In the past, D&Cs were done primarily in hospitals, but they have now moved out of the hospital setting into clinic or office settings. Ambulatory surgical centers are the best settings for a D&C, because they are geared toward serving patients who are coming in for half-day procedures. Your D&C should take about a half a day, including your arrival, the surgery, and your recovery time.

During the procedure, your doctor will use a speculum to see your cervix, which may be steadied with a tenaculum, a long-handled clamp. Next, your doctor will dilate your cervix, passing cylindrical cone-shaped metal instruments of gradually increasing size into your cervix in order to dilate it. This part of the procedure is accomplished very quickly. Once your cervix is dilated, your doctor will begin the curettage. A long metal instrument, the shape of which is rather like a lacrosse stick, is passed along uterine walls, which has the effect of scraping the uterine lining.

If cervical or uterine malignancy is suspected, a modification of a D&C, called a *differential dilatation and curettage*, is done. In this case, the cervix is scraped before the uterus to get separate cervical and endometrial tissue samples.

Normally, you will be able to go home within two hours after your D&C, although you should ask someone to drive you home. After the procedure, you will have some cramping, discharge, and bleeding similar to a period. Call your doctor immediately if you experience:

- bleeding that is heavier than would be on the first day of your period;
- a fever of 100.4°F or more;
- severe pain, especially if it's above your pelvic area;
- shoulder pain.

I strongly advise anyone having a D&C to consider a short-acting spinal or general anesthesia, as we don't yet have adequate ways to provide local pain relief for every person. Although some women may be able to tolerate a D&C without general anesthesia, I don't think pushing someone to the limits of her tolerance is necessary or even humane. But there are side effects of anesthesia such as nausea, vomiting, and headache. Be sure to talk to your doctor and your anesthesiologist before surgery to learn more about anesthesia.

Asherman's Syndrome

In Asherman's syndrome, scarring causes the uterine walls to become stuck together with the front wall of the uterus often adhering to the back wall. Asherman's syndrome can cause amenorrhea (no periods) and infertility. Depending on where the scar tissue is located, this condition can also predispose you to ectopic pregnancy, either because there is no place for an embryo to implant or because the opening of your fallopian tubes have become blocked by scar tissue. If you are not getting your periods because your uterine lining can't flow out through your vagina, you may develop retrograde menstruation wherein your menstrual flow moves backward through your fallopian tubes, a condition that is not only painful, but which can further predispose you to endometriosis.

Asherman's syndrome typically results from overly vigorous scraping, or curetting, of the uterus after a pregnancy termination or a pregnancy loss, or curettage of retained products of conception, such as a placenta that stays in the uterus at the time of delivery. It can also occur when the uterus is scraped while an intrauterine infection is present. All of these events seem to be particularly traumatic to the uterine walls, because they are soft, vascular, and prone to adhering.

Unfortunately, the more your uterus is curetted, for example, if you have had a number of D&Cs, the more likely you are to develop Asherman's syndrome. After about four or five such procedures, it's very likely that you will develop Asherman's.

Ironically, in the past, the same treatment that caused Asherman's syndrome was used to treat it, namely, curetting the uterus. Today, Asherman's can be treated hysteroscopically. Your doctor can see the scar tissue in the uterus directly and cut it away with scissorlike instruments until the uterus is reopened. After the procedure, a balloon device is kept in the uterus for a few days to hold the walls apart. Because infection can increase scar tissue, you will be given an antibiotic after surgery. You will most likely be put on a high dose of estrogen, because estrogen causes the uterine lining to proliferate and grow, making it more apt to heal correctly.

One of the risks after surgery is the increased likelihood of developing a placenta accreta, if you should get pregnant. In this condition, the placenta grows deeply through the uterine lining into the uterine wall. Often this condition is not discovered until delivery when it can necessitate a hysterectomy. This is a risk you obviously want to discuss with your doctor, should you require this surgery to treat your infertility. It may or may not be a risk that you want to take.

Endometriosis

The endometrium is the tissue that lines the uterus. Endometriosis occurs when implants of endometrial tissue grow in places outside the uterus, most commonly around the pelvis, the abdomen, the surface of the ovaries and bladder, the outside surface of the uterus, and the cul-de-sac—an area of the pelvis where the cervix, the top of vagina, and the rectum all come together. Rarely, endometriosis can occur in other parts of the body. It's been found in the outer surface of the lung, probably traveling through the diaphragm, and it's even been seen in the inner structure of the lung, perhaps arriving there through the bloodstream. It's been found in the umbilicus and not infrequently in the scars of women who have had cesarean deliveries. Endometriosis on the ovary can cause the formation of a cyst (fluid-filled structure) which, over time, accumulates old blood material from the endometrial glands in its lining. These types of ovarian cysts are called *endometriomas* or "chocolate cysts" after the thick brown fluid they contain.

The most prevalent theory about why endometriosis occurs is that it is actually a backflow of menstruation, called *retrograde menstruation*. Instead of leaving your uterus through the vagina, some uterine lining flows backward through the fallopian tubes, landing on other surfaces inside the peritoneum (the abdominal cavity). Retrograde menstruation is also more common in women who have a very narrow cervix, narrow enough that the endometrium doesn't flow out normally during menstruation. It can also occur in women who have a rare condition called a *blind uterine horn*, that is, a functioning uterus that is not connected to a cervix. Women with this condition only menstruate backward though their fallopian tubes. But you don't have to have either of these conditions to have endometriosis.

Your body doesn't reject these implants, because they are your own tissue. They cycle just as your uterus cycles in the menstrual cycle. They can grow, shed, and bleed inside your peritoneal cavity, causing irritation, inflammation, pain, and scar tissue. The inflammation and scar tissue are what contribute to infertility. The peritoneal cavity, the area around the reproductive organs, is fluid-coated. These fluids can mix with inflammatory fluids, the result being toxic to eggs, embryos, or fertilization. In addition, scar tissue can prevent the fallopian tube from doing its job of taking up an egg or transporting the egg or embryo into the uterus. However, some women have endometriosis without having infertility.

Because endometriosis can be staged just as cancer is staged, many people have misconceptions about the nature of endometriosis as something that progresses and eats away at the body. This is not true. While it

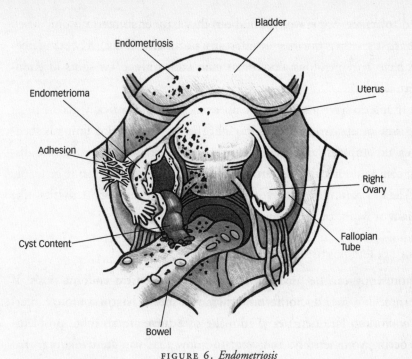

FIGURE 6. *Endometriosis*

Uterine glands found outside the uterus cause inflammation, scarring, and distortion of the normal reproductive anatomy.

is possible to have a small amount of endometriosis at thirty, say, and a lot more when you are thirty-five, endometriosis is not invariably a progressive disease. You can have a mild amount of endometriosis at twenty and no more by the time you are forty. And as a general rule, about 70 percent of the time, it does not come back when treated. This statistic is most improved after pregnancy, because pregnancy seems to have a beneficial effect on the course of endometriosis.

Some women have pain, especially around the time of menstruation (dysmenorrhea) and occasionally at the time of ovulation and during intercourse (dyspareunia), suggesting endometriosis, but many have endometriosis and no pain at all. Interestingly, the proportion of pain felt is not related to the amount of endometriosis you have, but instead is related to the location of the implants, how active they are, and your threshold for pain tolerance. Some women find out they have endometriosis only when they first see their doctors for infertility treatment. Conversely, some people have a tremendous amount of pain with only a few spots of endometriosis.

If you do have pain, it is usually cyclical, most classically occurring at the time of menstruation. It's thought that as your uterine lining is shedding, the implants are bleeding and shedding. It's sometimes hard to distinguish endometrial pain from ordinary menstrual pain, but generally periods so painful that they keep you from your ordinary activities, like school or work, can be a sign of endometriosis.

Treating Endometriosis

Laparoscopy can be used both to diagnose and treat endometriosis. If you're seeing your doctor for infertility, you should have a complete infertility workup (see Chapter 3) to make sure there are no other problems hindering your fertility. You want to know that you are ovulating, that your partner's sperm count is okay, and that your fallopian tubes are open. If your tubes are blocked, you may consider moving directly toward IVF. Endometriosis may affect IVF success.

Whether you will decide to diagnose and treat endometriosis or move directly to IVF depends on a number of factors, including your age. Removing the endometriosis and waiting to see if you get pregnant within the year may be reasonable for a woman in her early thirties, but when time is factor, IVF may be the best course.

Your doctor should be able to both diagnose and treat your endometriosis in the same procedure. A doctor should never perform a laparoscopy, simply look at your endometriosis, diagnose you, and then close. The goal of surgery is to remove scar tissue, restoring your anatomy to as normal a situation as possible. Scar tissue can be removed by cutting the tissue away, vaporizing the implants with a laser, cauterizing them with electrocautery, or by the other means. A harmonic scalpel (an implement with a tip that vibrates at ultrasonic frequency) can also be used to denature the implants—in other words, to change their properties. All of these methods work equally well.

An operative laparoscopy is generally done through multiple incisions in your abdominal cavity, known as multiple ports. Your surgeon will make anywhere from two to four ports, the largest of which will be just five to ten millimeters. Secondary ports are usually 5 millimeters or less, approximately the width of a No. 2 pencil. The surgical instruments, be they graspers or cauteries, lasers, harmonic scalpels, or scissors, are put through these auxiliary ports. When more than two ports are needed, more than one surgeon may be needed to accomplish the procedure. This may be your doctor and his or her associate, if you are treated in a private setting, or a surgeon and a resident in training if you are in an academic setting. If you are having your surgery with a general ob-gyn, your doctor may ask an RE to be available in the operating room for consultation.

The surgeon will survey your reproductive organs and bladder, identify the implants, and choose the appropriate tool to remove them. The laparoscopy itself can take about an hour to do, but it may take a second hour to treat the endometriosis, depending on what is found.

Side Effects and Complications of Laparoscopy. After surgery you may feel nausea from the anesthesia and bloating from the gas used to expand the abdominal cavity. Often, people feel shoulder pain caused by gas or irrigation fluid going under the diaphragm. Usually you will have some bleeding from having instruments put into your cervix, which is often done at laparoscopy to manipulate the cervix.

As with any surgery, there is a risk associated with general anesthesia. In about 1/100,000 cases death can result. There is a risk of injury to organs in the abdominal cavity, the most serious of which is damage to great vessels, such as the aorta, the inferior vena cava, trauma in the iliac arteries or veins, and puncture of the gastrointestinal or urinary system (the intestines, stomach, bladder, and ureter). All of these risks underscore the necessity of finding a surgeon who is experienced in laparoscopy.

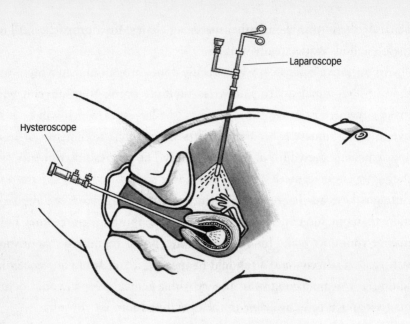

Laparoscope

Hysteroscope

FIGURE 7. *Laparoscopy and hysteroscopy*

Recovering After a Laparoscopy. Most people are back to work within days of their laparoscopy. I usually operate on Thursday, and I usually tell my patients that it's unlikely they will be back to work on Friday, but that they will be back by Monday. How quickly you recover really depends on how quickly you bounce back from surgery in general.

Getting Pregnant After Surgery for Endometriosis. You can start trying almost immediately, depending on where you are in your cycle.

BEFORE YOU HAVE SURGERY: CHOOSING THE MOST QUALIFIED SURGEON

Infertility care is a field like no other in medicine, resting at the intersection of our cultural fascinations with youth and high technology. It's sexy, it's costly, and it attracts dilettantes. Why? Reproductive medicine is both relatively simple and very difficult to practice. It's easy, because failure is inconspicuous. When a heart surgeon fails, the heart patient may die, but when a reproductive surgeon fails, the patient simply remains infertile. Now add the fact that many of the surgeries we have been discussing, specifically tubal surgeries, have only a 20 to 50 percent success rate, and you can begin to see why this field attracts doctors who are not fertility experts but who are willing to treat infertility patients. If the doctor fails, you simply don't get pregnant.

Reproductive medicine is difficult to do well. Your doctor must have the requisite knowledge and training to perform reproductive surgery and must be intent on giving you the maximum statistical odds of achieving your goal of conceiving. You should be utterly confident of your doctor's skill, expertise, and intentions. How do you know if you have the right doctor? How can you be assured that your doctor can expertly perform the surgery you need?

When seeking a reproductive surgeon, you must bear in mind that it is tough for the layperson to distinguish between a competent reproductive surgeon and someone who does not have the requisite experience to give you the best chance at succeeding. Naturally, you want a baby. Your need may be intense and urgent. But be aware that you are entering a minefield. There are many fertility doctors who concentrate more on PR than practice. When choosing someone as important as your surgeon, be careful and do your research.

Laparoscopic surgery, hysteroscopic surgery, and microsurgery to treat infertility are difficult surgeries to accomplish. In this chapter, I've mentioned that techniques to treat obstructions to the fallopian tubes and reversal of tubal ligation require expertise. Not every surgeon is skilled in using these techniques. Many ob-gyns are trained to treat fibroids with hysterectomy. As pointed out earlier, hysterectomies are sometimes recommended when doctors don't feel comfortable treating myomectomy (a surgery to remove fibroids).

Reproductive surgery is a dying art. Surgery for infertility is far less common today than it was twenty years ago. One reason for this is the advent of in vitro fertilization, which makes it possible to bypass problems like blocked fallopian tubes. But the truth is, low reimbursement for surgery is a second reason why fewer surgeries are performed. Your doctor is making up to 75 percent less doing reproductive surgery than in the past. The incentive to learn how to perform these surgeries effectively is waning. Reproductive endocrinologists do fewer of these surgeries, and fewer doctors-in-training witness them, leading to less education in delicate reproductive surgical techniques.

Insurance companies can't easily deny coverage for surgeries when they have a diagnostic component, as many reproductive surgeries do, but many insurers don't cover assisted reproductive technology (ART) procedures like IVF. This can either translate into unnecessary surgery or surgery that is the second best alternative for someone who needs an ART procedure. Consider that the same companies that deny coverage for IVF generally provide extremely low reimbursement for surgery. Get a written predetermination of your benefits for surgery from your health insurance company. That determination should show you what your doctor will make doing your surgery. Ask your doctor how long your surgery will take. Now compare the surgery reimbursement to the cost of your office visits. Is your doctor making more on office visits than surgery? Let's say your doctor is going to make $500 for two to three hours of surgery. Would there be greater economic incentive for your doctor to do something else with those two to three hours? This is an unfortunate, but common, calculation.

Low fees and less expertise in reproductive surgery put the reproductive surgery patient in a perilous situation. If you need surgery, or surgery is your only alternative, you must be vigilant in conducting a thorough search for a good surgeon. Otherwise, it is possible that your surgery may not be delivered with the maximum amount of effort or skill.

Here is what you can do to distinguish between a competent reproductive surgeon and a doctor who doesn't have the necessary skill. Ask your doctor:

- *What training do you have to perform the surgery I need?* One cannot be a self-declared expert. At minimum, your doctor should have subspecialty training either as a reproductive endocrinologist or as someone with pelvic surgery training beyond the four years of a residency program in obstetrics and gynecology. A surgeon must have the requisite knowledge in surgical skills and principles, but must also have experience with laparoscopic equipment, which can be fragile and finicky. Where surgery is concerned, your doctor's qualifications, reputation, and explanations really matter. Your doctor should be able to explain your surgery, clearly and thoroughly answering your questions about what will happen.

- *How often do you do these procedures? Is this the only kind of surgery that you do, or do you do a range of gynecological surgeries?* A doctor should not only be experienced in the surgery you are considering, but should focus on the type of surgery you need. A doctor who does a range of gynecologic surgeries, such as bladder repairs and hysterectomies, is unlikely to be committed or interested in one type of surgery, such as laparoscopy.

- *How long does this operation I'm considering take and how much time are you going to spend doing it?* Infertility surgery doesn't have the same end-point as other surgeries. For example, an operation to remove a gallbladder ends when the gallbladder is removed. Infertility surgery is far less definable, because there are various factors that enter into a judgment call about the best course of action. How much time does your surgeon have to get the operation right? Are you going to be squeezed in between the doctor's other obligations? A laparoscopy should take at least one hour. The procedure can take an hour or longer for surgery to correct problems like endometriosis or a blocked fallopian tube. Be concerned if your doctor assures you that it will take less time.

- *If your operation will be done at a hospital or outpatient facility, why did your doctor choose that facility?* A good answer is that the equipment is excellent or that the doctor and a dedicated team perform a lot of the surgeries you are going to have at the facility. You should be wary if the doctor says that he or she doesn't do a lot of work at the facility you're heading toward or that the equipment is lacking.

Meet with your doctor before surgery. When you go in for surgery, you'll be signing a number of consent forms, such as general consent forms required by the facility, insurance forms, and a health-care proxy. One of those forms will be your surgical consent form. This isn't something that should be waved in your face as you are wheeled toward the operating room. You, the specific patient, will undergo a specific operation, and you have a right to complete information about that operation before it happens. Meet with your doctor at a time when you are not in the examining room or in the surgical center, when you are seated and dressed in your doctor's office. Listen to the way your doctor talks about your procedure. Are all the facts explained to you in a way that makes sense to you? Or is your doctor just schmoozing you, patting you on the head, and providing you with more reassurance than facts? Is your doctor telling you that you're going to feel great after surgery? This isn't true with any surgery. If you're put to sleep, you're going to feel lousy when you wake up, even if no one operates on you. Sometimes your doctor won't be able to tell you precisely what will be found at your operation or exactly what will be done, but your doctor can guesstimate the possibilities with a reasonable degree of certainty. It's a very bad sign if your doctor won't be specific or doesn't want to discuss your operation with you.

Develop a game plan with your doctor. You don't want to encounter what is sometimes referred to as a "peek and shriek" situation where your doctor opens you up and is surprised by what he or she sees. It's crucial that your surgeon has discussed these various possibilities with you before you hit the operating room because, if you haven't talked about them, your doctor is going to have to make judgment calls based on his or her own imagination with no input from you, the patient. Somebody who discusses a number of different possible scenarios with you has obviously thought specifically about your case, and is inviting you to give your input

WHAT EXPERT DO YOU NEED WHEN?

If you are having any tubal anastomosis (tubal reversal), vasectomy reversal, or any type of sperm-retrieval procedure (see Chapter 9), you need a surgeon versed in *microsurgery*.

If your procedure is laparoscopic, you need an expert in *laparoscopic surgeries*. Are you getting a procedure to unblock fallopian tubes? Then make sure your doctor operates on fallopian tubes frequently. Do you have endometriosis? How experienced is your doctor in treating endometriosis?

as to what you want done with your body. This is the appropriate way to plan surgery.

Surgery is serious, but this doesn't mean you should avoid it. Most of the time when a doctor recommends surgery, it's the right recommendation. But you must be confident in your doctor's abilities. After all, you are in charge of your health care. You have a right to complete information about the services you are receiving and to the best care possible to protect and improve your fertility.

In the next chapter, we will look at causes of male factor infertility. It's not uncommon for a couple to have both male and female factor infertility. By reading the following chapter, you will get basic information about common causes of male factor infertility. In Chapter 9, which covers IVF, you will also get information about ICSI, a procedure that can be used to help men with no sperm in their ejaculate to become fathers.

6 | Get the Right Treatment: For Men

SINCE THE ADVENT OF ASSISTED REPRODUCTIVE TECH-nology in the late 1970s, phenomenal breakthroughs have been made in the treatment of male infertility. Medicine has truly pushed the limits of what is possible with techniques like intracytoplasmic sperm injection (ICSI) and sperm retrieval procedures that allow men with no sperm in their ejaculate at all to father a child. With ICSI, a single sperm can be injected into an egg to create an embryo. Sperm retrieval procedures can find sperm for ICSI in men who only recently would have been considered sterile. (We will cover ICSI in Chapter 9.)

Before you delve into this chapter, be sure to look at Chapter 3. There we discuss the components of the most important test for male infertility—

the semen analysis. Knowing about the semen analysis will help you to use this chapter most productively.

START WITH YOUR SEMEN ANALYSIS

If your semen analysis is abnormal, your next step will be to do a second semen analysis. Occasionally, a man's sperm count can be lowered temporarily. This can happen if you ejaculated more than once on the day you did your analysis, if you had a high fever, a viral infection, testicular trauma, or if you were exposed to negative environmental factors, such as heat, for example, if you had a recent steam bath or hot tub, or if you work near a heat source.

Your sperm motility (movement) can also appear to be impaired due to problems with collection or handling of your specimen. Sperm is very sensitive to temperature and should never be left at room temperature. You might suspect collection problems when the shape (morphology) of your sperm is normal and your sperm count is normal, but the motility (movement) is very low. This is certainly something that should be investigated carefully at a second semen analysis.

Your second analysis should be done at least a month apart from the first. If you wanted to be very technical about it, you could schedule your second analysis seventy-six days away from the first, because that is how long it takes for an immature sperm cell to mature. In this case, the second analysis would test semen from a completely different time period than the first analysis.

IF YOUR SECOND SEMEN ANALYSIS IS ABNORMAL

If your second semen analysis is abnormal, your next step depends on the severity and type of abnormality found at your second semen analysis. Most men who suffer from infertility have a low sperm count with no discernible reason, but in some cases, the reason can be understood. An abnormal semen analysis may result from an underlying problem that can be fixed. Whether or not you may want to consider repairing your underlying problem depends on a number of issues, including the age of your female partner. The older a woman is, the less fertile time she has to wait and see if treatment for an underlying sperm problem is successful. You and your partner may weigh treatment of your male factor issue against infertility treatment with intrauterine insemination (IUI) or in vitro fertilization (IVF), which we will talk about in Chapters 8 and 9. In any case, your next step will probably be to see an infertility urologist for further consultation.

> *I had a softball accident a while ago. I was very concerned. I wondered if it had an effect. I took a sperm sample and rushed that to the lab. I was thinking, maybe it is me. Are they alive? Are they dead? All these things go through your head.* —BILL

SEEING THE UROLOGIST: WHAT TO EXPECT

Some men begin treatment by going directly to the urologist, as may happen when you are seeking a varicocele repair or vasectomy reversal. Others begin infertility care with visits to a reproductive endocrinologist who can then refer them to an infertility urologist. If possible, see a fellowship-trained urologist who specializes in treating male infertility. You may be referred to a urologist, if:

• your second semen analysis is poor;
• you have problems with erection or ejaculation;
• there is evidence of infection;
• you have a history of a scrotal mass or pain;
• you have a history of delayed sexual development.

Your reproductive endocrinologist can streamline your visit to the urologist by making sure that you have copies of your semen analysis—ideally two, if the first was abnormal—and copies of any blood work before you see the urologist. It can take a few days to a week to get the results of your initial blood work. In the meantime, it can take that long to get an appointment with the urologist. Having copies of your semen analyses and your blood work in your hand to give to your urologist allows you to forgo a second visit. Otherwise, the urologist is going to do a physical exam and send you out for blood work, which will require you to wait another week to return for a second appointment.

On your first visit, your urologist will palpate (feel) your testicles, feeling for a varicocele (varicose vein), which can impede your fertility; evaluate your testicular volume (size) to see if there is a discrepancy from side

BEFORE YOU HAVE CHEMOTHERAPY OR RADIATION THERAPY

Chemotherapy and radiation therapy can be toxic to the germ cells in the testes (testicles) just as they can be toxic to any rapidly dividing cells, such as the cells that make blood, the bone marrow cells, and cells that make hair. This is why hair falls out during chemotherapy.

After a cancer diagnosis one's focus is on survival and on the treatment of the cancer. Banking sperm to ensure future fertility is often overlooked. Yet one of the fortunate by-products of the proliferation of IVF clinics around the country is that there are now many facilities where one can bank sperm. If you have been diagnosed with cancer, you can freeze and store your sperm and create your family by using intrauterine insemination or IVF in the future.

If you did not bank sperm before treatment, all hope may not be lost. Men who were azoospermic after treatment with radiation sometimes spontaneously become sperm positive again, even five years or more after treatment. I have had several patients who were azoospermic after being treated for Hodgkin's disease, whose wives initially got pregnant with donor insemination and then became pregnant with their husband's sperm without intervention years later.

to side, which can also indicate varicocele; and examine your prostate through a rectal exam. If there is any doubt about your physical examination, your doctor will order an ultrasound of your testes, called scrotal sonography. This is an excellent way of confirming the results of your physical examination and finding a varicocele.

Your hormones may be measured through blood tests, if they haven't already been. The most important hormones to be measured include:

- Follicle-stimulating hormone (FSH). (The testis is the equivalent of the female ovary, and a high FSH in a man is like a high FSH in a female, suggesting a problem with the gonad's ability to produce sperm cells.)
- Testosterone, a very good indicator of whether or not your testes are getting adequate hormone stimulation and reception.
- Prolactin levels, which can indicate a rare but usually benign pituitary tumor.
- Luteinizing hormone (LH) and estradiol, which are often sampled but really add almost nothing to the tests above.

Your urologist will ask you about:

- the frequency and timing of intercourse;
- whether you have had previous children and whether you had difficulty conceiving;
- whether you had a vasectomy and how long ago it was done;
- your childhood illnesses;
- your sexual history, including your history of sexually transmitted diseases;
- possible exposure to environmental agents that might affect your fertility, such as heat;
- medications you are taking;
- nutritional supplement use.

AZOOSPERMIA: WHEN YOU HAVE
NO SPERM COUNT

Azoospermia is the term used for absence of sperm in the ejaculate. Generally speaking, doctors categorize azoospermia as either obstructive or nonobstructive. *Obstructive azoospermia* means that you make normal sperm but a blockage of some kind is preventing it from getting out of your body. *Nonobstructive azoospermia* describes azoospermia that is due to hormonal problems or problems with sperm production in the testicle. As a final issue, you may hear the term *aspermia,* which is a bit of a misnomer. Men who have aspermia produce no ejaculate. This suggests a condition called retrograde ejaculation. We'll discuss all of these conditions shortly.

Nonobstructive Azoospermia

There are two types of nonobstructive azoospermia, azoospermia caused by hormonal problems and that caused by problems that originate in the testes.

When the Problem Is Hormonal

Just as the brain tells the female ovary to produce hormones and gametes (eggs), the hypothalamus and pituitary in the brain stimulate hormone and sperm production in the testes, or testicles. Azoospermia caused by problems with hormonal stimulation of the testes is sometimes called *pre-testicular azoospermia.* Men with pre-testicular azoospermia may have a problem either with the pituitary, the hypothalamus, or with the hormones that stimulate the testes, namely GnRH or FSH and LH. (See Chapter 2 for a discussion of the way in which these hormones affect sperm and testosterone production.)

Kallman's syndrome is a rare disorder in which the hypothalamus fails to produce gonadotropin-releasing hormone (GnRH), the hormone that tells the pituitary to secrete follicle-stimulating hormone (FSH) and luteinizing hormone (LH) to activate testosterone and sperm production.

The way Kallman's syndrome is treated depends upon a man's stage of life. The most efficient way to treat Kallman's syndrome during adolescence and prereproductive life is to replace testosterone. A young boy who isn't going through puberty normally may be diagnosed with Kallman's syndrome and treated with testosterone so he can complete puberty. Testosterone replacement will make him stronger, more muscular, and allow him to have erections and sexual function.

Later on in life, when he wants to have children, he is going to have to switch to a testicular stimulant, the most common of which is FSH, in addition to LH. (This hormone is generally delivered through injections of human chorionic gonadotropin [hCG], which behaves like LH, although LH itself can also be used.) Injections are given subcutaneously three times weekly, generally over the course of three to six months. The subcutaneous delivery makes it possible for men to self-inject. Men with Kallman's syndrome do have primitive sperm cells in their testes waiting to be stimulated with these hormones, but it can take several months to produce enough sperm for reproduction. If you are taking FSH and hCG, you will also begin to produce testosterone, receiving all of testosterone's effects.

Giving continuous GnRH to activate the pituitary's secretion of FSH and LH is another way to treat Kallman's syndrome, but is less practical than injections because it requires a continuous infusion pump.

Another potential cause of pre-testicular azoospermia is a pituitary deficiency caused by a typically benign pituitary tumor, although this is relatively rare in men. Detected by consistently elevated levels of prolactin in the blood, these tumors, called prolactinomas, interfere with testosterone production, but can be treated with bromocriptine, a pill that blocks the release of prolactin and shrinks the tumor. The effect is sustained as long as you are taking the drug, but reverts back when the drug is discontinued. Signs of a pituitary tumor include headaches, double vision, and occasionally a reduced field of vision, erectile dysfunction, and gynecomastia, which is the development of breasts in the male.

When the Problem Originates in the Testes

Total absence of sperm and sperm precursor cells may indicate a chromosomal problem, such as Klinefelter's syndrome or testicular failure where the testis has been destroyed, for example due to mumps orchitis (inflammation of the testicles). During the mumps, an overwhelming viral infection in the testis can essentially wipe out all of the testis's germ cells.

High levels of follicle-stimulating hormone (FSH), small testes, and no sperm in the ejaculate suggest Klinefelter's syndrome. This is a condition in which men inherit an extra X chromosome. Ordinarily, a man will have one X and one Y chromosome, written as 46XY, whereas men with Klinefelter's syndrome have an extra X chromosome, written as 47XXY.

Men with Klinefelter's syndrome may have isolated pockets of sperm within their testes. Some of this sperm can be surgically recovered and used with in vitro fertilization (IVF) and ICSI. (See Chapter 9.) However, many men with Klinefelter's syndrome do not want to take the risk of passing on a chromosomal abnormality to their children and prefer to use donor insemination. If you have signs of Klinefelter's, a *karyotype*, which is a profile of your chromosomes, should be done for diagnosis.

Men with no spermatocytes (germ cells) have a condition known as *Sertoli-cell-only syndrome (SCO)*. Sertoli cells line the seminiferous tubules, the tiny, coiled tubules in the testis. There, each Sertoli cell supports a sperm cell in its development. Men with SCO have Sertoli cells but no immature sperm cells between the Sertoli cells. If you are a man with SCO, you will have normal function, normal hormone levels, and normal ejaculations. You may just discover that you have SCO when diagnosed at a testicular biopsy. Today, even men with SCO may have small pockets of sperm-positive areas, allowing surgical sperm retrieval. This microsurgical technique is called testicular sperm extraction (TESE). We talk about TESE in Chapter 9.

CRYPTORCHIDISM: UNDESCENDED TESTES

The testes descend from the abdomen to the scrotum during fetal life. When the testes fail to descend, a lack of fetal testosterone may be one of the reasons why. If, after birth, an infant's testicles fail to descend spontaneously, they can be brought down surgically or medically. If a testicle isn't brought down into the scrotum by age two, its sperm- and testosterone-producing capacity will be impaired, and the testicle will be prone to tumor development. Most often doctors treat this condition, called cryptorchidism, surgically, but the testes may also descend by treating an infant with human chorionic gonadotropin (hCG), which acts like luteinizing hormone (LH), helping to stimulate testosterone production. If you have a history of cryptorchidism, you are at an increased risk for problems with sperm production, even if the cryptorchidism was successfully treated.

Fortunately, most men with a history of cryptorchidism are merely oligospermic, meaning they have lower concentrations of sperm in their ejaculate, but are not azoospermic (no sperm). Even a man who is in fact azoospermic because of cryptorchidism may still have sperm in his testes that can be retrieved for IVF/ICSI.

Obstructive Azoospermia: When Sperm Can't Exit the Body

When you have an obstruction or an ejaculatory disorder, you may have perfectly normal sperm that can't leave your body. Conditions that prevent delivery of sperm can include anything from an abnormality known as congenital bilateral absence of the vas deferens (CBAVD), a vasectomy, severe infections, or an injury during an operation, such as a hernia repair. For example, it is possible for a surgeon to mistakenly sever the vas deferens (the tubes that connect the testicles and the epididymis to the ejaculatory ducts) during a hernia repair. This is more likely to happen during hernia operations on children, because of the smaller size of these structures.

Vasectomy and congenital bilateral absence of the vas are two classic causes of an absence of sperm in the ejaculate. Ejaculatory duct obstruction is much less common. In Chapter 9, we will look at a range of methods to help men with obstructions retrieve sperm for IVF. We will also discuss the option of vasectomy reversal later in this chapter. For now, here is an overview of conditions in which a man may actually produce sperm yet have none in his ejaculate.

Vasectomy

Vasectomy is a procedure in which the vas deferens is cut, tied, clipped, or cauterized as a means of birth control. Although this should never be the original intent before vasectomy, a vasectomy can be reversed. Vasectomy reversals can be particularly beneficial for men with younger partners, because time is needed before the reversal heals. You are more likely to have success with a reversal if your vasectomy was recent, that is, done less than three to five years ago. The older your vasectomy, the less likely you are to be a good candidate for a reversal.

Some couples may find themselves contemplating the pros and cons of vasectomy reversal or IVF/ICSI.

Vasectomy Reversal. If you are considering a vasectomy reversal, the first issue to think about is your partner's age. As with varicocele repair, vasectomy reversals are ideal for men with relatively recent vasectomies and partners aged thirty or younger. There are two reasons for this. One is that vasectomy reversal takes time to heal and result in sperm production. It may take anywhere from one to three months to a year or even longer before you will have adequate sperm in your ejaculate. If your partner is reaching an age when her fertility is beginning to decline, beginning at thirty and certainly at thirty-five and older, IVF or IVF/ICSI are better choices for conception. (See Chapter 9.) If your partner is thirty or younger, the worst-case scenario is that, having failed a vasectomy reversal, you can try again with IVF a year or two later. But if your partner is thirty-seven or older and your reversal is unsuccessful, you may be trying again when she is thirty-eight or thirty-nine, a time when her fertility is markedly diminished and the risk of failure with IVF is greater. Vasectomy reversal is an ideal solution for younger couples who have no additional fertility problems and who are planning to have children in one or two years' time after the reversal. The second issue is whether you will be able to reconnect your vas deferens, or whether you will have to connect your vas deferens to your epididymis to open your vasectomy again.

Freezing Sperm at Your Vasectomy Reversal. You can and should freeze sperm at a vasectomy or vasectomy reversal, if sperm is present. Having sperm available for IVF or IVF/ICSI is crucial if:

- your vasectomy reversal fails;
- your sperm count lowers after a reversal or closes down;
- you want to maintain the option of having IVF/ICSI in case the vasectomy reversal fails, or you want to be assured of being able to have other children in the future with IVF/ICSI.

Choosing Between Vasectomy Reversal and IVF/ICSI. If you and your partner are good candidates for vasectomy reversal and are planning to have more than one child, a vasectomy reversal may be your first choice. But if this is not the case, or if you find no sperm at your vasectomy reversal, other options come into play, such as testicular sperm retrieval with IVF/ICSI at the same time or freezing sperm and doing IVF/ICSI with your partner later. (See Chapter 9 for more on these procedures.)

Antisperm Antibodies. If you have had a vasectomy, chances are you have antisperm antibodies. After a vasectomy, the normal barrier between the sperm and the bloodstream is broken. Having never encountered a sperm cell before, your immune system interprets the sperm cell as a foreign body, making antibodies to attack the sperm cell just as it would a virus or other foreign invader. Of men who have vasectomies, about 70 percent have antisperm antibodies.

Antibodies can attack the surface of the sperm, damaging the sperm and hurting its ability to move or bind with an egg. While having antisperm antibodies does not absolutely mean that you can't get pregnant, there are some techniques designed to try to separate the antibodies from the sperm.

One idea is to try to ejaculate into a sterile container containing sterile sperm-washing medium to dilute the antibodies. Sperm comes from the testes, and most of the seminal fluid comes from the seminal vesicles. Sperm and seminal fluid mix in the ejaculatory ducts almost at the moment of ejaculation. It is thought that you might be able to dilute the presence of antibodies if just beyond the moment sperm and seminal fluid recombined the ejaculate is received into a culture medium in which the antibodies are less able to bind to sperm cells. Some antibodies are tenacious and can't be diluted out, and although sperm production in culture media is not a proven technique, it does no harm. Even without this technique, sperm is immersed in culture media at sperm washing before IVF or IUI.

Congenital Bilateral Absence of the Vas Deferens

Almost all men who have cystic fibrosis have congenital bilateral absence of the vas deferens (CBAVD), and there is a strong association between CBAVD and men who carry a mutation of a gene related to cystic fibrosis, called the cystic fibrosis transmembrane conductance regulator, or CFTR, gene. About two-thirds of men with CBAVD have mutations of the CFTR gene.[1] Your urologist will be able to quickly ascertain if you have no vas deferens, because they can be easily felt within your scrotum.

If you have CBAVD, sperm can be retrieved from your epididymis using a technique known as microsurgical epididymal sperm aspiration (MESA) and used in IVF/ICSI. (See Chapter 9.)

Female partners of men who have or carry the gene for cystic fibrosis should also be tested for this hereditary disease before conceiving, as there is a 4 percent risk of anyone in the general population carrying the gene. If your partner also carries the gene, your embryos can be screened through a process known as preimplantation genetic diagnosis (PGD) in which a single cell is taken from an embryo and tested for the gene. This allows your doctor to select only healthy embryos for implantation. If your wife or partner does not carry the gene for cystic fibrosis, there is no risk of passing the disease on, as cystic fibrosis occurs only when a child inherits two copies of the gene, one from each parent. There is a 50 percent chance the child will carry one copy of the gene, but this is not a danger to the child's health.

Ejaculatory Duct Obstruction

The ejaculatory duct is a tubular structure that starts at the vas deferens, runs by the prostate, and empties into the prostatic urethra. Ejaculatory duct obstruction is a rare condition associated either with congenital Mullerian duct cysts or chronic inflammation of the ejaculatory duct due to chronic, recurrent prostatitis. (Mullerian ducts are the embryonic ducts from which male and female reproductive tracts arise.) No sperm in the ejaculate and low volume of ejaculate are signs of ejaculatory duct obstruction. This relatively rare form of obstructive azoospermia or oligospermia (low sperm count) can sometimes be corrected by surgically removing the obstruction.

TESTICULAR BIOPSY: ALWAYS FREEZE SPERM AT YOUR DIAGNOSIS!

A surgeon may recommend a testicular biopsy for a range of diagnostic reasons, including possible obstructive azoospermia, elevated FSH levels, and no sperm in a man's ejaculate, among other indications. It makes a great deal of sense not only to get a diagnosis at a testicular biopsy but, if sperm is found, to take that sperm and freeze some for use in IVF/ICSI later on. This can also be done at vasectomy, vasectomy reversal, and varicocele ligation, which we will talk about in this chapter. Before scheduling a testicular biopsy, be sure that the facility can diagnose as well as freeze sperm.

OLIGOSPERMIA: WHEN YOU HAVE A LOW SPERM COUNT

Oligospermia is the medical term for a low sperm count, which can be severe, as in the case of sperm concentration of less than 5 million/milliliter, or borderline, which is described as counts of between 10 and 20 million sperm. Sperm counts of 5 to 10 million are considered somewhere between borderline and severe.

As pointed out earlier, there is often no clear reason for a low sperm count, yet there are options for overcoming infertility even if the reason is unclear. We will talk in Chapters 8 and 9 about IUIs and IVF/ICSI to overcome fertility problems. In this chapter we will look at causes that can be detected and corrected.

If your sperm count is less than 5 million, you definitely need a urological exam. There is an increased risk of testicular tumors in men with severe oligospermia, and for that reason alone it's very important that a urologist examine you. Low sperm counts can also signal:

- A varicocele, a varicose vein in the scrotum that can interfere with fertility. (See the section "Varicoceles" on page 153.)
- A prolactinoma, a rare but usually benign pituitary tumor that can be treated with medication.
- Low testosterone. A testosterone level below 200 nanograms can also be treated with a fertility drug taken in pill form called clomiphene citrate. The pill is taken daily for six months. In women, clomiphene citrate stimulates ovulation. In men, clomiphene increases testosterone without reducing sperm count by causing the pituitary to increase the output of follicle-stimulating hormone (FSH) and luteinizing hormone (LH), the hormones that stimulate testicular testosterone and sperm production.

WHAT ELSE MIGHT BE WRONG?
REVIEWING YOUR SEMEN ANALYSIS

If you have had a semen analysis, you know that the analysis covers several components. If you are unfamiliar with the features of a semen analysis, take a look at the section "The Semen Analysis" in Chapter 3.

While sperm count (concentration) is the most important aspect of your semen analysis, other features of your semen analysis can affect your fertility. These include motility, morphology (shape), and volume.

Second to concentration (count), motility (movement) is most important to fertility because you will need at least 5 million motile sperm from a sperm wash (see Chapter 8) to do intrauterine insemination (IUI). Motility can be affected by external circumstances, such as the mishandling of a specimen. But motility problems can also be caused by conditions like Kartagener's syndrome. Kartagener's syndrome is a defect in the cilia and microtubules that causes sperm to be immotile. The ciliary motion of the cells lining the bronchial trees in the lungs are also affected, predisposing men with Kartagener's to pneumonia and chronic lung disease. Normally, it takes some motility for sperm to get beyond the cervix and through the uterus to fertilize the egg in the fallopian tube. Intrauterine insemination (IUI) can help people with impaired sperm motility by helping couples to get past the first hurdle of the cervix. If you have both low volume and low motility, insemination is definitely the best first course of action.

Morphology refers to the shape of the sperm, that is, the shape of the head, neck, and tail. Even in men with perfectly normal sperm counts, morphology levels—that is, the percentage of normally shaped sperm—can be as low as 14 percent. Morphology defects often suggest a varicocele. (See page 153.)

Most of the volume of the semen comes from the seminal vesicles. A low volume can mean that you are not producing as much fluid from your seminal vesicles as you normally would, and it's possible that you aren't adequately depositing your semen during intercourse. If your volume is low, but your postcoital test is normal, you are probably fine—but if your postcoital test is abnormal, there is a good chance that you can benefit from intrauterine insemination.

Intrauterine insemination can help men with low volume, low concentration, and/or low motility. While it's not uncommon to have low volume and no other problems with your sperm, it's also not uncommon to have a low sperm count and low motility. As pointed out, morphology problems are often isolated, most often connected to a varicocele.

OTHER CONDITIONS THAT CAN HARM MALE FERTILITY

Other problems can affect male fertility, including retrograde ejaculation, hypospadia, and erectile dysfunction (impotence).

Retrograde Ejaculation

Retrograde ejaculation is a fairly common disorder in which semen doesn't exit the body on ejaculation but instead flows backward into the bladder.

Retrograde ejaculation can be the result of neurological damage or medication. The two most common conditions associated with neurological damage that can cause retrograde ejaculation are diabetes and spinal cord injury. With these conditions, you may lose the reflex that normally closes the bladder during orgasm in order to prevent semen from getting into your urine. Drugs used to treat benign prostatic hypertrophy, the most common type of enlarged prostate in older men, can also cause this condition. Alpha-adrenergic antagonists, such as tamsulosin (Flomax), relax the sphincter action that prevents seminal backflow into the bladder at orgasm. You may ejaculate little or no semen and have semen in your urine, which can appear milky or cloudy.

Retrograde ejaculation can sometimes be treated with an adrenergic agonist like Sudafed and the antihistamine Ornade. Adrenergic agonists contract the sphincter that prevents backflow. Sudafed promotes normal ejaculation, and Ornade relaxes the bladder. Failing this, sperm can be recovered directly from post ejaculatory urine to be used during inseminations or IVF.

Before your sperm can be collected from your urine, you may be asked to take an antacid medication like Alka-Seltzer to buffer the acidity of your urine. Getting your urine pH to the desired level of 7.4 is a matter of trial and error. You can test your pH level at home. Once you reach the right balance, your doctor will collect urine from you to see whether or not you have motile sperm. When you're ready to collect sperm for insemination, your doctor will ask you to empty your bladder, ejaculate, and empty your bladder once more. The sperm will be collected from this second void.

Hypospadia

If you have hypospadia, a congenital condition in which the urethra is not at the tip of your penis, where it normally is, you and your partner may need insemination to assist in fertilization. Sperm that are able to get as far as the penile urethra are fully matured, so your fertility issue is likely to be simply a matter of delivering the sperm to your partner's cervix. This is where simple intracervical inseminations can really help. (For more on this topic, see Chapter 8.)

Erectile Dysfunction

Erectile dysfunction is a contemporary term for what used to be known as impotence. It refers to the inability to achieve the vascular engorgement of the penis that is known as an erection. The causes of this problem can be circulatory, neurological, or psychological.

You've probably heard of Viagra and other drugs to treat erectile dysfunction, or impotence. These drugs work by increasing blood flow to the penis, causing blood to be trapped in the penis, which is what causes an erection, and allowing for penetration. None of these drugs have either a positive or negative effect on fertility or sperm quality. Viagra and Levitra are short-acting drugs, taken within an hour of intercourse. Cialis can allow for the possibility of erections for up to two days. If you have significant heart disease or you are taking nitrates, you should not use these drugs. The general rule is that if you can climb two flights of stairs without duress, you can probably withstand sexual activity.

VARICOCELES

The veins in the lower part of your body have valves. Varicose veins are a congenital weakness of the valve in the vein. The tendency toward varicose veins, or varicocele, is to some degree inborn, and once you have a varicosity, it tends to worsen with time.

A varicocele is a varicose vein in the scrotum. This typically happens in the left testicle, because the venous drainage of the left testis is more prone to obstruction. Varicoceles are fairly common, affecting about 15 percent of all men. A varicocele can impede blood flow from the testis, raising the temperature of the testis and potentially damaging sperm. The optimal temperature for spermatogenesis is about 2°F lower than the temperature around your heart. Blood that is higher than this temperature can impair sperm production.

The larger the varicocele, the more likely it is to be associated with infertility and testicular atrophy (shrinkage). A left testicle that is smaller than the right may be an indication that a varicocele has damaged the seminiferous tubules, which is the sperm production apparatus inside your testicle. Thus, the more atrophied your testicle is, the more likely it is that your fertility has in fact been impaired.

Most people with small to moderate varicoceles have no symptoms, while people with larger varicoceles may notice a sense of heaviness or discomfort in their scrotum. Often, you can feel the varicocele itself, which has been described as feeling like a bag of worms. Although varicoceles can be detected on physical examination of the scrotum alone, doctors may sometimes use ultrasound to further define an inconclusive physical examination. This is most likely to be the case when you have a small varicocele. If you have a varicocele that isn't affecting your fertility and can't be felt on examination, you don't need an ultrasound.

If your varicocele is palpable and your semen analysis is abnormal, the varicocele can be treated surgically. As with other issues of male infertility, IVF may be your first line of treatment, depending on the age of your female partner and any fertility problems that she may have. Although varicocele repair can potentially give you long-term fertility allowing for conception without any medical intervention in the future, if your partner needs IVF to get pregnant because, for example, she has blocked fallopian tubes, IVF will be the best course of action to treat your infertility as a couple. Before considering any type of procedure to resolve a varicocele, your partner should have a thorough fertility workup to ensure that her ovaries are functioning and her tubes are open.

If you are young and not in a relationship, you may decide that you want to treat your varicocele so that you can father children in the future. Varicocele repair is best suited for men with younger partners who have time to wait and see if the varicocele repair was successful and who do not have additional, urgent fertility problems.

Treating Significant Varicoceles: Surgery or Embolization

There are two ways to treat varicoceles that are significant enough to interfere with your fertility: surgically or with a nonsurgical method called percutaneous (through the skin) embolization, which is performed by an interventional radiologist, a doctor who specializes in guiding catheters through small vessels in the body, such as blood vessels, using imaging techniques like X-ray and ultrasound.

The first option, varicocelectomy, is a surgical operation to ligate, or tie off, the varicocele to keep blood from pooling in that vein. You are likely to be a good candidate for a varicocele ligation if:

- your partner is under thirty-seven;
- you have a varicocele that can be felt;
- your testicles are noticeably different in size;
- you have an abnormal sperm count;
- you have infertility.

In the second option, percutaneous embolization, the interventional radiologist will use a catheter and contrast dye to visualize your venous system and guide the catheter toward the affected vein. An agent, such as coil or balloon, can be used to block the dilated vein. Embolization is less invasive than surgery and may have the advantage of allowing the radiologist to visualize the dilated vein, its occlusion, and the subsequent effect, if any, on surrounding vessels. While embolization may be preferable because of its less invasive nature, it is not available everywhere, and so there is still a place for the standard surgical approach.

Waiting to Find Out if Treatment Worked

Success treating a varicocele means either seeing an improvement in your semen analysis and/or having a pregnancy. If you have had varicocelectomy, you should anticipate waiting about twelve months, while having a semen analysis every three months, to detect improvements. If by six months, you don't see any improvement at all, you might start discussing IVF with your partner and doctor. On the other hand, if you are better at six months than you were at three months, and better at nine months than you were at six months, you may not need IVF. It might be better to wait until a year has passed to consider other strategies.

Again, the time needed to gauge the success of a varicocele repair is why the procedure is better suited to couples with time to wait and see if the treatment was effective. Remember that female fertility is much more age-dependent than male fertility, and if a woman is thirty-seven or older, she is much less likely to be as fertile as she was when she was younger.

There are solutions to low and even no sperm count, but before you travel down the road toward treatment of male infertility, make sure that your partner does not also have infertility. The treatment that is right for you—as a member of a couple—depends very much on her reproductive health status. If you are a man reading this chapter, you can help your partner by having a semen analysis, and learning more about male fertility issues as well as about the treatments she may be undergoing so that you can be supportive in your relationship. Remember, your goal is parenthood, where you will both be cooperating on a daily basis to raise healthy, productive children. Working together now can be the beginning of an effective partnership wherein each person's concerns are heard and considered.

7 | Fertility Drugs

WHEN YOU FIRST LEARN ABOUT INFERTILITY DRUGS, you may be overwhelmed by the variety of acronyms and brand names that you hear. But once you have a general sense of how these drugs work and when you will need them, you will be much less intimidated. This chapter will give you information about the drugs you may be using, how to take them, and side effects to watch out for so that you will know what to expect as you go through treatment. You may be taking fertility drugs to:

- Help you ovulate, if you don't ovulate at all. Fertility drugs may help you to ovulate more consistently if your ovulations are irregular;
- Help you to ovulate on the side of your open fallopian tube when the other fallopian tube is blocked;

- Help you to increase your chance of success with monthly intrauterine inseminations (IUI) by getting you to produce multiple eggs each month for fertilization;
- Help you to produce three or more eggs for in vitro fertilization (IVF) each cycle. Within limits, the more eggs that you have to choose from, the better your chances are of having viable embryos for implantation.

CLOMIPHENE CITRATE (CLOMID, SEROPHENE)

Clomiphene citrate was one of the first medications used for ovulation induction, also known as ovarian stimulation. It is the most common and least expensive fertility drug used to stimulate ovulation in women who do not ovulate or who ovulate infrequently. Clomiphene works by fooling your pituitary into putting out more FSH, but does not act directly on your ovaries. If you ovulate infrequently, monthly doses of clomiphene will help regulate your cycle. When you are already ovulating regularly, clomiphene may also help you to ovulate more than one egg at a time, called multiple ovulation. If you fail to ovulate or get pregnant on clomiphene citrate within three to six months, you may decide to switch to injectable FSH.

> *My husband and I started trying to get pregnant after we got married. I just had a feeling inside that there was something wrong. I just knew. My regular ob-gyn didn't take me seriously because of my age. I was twenty-two. She said we had to wait a year. I knew something wasn't right, so I switched to a different ob-gyn, and she was great. She started me right on Clomid, because I was not ovulating. She took the time to listen to all of my concerns.* —RUTH

Candidates for clomiphene citrate include women who:

- don't ovulate;
- ovulate infrequently;

- need bilateral ovulation (ovulation from both fallopian tubes);
- are enhancing IUI with superovulation. (We will talk about this later in the chapter.)

Except for women with PCO, clomiphene has several advantages over injectable drugs as a first line of treatment for most women:

- Clomiphene is relatively cheap and is often covered by drug plans in health insurance policies. Many insurers that do not cover injectable medication will cover oral medications.
- Clomiphene requires much less monitoring than injectable FSH.
- Clomiphene is associated with a lower risk of multiple pregnancies. There is a 5 percent risk of multiple pregnancies on clomiphene versus a 20 percent risk with injectable FSH.

Clomiphene is taken in pill form for five days, causing ovulation approximately one week after the last pill. It should be administered on a month-to-month basis with ongoing examination. Ideally, you should be monitored with ultrasound monthly while on clomiphene. With ultrasound, your doctor can see that you are ovulating and determine precisely whether your ovulation is single or multiple, bilateral or unilateral. At each cycle, you should be monitored to:

- Verify that you are ovulating;
- Check that you don't have ovarian cysts;
- Make sure that you're getting the right dosage of clomiphene;
- Double-check your pregnancy test. Occasionally, a woman may be pregnant despite getting what seems to be a regular period;
- Get an ultrasound at midcycle as well, if possible. This will help assess your response to the medication and time ovulation. Or, you can have your LH levels checked with a blood or urine test. Checking your progesterone levels approximately two weeks after your last clomiphene pill will also confirm that you have ovulated.

Clomiphene is given only for short periods of time for two reasons, one being that most pregnancies assisted by clomiphene occur within the first four months of clomiphene use. Continuing the drug for eight or twelve months provides no further benefit. In addition, one study suggests that the use of clomiphene for twelve months or more may be associated with borderline ovarian tumors.[1] With these two pieces of information in mind, most practitioners do not recommend using clomiphene for more than about six months with an exception for women who have had previous pregnancies with clomiphene, because the data on borderline tumors only applies to women who have not had children.

Clomiphene has side effects. Women using clomiphene citrate often report mood swings that can be severe enough to interfere with their relationships. Other side effects include bloating and pelvic pain. Women who have never ovulated may experience pelvic pain more profoundly than women who do ovulate simply because women who haven't ovulated are less accustomed to the discomforts of ovulation. Visual blurring is a rare side effect of clomiphene citrate. It's certainly very disconcerting when it happens, but it is temporary and not a long-term health risk. If you do experience visual disturbances on clomiphene citrate, you should move on to another medication.

Women are often given too much clomiphene. Many physicians sequentially raise the dose of clomiphene each month with the mistaken idea that more clomiphene will promote more response. This is only true if you are not ovulating at all on a lower dose. If you are ovulating at a low dose of clomiphene, increasing the dose won't generally change your response. Clomiphene has a kind of threshold effect. Once you reach your threshold dosage, you will either ovulate or you won't. More is not better.

Human chorionic gonadotropin behaves like LH, prompting the final phase of egg maturation and release. Most people taking clomiphene will not need a trigger shot of hCG to start ovulation, because most women will have their own natural LH surge on clomiphene. However, with monitoring by ultrasound at midcycle, a well-timed hCG shot can help control the day of ovulation.

Combining Metformin and Clomiphene to Treat PCOS

For years, clomiphene citrate was the first choice for women with poly-cystic ovarian syndrome (PCOS). Recently, however, an insulin-enhancing agent called metformin (Glucophage) has become the first line of treat-ment for women with classic PCOS. Not only do about half of women with true PCOS start ovulating on metformin, but when they do, they continue to ovulate each month without the need for the monitoring that is required when taking clomiphene. Women are also less likely to mis-carry on metformin. If you are taking metformin, you may not need in-seminations as many women do when on clomiphene, because metformin doesn't diminish cervical mucus as clomiphene does.

Clomiphene enhances metformin's action, because insulin increases the ovary's sensitivity to FSH and LH. Although you should probably be started on metformin first, if you have PCOS and are on clomiphene, metformin can be added, helping you to ovulate when you are not having success with clomiphene alone. Or, if you don't ovulate on metformin alone, clomiphene citrate can be combined with metformin as a second line of treatment.

Clomiphene Alternatives

Letrozole is yet another drug being added to the list of treatment options for PCOS, and it may ultimately replace clomiphene. Letrozole is what's called an aromatase inhibitor. It blocks aromatase, the last enzyme in the pathway in estradiol production, thereby lowering the amount of estrogen in your system and increasing your FSH levels. An advantage may be fewer side effects, such as moodiness. If you have had three cycles of clomiphene citrate and you did not respond or did not get pregnant on clomiphene, you may want to ask your doctor about trying letrozole.

The use of letrozole is becoming complicated. Although it is being in-creasingly used for ovulation induction, it is not FDA-approved for that use, and the company that manufactures it does not want it used for this purpose.

(They have a much bigger market for its use in breast cancer.) Furthermore, letrozole is a dangerous drug if mistakenly given during pregnancy.

Taking Clomiphene for Intrauterine Insemination (IUI)

Women taking clomiphene often wonder if they'll need intrauterine insemination (IUI—see Chapter 8) and what the advantages may be. Even if you aren't planning inseminations, you may need them if you are taking clomiphene. Because it's an antiestrogenic agent, clomiphene directly affects the cervical glands that produce mucus, causing many women to make less cervical mucus than usual, hindering sperm transport into the uterus and to the fallopian tubes, where fertilization takes place. Before taking clomiphene, you and your partner should have a postcoital test and recheck your postcoital test again after taking clomiphene to make sure that your cervical mucus is hospitable to your partner's sperm. (You can read about this test in Chapter 3.) If your postcoital test shows a problem with your cervical mucus–sperm interaction, your doctor may recommend IUI.

Before the widespread use of IUI, some practitioners gave women estrogen to counter this effect of clomiphene citrate, but IUI is actually a much more efficient solution. With insemination, you have the advantages of being able to bypass cervical mucus, of timing your inseminations precisely prior to ovulation, and boosting pure sperm beyond your cervix into your uterus.

Inseminations can also ease relationship issues that arise when couples have to have intercourse on demand for conception. With IUI, sperm can be frozen and used at the best time for fertilization. Couples don't have to have frequent intercourse before ovulation, as they must without IUI. For these reasons, it is common practice for physicians to offer IUI to people using clomiphene whether or not a woman's partner has an abnormal semen analysis.

Intrauterine insemination (IUI) is one of the best ways to address moderate (as opposed to severe) sperm problems, which may be addressed with IVF/ICSI. But fertility drugs, such as clomiphene or injectable FSH, do not by themselves help couples with male factor infertility. This may seem obvious, but many people get confused about this because fertility drugs are often added to IUI. Ovulation induction (ovarian stimulation) is meant to help you ovulate or make multiple eggs at each cycle. Generally speaking, you can't overcome a very low sperm count by getting a woman to make more eggs.

Emotional and Physical Effects of Clomiphene

About half of all women who take clomiphene citrate will experience unpleasant mood swings. Generally, you will start to experience moodiness right away, when and if you have this side effect. The best way to cope with mood swings is to be prepared in advance and to let your significant other know that clomiphene is the likely cause of changes in your temperament.

Physically, you may not feel much difference in your cycles. You may have some midcycle pain. On the other hand, if you have not been ovulating, ovulation may be noticeable. As your follicles grow, they will account for almost half of the ovary's volume. You may actually feel a twinge when the ovary ruptures. A few days later, after your progesterone level rises, you may feel bloated, because progesterone relaxes your muscles. Your breasts may feel different, because progesterone temporarily enlarges your breasts. You may notice premenstrual changes—again, ranging from mood to appetite changes. If you don't become pregnant, you should get your period about two weeks after you ovulate, at which point you may get cramping.

> *I reacted to the drugs with vehement mood swings. It would get to the point where my husband and I would be shouting at each other, "Who are you? I don't even know who you are anymore!" Years ago, when I was much younger, I tried birth control pills. They made me very crazy too. I knew the hormonal medications were going to set me off.* —CYNTHIA

I had 8 cycles on Clomid with my ob-gyn. I had mood swings and hot flashes. It was horrible. I just didn't feel like myself. But once you start thinking you might be getting somewhere, you get so excited. I said, "I'll take whatever I have to take." I considered it good pain, pain that was getting us closer to our goal of getting pregnant. —LANNIE

If You Don't Ovulate or Don't Get Pregnant on Clomiphene

Allow at least three and no more than six months before deciding whether to try other options to help you ovulate. If you have had a complete fertility workup and everything is normal, but you haven't ovulated on three cycles of clomiphene or gotten pregnant after six ovulatory cycles of clomiphene, your next step may be to go on to injectable FSH. (Also see "Are You on the Right Treatment Path?" on page 177.)

The Risk of Multiple Pregnancy with Clomiphene

Many people are concerned about the risk of multiple pregnancies when taking clomiphene citrate. The risk of multiple gestations with clomiphene citrate is approximately 5 percent, and the vast majority of these multiple gestations are twins.

INJECTABLE FSH

Follicle-stimulating hormone (FSH) is key to the growth of your follicles. It stimulates the ovary to develop follicles and mature eggs. When you are undergoing IVF, you will be given what's known as injectable FSH. Very simply, injectable FSH works by increasing the amount of FSH in your body, stimulating the ovary to activate a number of follicles, each one of which contains an egg. Rather than producing a single egg each month, you will produce many more than you normally do.

As its name implies, injectable FSH is injected subcutaneously (under the skin) to stimulate ovulation. It can be used to increase the number of eggs you make each month from one egg to two or three eggs, for example, for what's known as *superovulation,* used in conjunction with IUI or intercourse. (See page 166.) Or, it can be used more aggressively with IVF to help you to make more eggs, giving you the best chance of creating enough embryos to choose from for implantation. Every woman undergoing IVF will be treated with injectable FSH.

Today, most FSH medications are made from a process called recombinant DNA technology where genes for hormones are transferred into other cells. These cells serve as hormone "factories," producing hormones for use in medications. Most physicians use injectable FSH made by recombinant DNA technology. Brands names are Follistim (follitropin beta, manufactured by Organon) and Gonal-F (follitropin alpha, manufactured by Serono). From a clinical perspective, there is no difference between these drugs and most doctors are comfortable using both.

Although it is initially expensive to develop recombinant DNA technology, in the long run it's cheaper and more efficient from the manufacturer's point of view than the classic method of extracting FSH from the urine of menopausal women, which contains extremely high levels of FSH. Human menopausal gonadotropin (hMG), brand-named Pergonal, is the grandmother of all the classic FSH preparations, but is no longer available in the United States.

Until recently, Repronex was the only such FSH medication available in the United States. But Ferring, the company that makes Repronex, now offers Menopur, a highly purified urinary preparation. This preparation is just as effective as recombinant medications, and it contains FSH and LH, which may be key in helping some women who do not do as well on FSH alone. Menopur can be injected under the skin.

There are no generic FSH brands, and all FSH drugs are injectables. None are active orally, because they are essentially proteins that would be digested if taken orally.

Who Are Candidates for Injectable FSH?

- women undergoing IVF
- women who did not ovulate on three to six months of clomiphene citrate
- women who did not get pregnant on three to six months clomiphene citrate
- women undergoing IUI with superovulation
- women who ovulate on only one side (unilateral ovulation)
- women with hypothalamic amenorrhea. (These are women who don't ovulate or menstruate, typically women with very low body weight, athletes, and women with anorexia nervosa.)
- women with low levels of both FSH and LH

Who Should Not Take Injectable FSH?

Women who have estrogen-dependent tumors, such as breast cancer, should not use injectable FSH, because it increases estrogen levels. Importantly, women with unresolved breast cancer should be advised against pregnancy, which can exacerbate these types of cancers.

How Injectable FSH Works: An Overview

The best way to explain a possible ovarian stimulation drug schedule is to first show you a bare-bones stimulation cycle and to show you what elements may be added, depending on whether or not you are trying to get as many eggs as possible for IVF. For instance, if you are having ovulation induction for intrauterine insemination (IUI), you don't want to make ten eggs. If you were having IVF, you might. Generally, stimulations for IVF are far more aggressive than stimulations for superovulation, where you might want to make two to three eggs a month rather than a single egg each month. (See the box "Using Injectable FSH with IUI: Superovulation," on page 171.)

The IVF Drugs

If you are having IVF, you may be on a schedule of:

- birth control pills to place the ovaries in a resting state, ready to receive stimulation;
- injectable FSH to stimulate growth of multiple egg-producing follicles;
- human chorionic gonadotropin (hCG) to trigger ovulation;
- a gonadotropin-releasing hormone analog to shut down the ovaries before your natural LH surge. (See Chapter 9.)

"How Injectable FSH Works: An Overview," on page 166, will give you a good sense of what these drugs do and how they fit into your treatment.

Normally, your natural FSH causes one follicle to develop each month. Once it reaches critical maturity, critical size, and a critical estradiol level, it promotes an LH surge that will cause final maturation and the release of the egg soon thereafter. With ovarian stimulation, we want to stimulate the ovaries to outperform their usual capacity for one monthly egg.

The simplest augmentation of your normal cycle is to give you 225 units of injectable FSH for IVF (or 150 units for superovulation) for seven to twelve days, to create much higher levels of FSH in the bloodstream and the ovary to override your natural system and cause several follicles to develop.

Most often, injectable FSH will confuse your LH surge. So it's usually necessary to give another medication to emulate the LH surge, typically hCG, the same hormone measured in a pregnancy test. Recently, a recombinant form of LH called Luveris was approved for marketing in the United States. At the time of this writing, it remains to be seen whether Luveris will be used to trigger ovulation.

As a general rule of thumb, your doctor will give you an hCG shot to promote an LH surge about thirty-four to thirty-six hours before your timed intercourse, IUI, or your egg retrieval for IVF. The usual hCG dose is 10,000 units.

So what can we add to this simple structure? Your doctor may pretreat you the month before your cycle with birth control pills to suppress FSH and LH. When you stop taking birth control pills and you get your period again, your uterine lining will have shed and your ovaries will be in a resting state, ready to receive stimulation. This is the best place to start ovarian stimulation. When all your follicles are small and resting, several follicles can begin to grow at the same time. The eggs they contain will be at the same state of maturity at the time of your egg retrieval.

Getting your ovaries to a baseline state before stimulation and controlling timing is very helpful to both patient and clinic. When you consider how much is involved during the two weeks when you have the most office visits for monitoring, it's good to know which two weeks these will be. Some people worry that birth control pills will have a negative effect on their next cycle, but there is really no good evidence of that. There is also no evidence that taking birth control pills will make you more difficult to stimulate. The only people who should not take birth control pills are people with high blood pressure or those with other contraindications, such as smoking.

Another addition would be to address the possibility of LH surging prematurely before you are ready for the hCG shot. The premature activation of eggs is disastrous to an IVF procedure. If the egg is in the wrong state of maturity or can't be retrieved from the ovary to be combined with sperm in the laboratory, you cannot have your procedure. Once an egg is released from the ovary, it's very hard to find. One thing we can do to prevent this from happening is to give a GnRH antagonist, such as Antagon or Cetrotide (see Chapter 9), toward the end of ovarian stimulation when LH might start to appear naturally. Not only will the GnRH antagonist prevent this from happening, it will allow your doctor to delay the hCG shot, if needed, to push the ovaries a day or two further to get as many follicles as possible. A GnRH agonist, such as Lupron, can also be used, but the advantage of an antagonist is that it can shut down the ovaries very quickly, within hours. (You will learn more about GnRH antagonists and agonists Chapter 9.)

> *I had to be on birth control pills the month before I started. This is a very odd experience when you are trying to conceive. I was put on Lupron, which basically puts you into menopause. You get hot flashes, and you feel horrible. Lupron shuts down your whole hormonal system. Then they start it up again. You get a rush of estrogen. I got very jittery. Then I was on proges-terone. With progesterone, you may not get your period. On progesterone I always had "simulated" pregnancies, complete with symptoms, including bloating and nausea. My skin broke out. Time went very slowly.* —CINDY

Taking Injectable FSH: More Is Not Always Better

A course of FSH injectables is generally one subcutaneous shot a day taken for seven to twelve days. This may be repeated on a monthly basis. There are two important things to remember about the dosage of injectable FSH: there is a direct relationship between the amount of FSH you take and the amount of ovarian response you receive, but once you reach certain high doses, more is not better. Beyond about 450 international units (IU), or 6 ampules of injectable FSH, it's unlikely that you are going to respond to a higher dose. If you *aren't responding to FSH,* a higher dose won't hurt you, although it's unlikely to help you ovulate. Often, people who don't respond to FSH wind up on very high doses to no one's benefit but the drug company, given that 450 units of injectable FSH can easily cost $300 a day. Doubling that is unconscionable from a financial perspective and dubious from a medical point of view. The only time to increase the dosage beyond this point is when someone's body size is very large.

While high doses of FSH can't hurt you when your ovaries are not re-sponding, high doses of FSH can kill you if your ovaries *are* responding. Rarely, women experience *severe* hyperstimulation. This is not the normal hyperstimulation, which is the goal of treatment, but a potentially very dire medical condition. Your doctor should inform you of the risks and symptoms of hyperstimulation before you take this drug. (See "Before Taking Injectable FSH: What You Should Know," on page 175.)

If you are not responding to injectable FSH, you should begin to consider other options. Not responding may mean that you have a limited ovarian reserve or that you are simply not getting ovarian activity in response to this agent. Remember, women are not really meant to produce more than one egg a month. Ovarian stimulation is an artificial situation to which some women just don't respond. If the problem is not one of diminished ovarian reserve, then further attempts should be made to address all other correctable infertility factors, such as endometriosis. (See Chapter 5.)

Monitoring Your Ovulation with Injectable FSH

When taking injectables, it's crucial to know how many egg-containing follicles are developing in your ovaries and when they are likely to mature. If you are using IUI or having intercourse, you want advance notice of when you are likely to ovulate so you can try for conception or time your insemination *before* your eggs are released. Precise timing is even more critical to egg retrieval for IVF.

Your doctor will monitor your stimulation and determine when you are likely to ovulate by using ultrasound and testing your blood estradiol levels. Ultrasound shows the size and number of your follicles. Your estradiol level is then correlated to the number and size of those follicles, giving your physician an indicator of when your eggs are likely to be mature.

You will be given a trigger shot of hCG to promote ovulation, because you won't have an LH surge on your own. If you are taking injectable FSH, you should plan to be available for five to seven *daily* doctor's visits for ultrasounds and blood estradiol levels during your regimen.

Mature eggs are contained in follicles that are somewhere between 15 to 20 millimeters or 1.5 to 2 centimeters in diameter. You will generally get your trigger hCG or LH shot when your largest follicle is somewhere between 15 to 20 millimeters and when your corresponding estradiol level is appropriate. You should ovulate within thirty-six to forty-two hours after your shot. If you are having IVF, your egg retrieval should be scheduled thirty-four to thirty-six hours after your shot. Retrieval has to be done on time, because once the shot is given, the egg will start to leave the ovary.

Using Injectable FSH with IUI: Superovulation

Normally, women ovulate one egg per month with one chance each month of fertilizing that egg and getting pregnant. Imagine if you made two to three eggs a month. You might have two to three times the chance of getting pregnant each month with insemination or intercourse. That's the concept behind superovulation or controlled ovarian hyperstimulation (COH). Unlike clomiphene citrate, which works indirectly, the more injectable FSH you take, the more your ovaries respond, because it works directly on the ovary. If your ovaries are capable of responding to 150 units of injectable FSH, they may respond more to 225 units, although there are limits to this, as we discussed earlier. With superovulation, you will begin your treatment with a modest dose, generally 150 units. (Women undergoing IVF start with much more, typically 225 to 300 units.)

With superovulation, the chance of having a multiple pregnancy is about 20 percent. The risk is much higher than with clomiphene citrate. With IVF, you can control the number of embryos you transfer to your uterus. However, the risk of having high-order multiple pregnancies (carrying more than twins) depends very much on your age, with the likelihood being higher for younger women than older women.

Many women choose superovulation over IVF even though IVF is two and a half times more likely to result in pregnancy than superovulation and carries a lower risk of high order multiple births. Yet if a woman stimulates very well on superovulation, making not just two to three follicles, but a much higher number, as might be the case for someone with PCOS, she might be better off going directly to IVF, because she now has a large number of eggs from which to make embryos. Her risk of high order multiple births with IVF is much lower, because a woman who puts back no more than two embryos in her uterus for implantation is at most going to have twins. The other embryos can be frozen for future embryo transfer attempts, if she wants more children.

Of course, insurance and finances are a big issue with IVF. Many insurers that cover injectables and inseminations don't cover IVF. You may even have to fail three cycles of superovulation to qualify for coverage for IVF. Unless you have had previous success with superovulation, you might consider doing no more than three cycles of superovulation before moving to IVF, if insurance and money issues don't stand in your way.

Making Injections Easier

If you are one of those people who are squeamish about shots: don't despair. You are definitely not alone. There are tricks and tips to make it easier. No matter how afraid you are, you will quickly become adept at giving or receiving shots as you practice. There are two types of shots: subcutaneous, the method through which most medications are given, and intramuscular injections. Progesterone can be given intramuscularly or through vaginal suppositories. Gonal-F and Follistim (injectable FSH) now come as an injectable pen, making the shot easier to do. But if you are mixing medications, you will probably still be using needles. Here are some tips:

- Be sure to take any patient education courses available to you to help you learn how to give or receive an injection. Practice on oranges or grapefruits. Their skins are actually close to the consistency of human skin.

- Realize that the subcutaneous shot only takes a second. It will sting a bit like a pinprick or a bee sting, and then it will be over.
- Getting a shot gets easier each time you do it.
- Find out if there is someone in your family, a friend, or even a neighbor who has been through this. Can this person give you tips? Can she help you? Your partner may be able to give you shots, but sometimes partners are unavailable for practical or emotional reasons. Your IVF program can teach anyone you want to give you your shot safely and effectively. As well, nurses sometimes make themselves available on their own time for a small fee.
- IVF programs often arrange for patients to visit their local emergency rooms to get their hCG shots at night.

Make sure you pinch your skin when you do it. They have a class to help teach you how to do the shots, but they don't teach you to pinch. It makes it less uncomfortable, if you pinch your skin. —JILL

Getting an Intramuscular Injection

The best place for an intramuscular injection is in the upper outer quadrant of your buttocks. This is preferable to using your thigh muscle, although women who have to give themselves injections use the thigh muscle. You are going to be a little sorer if you give yourself a shot in the thigh. That's why it's best to try to find someone to give you the shot instead. When receiving intramuscular shots, try these tips:

- While your partner is drawing up the medication, drape an ice pack over the site and count to five using the old "1 (1,000); 2 (2,000) . . ." method. Take the ice pack off and get in the following posture for the shot: If you are going to have the injection in the upper outer quadrant of your right buttock, when standing, lean into your left leg and turn the right leg inward. This relaxes the gluteus muscle and makes the shot less painful.

• After the shot, gently rub the muscle and place a heating pad over the spot to lessen soreness.

There can be so many instructions to giving and receiving shots that the whole process can seem overwhelming. Some aspects of giving a shot really matter and some you may not need to lose sleep over. Remember these things:

• Create a clean environment. You have don't have to be sterile in scrubs and a mask, but cleanliness is important. Clean the surface that you are using to set up your medications with an alcohol pad or bactericidal soap. Wash your hands. Before inserting a needle into the rubber stopper, make sure the stopper is clean by wiping it with an alcohol pad.

• Air bubbles are a concern, but should not be an obsession. If the air bubble displaces the medication, it's a problem. Tiny, almost microscopic, bubbles should not worry you.

• Make sure you are using the right needle. Believe it or not, some patients getting subcutaneous shots do make the mistake of giving themselves an injection with the bigger mixing needle. They don't usually make this mistake twice.

• Tighten the needle before injecting so that the fluid does not escape.

• Relax. One of the ways you and your partner or friend can share the experience is to create some "down" time before the shot. If you can, rest while your partner draws up the medication, listen to music, focus your eyes on a spot on the wall, and imagine yourself in a relaxing environment. The shot will be over soon.

From your partner's point of view, it's very hard to give someone you love this big needle; it's very hard. At my doctor's office, there was a nurse avail-

able to give patients injections. It may be worth the extra money to have someone else give you your daily injections. —DINAH

I felt more in control learning how to give myself shots, mixing the medicines, praying and meditating about this child who was going to come to me. I visualized the shots as nourishing the physical part of this person who was going to come to me, so the soul could possess something physical and come here. —BARBARA

The intramuscular injection of progesterone is awful. It's an oil-based solution. It's a very large needle that you have to stick in your derriere. I gave it to myself once in my leg, but usually the husband gives it to the wife. I would have no patience because my hormones were flying all over the place. He would say, "I don't want to hurt you." I would say, "Guess what? Childbirth hurts more. Give me the shot." But it would bother him that he had to give me this shot. He did it, and he was actually pretty good at it. —PAM

Before Taking Injectable FSH: What You Should Know

Before you take these drugs you should be aware of two possible but opposite adverse results: not stimulating at all, or hyperstimulating, which in its most severe form is a medical emergency. Here we will look at both of these possibilities.

No Response to Ovarian Stimulation

As we move along in the discussion of ovarian stimulation, it's important to recall that we are engageding in *assisted* reproduction. Women's bodies are not designed to produce more than one egg a month, and some women may simply not respond to ovulation induction. Even some women who have regular cycles may produce no more than one egg a month on fertility drugs. The following are indications that you are most likely to respond poorly to fertility drugs:

- the older you are
- the higher your day three FSH/estradiol level. (See Chapter 3 for a description of this test.)
- the smaller your ovaries are
- the fewer follicles you have in your ovaries
- the more ovarian surgery you have had
- you have severe endometriosis

While you may be more likely to have a poor response if you are older, young women can also be poor responders. Before starting IVF, talk to your doctor about whether or not you are a good candidate for fertility drugs. Even if you are a possible poor candidate for stimulation, it's reasonable to try stimulation with the proviso that if you stimulate well you'll continue on to IVF, and if you don't, you will cancel your IVF cycle.

Some women are counseled about the risk of a poor response before starting IVF, and some women only find out that they don't respond well after the fact. Tragically, some women with only limited response may be guided into believing that while they don't have a significant response, their minor response may lead to success. Certainly, two doctors may see poor stimulation differently. One may see doom where the other sees hope. While a handful of patients may succeed with a minimal response, most don't.

If you are not responding to injectable FSH at 450 to 600 units per day, you are most likely not going to respond. This may mean that you are not a candidate for IVF, because you must make a number of eggs for IVF to be an efficient and viable option. If you have blocked fallopian tubes or your partner has a very low sperm count, you could be in a very tough situation, because you absolutely need IVF. When you have only one or two eggs, however, the procedure becomes so inefficient that another alternative, such as donor eggs (see Chapter 12), should be considered sooner rather than later. When you first realize that you may not be able to do IVF, you may feel defeated, but remember that you are doing this to become a family. You *can* have a child, but it may not be with the method you first intended. In Chapter 12, we will talk about making the decision to quit fertility treatment and about other methods for creating your family.

Severe Ovarian Hyperstimulation and Other FSH Side Effects

Hyperstimulation is a disorder in which the ovaries becomes so enlarged that they cause discomfort and bloating in its mild form and a life-threatening condition in its most severe form. Your ovaries are making many more follicles than they would in normal reproductive life. Not only can this be painful, it can be dangerous, stretching the surface of the ovary and the blood vessels on the ovary to such a degree that they leak. When the ovary leaks, it leaks fluid into your abdominal cavity. The enlargement of your ovaries and the pressure on your stomach can make you feel nauseous. In severe cases, fluid can travel under the diaphragm, even leaking into the thoracic cavity, which contains the heart and the lungs, causing shortness of breath or inability to breathe deeply.

When you are hyperstimulating, the ovaries also secrete exceedingly high levels of estradiol and progesterone. Progesterone is a hormone that can relax the muscles of respiration, contributing to breathing difficulties. High levels of estradiol can promote blood clots. Blood cells that don't leak through the vascular system can become concentrated, raising your blood count dramatically. And as your red blood cell count rises, the blood can become sluggish and concentrated, making it further prone to clotting. Blood clots can break loose in your vascular system and travel to other parts of the body, such as the lung, the blood supply to other organs, even to your brain. Women with severe ovarian hyperstimulation have had strokes; clots to their kidneys, causing kidney damage; or clots to their lungs, which can be fatal. Blood clots are the most common cause of death from severe ovarian hyperstimulation.

Ovarian hyperstimulation can be mild, moderate, or severe. In a milder case, you may be able to eat and drink and go to the bathroom relatively normally. You may have some mild pelvic discomfort, but no trouble lying down. You may even feel some fluid sloshing around in your belly. Your belly might stick out a little bit, and you may not be able to button your pants. Although you may eat less than normally, you will still be able to void and have bowel movements. In severe cases, you may experience shortness of breath, trouble taking a deep breath, panting, pelvic pain, nausea, or vomiting. *Always consult your doctor if think you may be experiencing hyperstimulation.*

If it is going to happen, hyperstimulation generally occurs a week after your shot of hCG, which triggers ovulation. It's very rare that hyperstimulation occurs without an hCG shot. Unless you are given the shot, which triggers the release of the follicle, your ovaries tend to regress to normal. Similarly, it's very rare for someone to be hyperstimulated by taking the hCG shot alone without prior FSH administration. Because of the renewed source of hCG from the pregnancy itself, being pregnant can compound hyperstimulation. Adding to the crisis in these extreme cases is the need to terminate the pregnancy—particularly tragic for someone who is trying so hard to have a baby.

Fortunately, hyperstimulation seldom happens without warning. Knowing that you are at risk and being aware of the signs of severe hyperstimulation is one of the best ways to avoid it. You and your doctor should confer early about your risk if you are:

- young (in your twenties or early thirties);
- have PCOS;
- don't ovulate regularly;
- have a large number of developing follicles or eggs.

If you are in all or any of these high-risk categories, your doctor must closely monitor your cycle. If you are getting extremely high estradiol levels and have many small follicles that show exquisite sensitivity to even low doses of FSH, you might consider not completing your stimulation cycle with an hCG shot. In expert hands, with close monitoring, these serious complications are almost always avoidable.

Side effects and complications are surely the downside of taking FSH. When taking injectables, you will have soreness at the injection sites. You may experience mood changes, although fewer women complain of mood changes with injectable FSH than with clomiphene citrate. You may feel pelvic fullness and some degree of bloating as your ovaries enlarge. But when it comes to side effects, it's vital to be aware of the possibility of hyperstimulation so that you can recognize the signs of moderate to severe hyperstimulation and get help before you experience a medical emergency.

Injectable FSH and Cancer

If cancer is a growth and you are taking a hormone that promotes growth, might this hormone promote cancer in the organ upon which it acts?

**BEFORE CHOOSING A DOCTOR OR CLINIC, ASK ABOUT
SEVERE OVARIAN HYPERSTIMULATION**

Ask your doctor what percentage of his or her cases involve hyperstimulation that requires hospitalization or paracentesis. The answer should be no more than 1 percent.

While this is a logical train of thought, we really don't know what causes ovarian cancer, but we are fairly sure it is not infertility drugs. Certainly, if high levels of FSH were to cause ovarian cancer with great frequency, there would be a very high incidence of ovarian cancer among menopausal women who, of course, have high FSH levels. While ovarian cancer is more common in older women, it is still a relatively uncommon cancer.

Moreover, there are absolutely no good studies to show even an indirect relationship between ovarian cancer and the use of clomiphene citrate or injectable FSH. Ovarian cancer is more common in women who have never had children. It's not surprising that there is a higher rate of infertility among women who never had children. This raises the question of whether these women had something wrong with their ovaries that predisposed them to both infertility and ovarian cancer. On the other hand, we know that ovarian cancer can occur in women who are fertile, as well. We do not know the cause of ovarian cancer, but there is very good evidence that ovarian stimulation is not a risk factor.

As suggested earlier, one study has suggested a relationship between clomiphene citrate and what are called borderline tumors. Borderline tumors are not cancer. Furthermore, borderline tumors are less likely to occur in women who took clomiphene, even a lot of clomiphene, if they had a child at some point in their lives. This may either mean that there is no true relationship between clomiphene citrate and borderline tumors or that having a child to some degree immunizes you against borderline tumors.

OTHER DRUGS THAT CAN HELP YOU TO OVULATE

There are several drugs that can indirectly help ovulation. If your ovulation problems are a secondary symptom as a result of another problem in your body, your doctor may prescribe one of these to treat the problem and help you ovulate.

- *Bromocriptine* (Parlodel) is used to treat women who don't ovulate because of high levels of prolactin. By mimicking the neurotransmitter dopamine, bromocriptine lowers prolactin levels so that a woman can resume ovulation. This drug does not act on the ovary and is only used for women with high levels of prolactin.
- *Dexamethasone/Prednisone* are corticosteroids given in very low doses to treat women who don't ovulate due to elevated adrenal hormones. Unlike many drugs, dexamethasone is usually not called by its brand names, but is just generally termed dexamethasone.
- *Metformin* works by enhancing the action of the insulin in women with PCOS. PCOS is generally treated by metformin first, clomiphene and metformin second, and then perhaps letrozole. However, most women who are not responding to oral medications may want to move to injectable FSH. Brand-named Glucophage, metformin is an off-patent drug and may also be called by its generic name of metformin. (For more detail about metformin, see Chapter 5.)
- *Letrozole* blocks estrogen synthesis, lowering the amount of estrogen in the body as does clomiphene citrate, and may be used to help women with PCOS ovulate. If you can't tolerate or don't do well on metformin, then using clomiphene alone or letrozole alone may be reasonable.
- *Tamoxifen* (Nolvadex), like clomiphene citrate, is an antiestrogen. It binds to estrogen receptors without an estrogenic effect. Tamoxifen is also used in treating breast cancer, but there is no relationship between breast cancer and the drug's use for infertility care.
- *Spironolactone* (Aldactone) is a drug used to treat high blood pressure,

CONSIDERING MAIL-ORDER DRUGS: PROTECT YOUR HEALTH

Because of the high cost of infertility drugs, many people are tempted to buy drugs through mail-order companies. But is it safe? Before you buy, it's important to remember that some drugs may not be manufactured in the industrialized world, where standards for quality are higher than in less industrially developed countries.

Many fertility drugs must be handled very carefully. Some must be kept at temperatures no higher than room temperature; others must be refrigerated. Shipped drugs that may sit on loading docks or under a hot sun may lose their potency.

Many drugs are dispensed as liquids. Powdered drugs that must be reconstituted are less subject to handling problems than liquid drugs.

but it also acts as antiandrogen (male hormone) and may help hyperandrogenic women ovulate. Although this drug is not in frequent use, it can be helpful for people who can't take metformin, don't respond to clomiphene or letrozole, have high androgen levels, and want to stick to oral medications only.

Now that you know more about fertility drugs and the way they work, you will be better prepared to understand how they work with intrauterine inseminations and IVF. In the next chapter, we will look at IUI and following that chapter visit the topic of IVF in depth. Being aware of how IUI and IVF work can really help you take charge of your infertility care. Depending on your treatment plan, you may be using IUIs before IVF or going straight to IVF. Because IVF has become the foundation of infertility care, you and your doctor run the risk of overlooking other diagnostic and treatment possibilities, such as when you have unrecognized endometriosis or when you have blocked tubes. When you read about IVF, you will also learn what can go wrong in an IVF stimulation cycle. Knowing the pitfalls ahead of time can help you really understand what to expect and avoid problems along the way, saving you time, money, and emotional pain.

8 | Intrauterine Insemination (IUI)

INSEMINATION IS A SIMPLE, LOW-TECH, AND RELATIVELY noninvasive fertility solution for some couples with specific fertility issues. Intrauterine insemination (IUI) is often the first line of treatment for women who don't have problems ovulating, although this technique can be coupled with fertility drugs in a technique called superovulation, which we talk about in Chapter 7.

Inseminations can be done in one of two ways: intra*cervically,* meaning that unprepared sperm is deposited at the end of the vagina near the cervix, or as intra*uterine* inseminations (IUI), meaning sperm is prepared and put beyond the cervix into the uterus. Today, the vast majority of inseminations are intrauterine inseminations.

Intrauterine insemination is a two-step procedure. Your partner's sperm or your donor's sperm goes through a process known as sperm washing, a procedure that isolates the most motile sperm to introduce into your uterus. In your doctor's office, you will undergo a relatively painless procedure in which your partner's or your donor's purified sperm is slowly infused into your uterus.

THE ODDS OF SUCCESS WITH IUI

Before considering IUI, you should know that you are ovulating, you should know that your fallopian tubes are open, and you should know that your husband or partner's sperm count is not severely abnormal. Importantly, if your tubes are blocked and you don't know it, you could wind up spending thousands of dollars and several months getting a treatment that won't work. Before you start IUIs, you should have had a hysterosalpingogram (HSG) to find out the status of your tubes. (See Chapter 3.) If your doctor doesn't offer you or tell you about this test, consider it a sign that you are not getting thorough and high-quality care.

The hardest part of IUI will be the two-week wait to discover whether you are pregnant or whether you get your period as usual. Without sounding too pessimistic, the best advice to anyone having IUI is to approach the procedure with the knowledge that more than 80 percent of the time it won't succeed. When you are using injectable FSH with IUI (superovulation), you have a 20 percent chance of conceiving each cycle. With clomiphene citrate or no drug intervention (called a natural cycle) the odds are lowered to 10 to 15 percent.

But isn't IUI assisted reproduction? With the all the initialisms used in artificial reproductive technology, it's easy to get confused about the difference between IVF and IUI. Intrauterine insemination (IUI) is a procedure in which you are boosting pure sperm beyond your cervix. In vitro fertilization (IVF) is an artificial reproductive procedure done "in vitro" (in glass, referring to the laboratory). A woman's eggs and a man's sperm are combined in the laboratory for fertilization, after which selected fertilized eggs called embryos are later placed in the woman's uterus to implant.

IVF can be used to treat a range of problems that IUI does not address. IUI is much more akin to natural reproduction.

There are many misconceptions about IUI. One of the most common is that it can be used to help women with tubal problems or couples with severely abnormal semen analyses. People tend to think of IUI as a low-tech version of IVF, which it is not. Hopefully, after reading this chapter you won't share this misconception.

To help you really understand the difference, let's look closely at both of the issues. In vitro fertilization (IVF) was invented for women without fallopian tubes and/or severely damaged tubes. Because they had no fallopian tubes, their eggs and their partners' sperm could not meet in the fallopian tube where conception normally takes place. Doctors had to think of a way to get around this major barrier to pregnancy, so they ultimately removed the egg from the ovary, combined it with sperm in the lab, and brought it back to the uterus. Later, when even further advances in IVF had been made, physicians began to wonder how to overcome severe male infertility, knowing that all it takes is one sperm to fertilize an egg. Ultimately, doctors were able to inject a single sperm directly into an egg, and intracytoplasmic sperm injection (ICSI) was born. It is now combined with IVF. (See Chapter 9.)

Intrauterine insemination, on the other hand, is assisted natural conception. Your doctor is just helping you past less dramatic fertility barriers, such as having thin or absent cervical mucus, which makes it hard for your partner's sperm to get beyond your cervix to swim toward your fallopian tubes to fertilize your egg. Although couples with borderline low sperm counts may benefit from IUI and sperm washing, men with severely low counts need the extra assistance that only IVF can provide. If 5 million motile sperm can be isolated after sperm washing, you might be able to use IUI to get pregnant. On the other hand, if fewer sperm are repeatedly isolated, IVF may be your best choice.

While the statistics for IUI seem less favorable than what you might experience if you were trying without intervention, you must remember that IUI is used to treat couples with infertility whose chance of conceiving may be far below the 20 percent chance a couple without infertility has of conceiving each month. Assistance can give people with infertility nearly the same chance of conceiving as fertile people, and this can be a terrific boon, considering some couples may have a low or no chance of conceiving without help.

WHEN YOU MAY NEED IUI

A postcoital test (see Chapter 3) is one of the best determiners of whether you really need IUIs. If you have a good postcoital test, you should have a lot of cervical mucus, the fluid that helps conduct the sperm through the cervix to the uterus and protect the sperm from the vagina's normally acid environment. On a postcoital test, sperm should be found living in the mucus. If your postcoital test is good, you don't need an IUI, but if your test is poor, you will be advised to do IUIs.

How does cervical mucus work? Estradiol stimulates the glandular cells lining your cervix to produce mucus. As your estradiol levels rise in the first part of your cycle, the cervix produces copious amounts of cervical mucus. Around ovulation, when estradiol has its maximum effect, your cervical mucus should be abundant, clear, and sticky. In your daily life, you may have noticed the presence of cervical mucus around the time of ovulation. If you don't, that's an indication that there may be something wrong.

What could go wrong? Some surgeries can permanently harm your cervical mucus, including procedures where the lining of the cervix is partially destroyed or removed, such as:

- LEEP, a procedure in which a looped electrode is used to remove the cervical lining;
- cryotherapy, freezing of the cervix where the lining is partially destroyed and sloughed off.

Clomiphene citrate (Serophene or Clomid) can definitely harm your cervical mucus because it's an antiestrogen that tells the pituitary to make more follicle-stimulating hormone (FSH). But as you make more FSH, you make less cervical mucus. Bacterial infections, such as bacterial vaginitis or chlamydia, yeast infections, douching, overuse of antibiotics, birth control pills, and sperm antibodies can also create what is called hostile cervical mucus.

Before the widespread use of artificial reproductive technologies in the 1980s, very few infertility doctors were engaged in large-scale intrauterine insemination programs. But in fact, IUIs could have been offered widely even thirty or forty years ago, because the procedure requires simple equipment. Yet IUI really didn't become popular until IVF became widely available.

Today, IUI, a once underutilized treatment, has become overutilized. Artificial reproductive technologies have changed the nature of infertility care and the orientation of fertility practitioners so profoundly that IUI is being offered to couples with no medical indication except the fact that the couple has infertility. This overuse has to a small degree been fostered by insurance companies who limit coverage to IUI and exclude IVF or insist on a certain number of failed IUIs prior to approval of IVF.

But there are times when IUI can definitely help couples overcome specific fertility problems, such as:

- when you have no or thin cervical mucus;
- when you are taking clomiphene citrate, which has a negative effect on your cervical mucus;
- when there is a negative interaction between your cervical mucus and your partner's sperm;
- when you are using frozen sperm;
- when your partner has retrograde ejaculation.

You can use intracervical insemination (ICI), which, like normal relations, simply involves depositing sperm at the end of the vagina at the opening of the cervix, when your partner has a physical anomaly, such as hypospadia that prevents him from depositing sperm high in the vagina, or when your partner has erectile or sexual dysfunction.

When using injectable FSH for superovulation, intrauterine insemination is often done in order to precisely time the introduction of sperm into your uterus before ovulation, giving you the best chance of conceiving after the effort of going through ovulation induction.

There are also times when IUI *may* help, such as when you are attempting to overcome the presence of antisperm antibodies. Theoretically, it makes sense to use insemination and sperm washing (see page 147) to dilute antibodies and boost the sperm higher in the reproductive tract, but it's never been shown unequivocally that IUI can overcome sperm antibodies in this way. On the other hand, IVF can help couples overcome sperm antibodies, because most people with this problem get pregnant using IVF. With IVF, you are not only washing the sperm as you do with IUI, but delivering the sperm right to the egg in high concentrations outside of the body and therefore away from the immune system.

IUI may help when your partner has a borderline sperm count. If your partner has a borderline sperm count and you are younger than, say, thirty-two years old, it is certainly reasonable to go ahead with IUIs. But if you are older, say, thirty-seven or thirty-eight years old, your fertility will decline significantly in the next twelve months. IVF may be a much better choice, because it can have a much higher success rate—up to 50 percent. You may not want to waste valuable fertile time undergoing treatments less likely to get you pregnant.

YOUR IUI STEP-BY-STEP (FOR AN UNSTIMULATED CYCLE)

In this section, you will get an overview of what it will be like to have an IUI. This overview does not include the protocol for ovarian stimulation, because not everyone having IUIs will go through stimulation. For more information about fertility drugs and ovarian stimulation, see Chapter 7.

In Chapter 2, we talked about your hormones, including luteinizing hormone (LH). It may be helpful to refer to that chapter, if you are unfamiliar with the concept of an LH surge. The surge of LH just before ovulation stimulates the final maturation and release of an egg. Being able to detect your LH surge will help you and your doctor to time your insemination.

Step 1: After Your LH Surge, Schedule an Appointment for the Next Day

As pointed out, timing is crucial to the success of your IUI. The best time to do an insemination is when your ovulation testing method shows that you have reached your LH peak. Your facility or doctor must be prepared to do your insemination any day of the week. You should be able to call your doctor's office when you reach your LH peak and schedule an insemination within the next twenty-four hours. If your clinic or doctor is not available seven days a week, choose another clinic.

You will ovulate twenty-four to forty-eight hours after your LH peak. You may be timing your ovulation with an LH kit (urine kit), an ovulation machine, or with sonograms (ultrasounds). If you are doing a urine kit, schedule your appointment the day after your peak result. Some ovulation machines calibrate your peak, telling you that the next day is the best day for insemination. This is fine as long as you are careful to check what the machine is actually measuring. Again, the best day for IUI is always the day *after* your most positive day.

Some women and their doctors use transvaginal ultrasound to time their IUIs. With ultrasound you can actually watch a follicle grow. On one day you will see a large follicle on the ovary, and the next day you will see that it has gone. You know you've ovulated. As you can imagine, ultrasound can be tricky to use as the only means of monitoring ovulation. If you have two ultrasounds two days in a row, you may still not know exactly when you ovulated. You may have ovulated between your ultrasounds. For example, if you ovulated right after your first ultrasound, by the time you have the second ultrasound (twenty-three hours later), you barely have

OVULATION PREDICTOR KITS (OPK)

Ultrasound adds to precision in timing an IUI, but should be used with other methods to target the best time narrowly. Before the use of ovulation predictor kits, many women used basal body temperature charts. Although they are cheap—all you need is a thermometer, a piece of paper, and a pencil—tracking your temperature until you see a rise in temperature (and hence a rise in progesterone) could only tell you that you had already ovulated. But ovulation predictor kits show you when you are having your LH surge, which rises and peaks *before* you ovulate. Most people ovulate between twenty-four to forty-eight hours after the LH surge or, to be more precise, twenty-four hours after the peak.

time for insemination. Most physicians combine ultrasound monitoring with testing for the LH surge, using either a blood or urine test.

Again, once you have your LH peak, call your doctor or clinic to schedule an appointment the next day. If you are using fresh sperm, you and your partner will need to coordinate bringing the sperm to the office or andrology lab, if it's outside your doctor's office. This brings us to Step 2.

Step 2: Bring Your Partner's Sperm and a Photo ID for Sperm Washing

Most infertility programs have labs in their offices to prepare the semen for IUI by sperm washing. If you are using fresh sperm, you and your partner should plan to bring the semen on the day of your insemination. You don't have to be there at the same time, however. Your partner can bring the sperm specimen to the lab in the morning, for example, and you can come in later that day for the insemination. Whatever arrangement you make, you, the laboratory, and the physician or nurse practitioner should be prepared to carefully check identification of the sperm at every stage of the process to be absolutely certain that it is your partner's sperm that is being used for your insemination. Be concerned about a program that does not include the following checks.

Your partner should bring a photo ID, such as a driver's license, along with his specimen. If you are coming in with your partner's sperm, you should bring ID and plan to come earlier than your IUI appointment, because sperm washing usually takes about an hour to do.

When you give the specimen to the lab with identification, the lab will log it for sperm washing. Semen is a mixture of sperm and fluid from the seminal vesicles and prostate gland. When "washing" sperm, we are essentially separating the sperm cells from this fluid to avoid the irritation or allergic reactions that can occur when unprepared semen is put directly into the uterus without first having gone through the cervix's natural filter.

To prepare the sperm, semen is put into a culture medium, which is a balanced solution of approximately 7.4 pH, and then separated in a centrifuge. Because sperm cells are the heaviest and most solid component of this mixture, they will go down to the bottom of the mixture. The top part is then poured off and the sperm is spun a second time to get a high concentration of sperm cells. Some doctors use what's called a *swim-up technique,* an aspect of sperm washing often used in IVF procedures. The isolated sperm are put into additional culture media after having been spun down. After a short waiting period, the culture media is taken off and spun once more to isolate sperm that are motile enough to swim up from the centrifuged pellet. This procedure makes the most sense in preparation for IVF and IVF/ICSI, when only select sperm should be used.

When the sperm is ready, you will then pick up the labeled specimen. The lab should recheck the label on your specimen with your identity. You will then bring the specimen and your paperwork into the examination room. Before drawing the specimen into the syringe, your doctor or nurse practitioner should recheck your identity and the label on the sperm and sign off on the paperwork.

If you are using donor sperm, the sperm bank will ship your sperm to your doctor's office with identifying information, including the number of the sperm bank and the number assigned to your specimen. This number is used instead of the donor's name. When you pick up the sperm at your doctor's lab, be sure to bring the number of the sperm bank and the identifying number of your specimen with you so that you can double-check your specimen's identity.

> *When you drop the (semen) sample off, you have to wait a half hour to get it washed. During that time, I would think to myself, "Did I have enough? Was it up to level? Did anything taint it in any way?" That was highly stressful for me. I thought positively about it, and when they came out with the vial and said, "Okay we have enough and this is how many [sperm] we have," I thought, "Whew, that's a relief."* —DAVID

Step 3: Having Your IUI

You will lie on the examining table just as you would for a Pap smear. A speculum will be gently inserted into your vagina and your cervix will be cleansed. The doctor or nurse practitioner will draw the specimen into a syringe. The amount of the specimen is usually between 1 to 5 milliliters of volume. An insemination catheter will be threaded through your cervix into your uterus and the specimen will be slowly injected. This may cause mild cramping.

Although most women prefer to lie down after an intrauterine insemination, it's not necessary. By the time the speculum is removed, the sperm is already in the fallopian tubes and may even have already traveled out of the fallopian tubes.

Sometimes there is backflow of the semen from the cervix, either because the specimen was large, because you had uterine contractions, or because the specimen wasn't put fully through the cervix. In these cases, your doctor may insert a cap against your cervix. The cap looks like a small

FRESH OR FROZEN SPERM FOR IUI?
WHAT ABOUT ANTIBODIES?

Unlike IVF procedures, where it makes no difference, IUI is more efficient with fresh sperm. Fresh sperm stays viable longer, giving you and your doctor a wider margin in which to time your insemination. Fresh sperm becomes even more important when your partner's semen analysis is abnormal. Normal sperm is more amenable to freezing than abnormal sperm. However, frozen sperm can solve logistical problems such as when you are trying for conception with a partner who is away frequently or when having sex for conception causes too much stress in your relationship. When you are using donor sperm, it must be frozen. The donor should be tested for genetic and communicable diseases. The sperm is frozen and quarantined, and the donor must be retested before the sperm can be released. (For more about donor sperm, see Chapter 12.)

Men with antisperm antibodies may want to try a technique to reduce antibodies. Sperm and seminal fluid mix at almost the moment of ejaculation. If antisperm antibodies are presumably to be found within the urethra, from which most of the ejaculate comes, theoretically it may be possible to remove some of the antibodies by ejaculating into a culture media, the idea being that if the mixing of antibodies occurs almost at the moment of ejaculation, perhaps just beyond that moment, if semen enters this sea of culture media, the antibodies will not bind to the sperm as avidly. Although this is a not a proven technique, there is very little harm in ejaculating into a sterile cup containing a sterile culture solution rather than into a dry cup and diluting the semen later with that solution.

sponge in a plastic bag connected to string, sort of like a tampon. It's used to keep sperm from flowing out. It's not necessarily a bad thing if your doctor doesn't do this, because again most of the sperm will have gotten high enough into the fallopian tubes to be effective.

Side Effects that May Be Felt After IUI

Inseminations can cause menstrual-like cramping. You may experience bleeding from irritation of the cervix or the uterus, which is sometimes unavoidable. You may also notice ovulatory discomfort, such as twinges of pain or bloating. Fever is a warning sign of infection, however, and you should call your doctor immediately if you have a fever of 100.4°F or more. An infection may be the result of a breakdown in the sterility of the IUI process, which can happen at the cervix, or in the sperm specimen, or in the process of preparing that specimen.

DO YOU REALLY NEED THOSE LAB FEES?

Most inseminations are done as intrauterine inseminations, that is, the sperm is put inside the uterus. But if you are having husband or partner inseminations for erectile dysfunction or because your partner is away from home too frequently for you to get pregnant with intercourse, you may not need or want intrauterine inseminations and may need only intracervical insemination where frozen sperm is deposited at the far end of the vagina near the cervix. Because the sperm is being placed in the vagina, and not beyond the cervix, sperm washing isn't necessary.

The assumption here is that were it not for logistical or physical issues, you would be normally exposed to your partner's sperm without intervention and so you don't need quarantine and preparation of sperm in the same way you would with donor insemination, the exception being for couples living with HIV. If you are having inseminations for the reasons above, you may be able to save a significant amount of money by not paying for the laboratory services involved in preparing the sperm for intrauterine insemination. You may not be offered an intracervical insemination unless you ask, as most physicians are geared toward IUIs. If you think you could benefit from intracervical insemination, ask!

Step 4: Coping with the Wait

Having to wait two weeks until you get your period or find out you are pregnant can create a great deal of anxiety to say the least. That's why I recommend reminding yourself that the odds are that it won't work. If you don't come to terms with the odds that dictate that IUI will fail eight out of ten times, you are going to be extremely disappointed. Remember that if you were a person without infertility trying to conceive without intervention, you would still have only a 20 percent chance of getting pregnant each cycle. It is understandably very hard to maintain this attitude and certainly tough to carry on after an insemination fails, but it is the best way to cope with this process.

As a standard of practice, clinics provide a pregnancy test two weeks after insemination regardless of whether a woman has had bleeding or not. If you have had a full period, you may want to decline the test. Still, you can have some bleeding, such as spotting or a light period, and still be pregnant.

WILL IT HELP TO DO TWO INSEMINATIONS PER CYCLE?

When inseminations are very well timed, there is no clear benefit to doing two in the same cycle. But my personal bias is based on the quality of the specimen. One insemination should suffice for a totally normal sperm specimen. On the other hand, it may be reasonable to do two inseminations two days in a row for someone with a frozen specimen or a specimen taken from someone with a borderline sperm count.

IS IUI REALLY MORE ECONOMICAL THAN IVF?

People tend to think of IUI as less expensive than IVF, but in some cases it can be even more expensive. Most couples will need six cycles of IUI to give it a fair chance. That amounts to six months of treatment. Whether you can save money with IUI depends on whether or not you need medication to ovulate, particularly injectable medications, which makes the whole process much more expensive, because of the costs of the drugs and monitoring. IUI can be less expensive than IVF when you don't need drugs and can do IUI simply by using home ovulation predictor kits to time conception, forgoing ultrasound. You may be able to do this if your cycles are very regular. The charts below show you the possible extremes in costs, based on estimated costs that may differ per clinic and geographical region.

If you use donor sperm, add $200/vial plus $100 shipping and handling. Assuming that you order donor sperm in batches of two 3-month supplies for six inseminations, you would pay at least $1,200, plus two times shipping and handling, amounting to $1,400.

The average base cost of one cycle of IVF is $10,000 without additional costs like ICSI, which can run between $500 and $2,500 dollars. (Remember, it is very possible that you will need more than one IVF procedure.) The price for IVF can rise dramatically if the male partner requires a surgical procedure to retrieve sperm, increasing anywhere from 50 to 100 per-

SIX CYCLES OF BASIC IUI WITH CLOMIPHENE

Insemination:	$150 x 6 = $900
Sperm wash:	$200 x 6 = $1,200
Home urine ovulation predictor kit:	$50 x 6 = $300
Costs of clomiphene citrate:	$150 x 6 = $900
One office visit and sonogram to renew clomiphene:	$300 x 6 = $1,800
One office visit and sonogram at midcycle to assess response:	$300 x 6 = $1,800
Total:	$6,900

SIX CYCLES OF IUI WITH INJECTABLE MEDICATION

Insemination—$150, plus sperm wash—$200	$350 x 6 = $2,100
22 amps of injectable medication @ $50 each:	$1,100 x 6 = $6,600
Human chorionic gonadotropin:	$50 x 6 = $300
4–6 office visits + 1 sonogram per visit:	$300 x 5 x 6 = $9,000 (For example, you may make 5 office visits)
Total:	$18,000

cent. In terms of success, and roughly speaking, two IVF cycles equal six FSH/IUI cycles, *if* your anatomy is normal.

WHEN IUI ISN'T WORKING

You should try no fewer than three IUIs and probably no more than six IUIs before thinking about moving on to another form of therapy. This is a statistical rule. As you've read, IUI has only a 10 to 20 percent chance of working, so it makes sense to give it time. On the other hand, if you tried six inseminations, you have reached the point when most people who are going to get pregnant with IUI will have gotten pregnant. It makes sense to move on.

If this is the case for you, you've probably reached the proverbial fork in the road between going forward with IVF and investigating the possibility that anatomical problems are the cause of your infertility. Could endometriosis be preventing pregnancy? Will you need laparoscopy, a same-day noninvasive surgery, to find out?

I usually speak with couples who have reached this point and suggest that one option is to do a laparoscopy and hope that it will tell us what's been going wrong. We can repair the problem—for example, endometriosis or adhesions—and you may not only have the answer to the question of what's gone wrong, but the solution to the problem as well. Once your endometriosis or adhesions are treated, you may be able to get pregnant without IVF. On the other hand, if your tubes are open (and we should already know the answer to that question at this point), the problems that we find at laparoscopy can be bypassed by IVF. IVF is a much more expeditious means of problem solving, because the likely results are apparent early. You will know within two weeks of your first IVF if you are likely to get pregnant with this method or not.

Once again, your age and your insurance coverage will to some extent dictate the road you choose. Women thirty-seven years of age or older may choose to go directly to IVF so as not to waste time waiting to find out whether they have endometriosis and whether surgery to correct it is going to be successful. Yet older women without coverage for IVF are in a difficult situation, because of the expense of IVF. If you are a younger woman without insurance for IVF, it is more reasonable to choose laparoscopy. As a last resort, some women and couples actually move to states where IVF is universally covered by health insurance, such as Massachusetts. We'll talk about insurance and financial concerns in Chapter 15.

A final concern is whether you have primary or secondary infertility. When you already have a child but are having difficulties having a second child, this is called secondary infertility. Since you've been able to conceive before, doctors tend to treat secondary infertility less aggressively, assuming that there is a lower impediment to your success a second time. If you are young and have a child, you might want to treat your underlying condition with the knowledge that you are likely to get pregnant once this problem is addressed.

In the next chapter, we will take an in-depth look at IVF. If you think you might ultimately use IVF, be sure to read this chapter for an overview of what it will mean to you medically, practically, and financially.

9 | In Vitro Fertilization (IVF)

First done successfully in 1977 in Great Britain, and shortly thereafter in Australia, in vitro fertilization (IVF) was developed to help women with no fallopian tubes become pregnant. Years ago, the proper treatment for ectopic pregnancy (a condition in which a pregnancy grows in the fallopian tube or elsewhere outside the uterus) was to remove the affected fallopian tube. After one ectopic pregnancy, there is a chance of having a second. In the past, many women who had more than one ectopic pregnancy lost both fallopian tubes. Doctors felt terrible that women were losing their fallopian tubes due to the treatment for ectopic pregnancy and began to investigate solutions to the problem.

Although the first IVF pregnancy was ectopic, the first IVF baby was born the next year in England in 1978. Since that time there have been steady advances in the field. As you will read in this chapter, IVF is a process that involves stimulation with fertility drugs to produce a sufficient number of eggs from which to choose for fertilization, close monitoring to time the release and retrieval of your eggs, and combination of your eggs with your partner's sperm (or donor's sperm) in the laboratory. Your fertilized eggs, called embryos, are then placed into your uterus for implantation and, hopefully, pregnancy.

Although originally intended to solve the problem of bringing egg and sperm together outside the fallopian tube, IVF now has many additional uses, including helping couples to overcome low or absent sperm counts and to help couples using donor eggs. Later on in this chapter, we will talk about the reasons why you might choose IVF, and we'll go into the details of the IVF procedure, termed an IVF cycle.

To get the most out of this chapter, first take a look at Chapter 7, where we talk about the fertility drugs used for IVF. In particular, you'll want to know about injectable FSH, which every woman undergoing IVF must take. While IVF can be complex, a basic understanding of your cycle and the way in which your hormones work will make this chapter much easier to digest. You can find more information about your cycle in Chapter 2.

> *For two weeks everyone needs a commitment—the doctor, the husband and wife, everyone involved. From the start of your cycle until you do IVF, you need that two-week period scheduled. It helps if someone can give you a calendar and say, "You need to come in on these days," so that you can have it laid out a week or two ahead of time.* —ANN

THE IVF CYCLE: A STEP-BY-STEP OVERVIEW

Before you begin treatment, you should have a thorough infertility workup. (See Chapter 3.) Your uterus should be evaluated by a hysterosalpingogram (HSG), by saline sonohysterogram (a test during which a saline solution is injected into the uterus, which is then seen on ultrasound), or by hysteroscopy within one year of your IVF cycle, but preferably

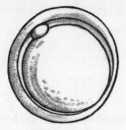

Mature Oocyte (Egg)

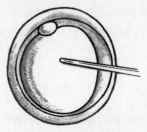

ICSI (Intracytoplasmic Injection)

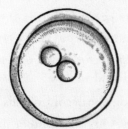

2 Pronuclear (Fertilized Egg)

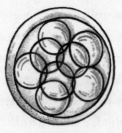

8-Cell Embryo

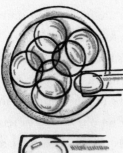

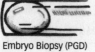

Embryo Biopsy (PGD)

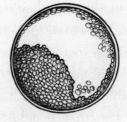

Blastocyst

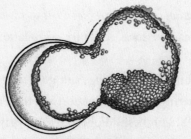

Hatching Blastocyst

FIGURE 8. *Fertilization and embryo development*

before beginning *any* treatment. Following is a step-by-step overview of what IVF will be like once you are ready to start.

Step 1: You Prepare for Stimulation

After you get your period, you'll begin birth control pills for no fewer than fourteen days and no more than twenty-eight days. Many women average twenty-one days, simply because there are twenty-one pills in a pack of birth control pills. Although it may seem strange to take birth control pills when you are trying to have a baby, birth control pills put your ovaries and uterus in a resting state, giving you and your doctor a kind of clean slate from which to begin stimulation.

After the twenty-one days, you'll stop taking birth control pills and get your period, usually within two to four days. On the second or third day of bleeding, you will go to your doctor's office for an ultrasound to:

- *Check your ovaries* to make sure that they are in a resting state and to get baseline measurements of any ovarian follicles or cysts.
- *Check your uterine lining* to make sure it is thin. Because you are going to rebuild your uterine lining during stimulation, it's best not to have residue of the old lining left. If a patient's uterine lining hasn't completely shed, and there is evidence of that on ultrasound in relation to very low estradiol and progesterone levels, which are associated with shedding lining, I will go so far as to evacuate that lining by D&C or aspiration.
- *Check your estradiol levels with a blood test* to make sure your ovaries are in a relatively inactive state, ready for stimulation.

As with everything in life, things can go wrong with your IVF cycle. Women with borderline ovarian function can have good and bad months when testing for FSH and estradiol levels. You may be one of the unfortunate women who tested well at entry into her IVF program but who shows high levels on the day she is supposed to start her drugs. You may have to defer the cycle or, depending on your history, you may be advised that IVF is not going to be the best choice for you. FSH levels are not as important in women under thirty-five, but in women thirty-seven or older they are critical.

Step 2: You Undergo Ovarian Stimulation

Most often your cycle will begin with injectable FSH (see Chapter 7), either a pure recombinant FSH, such as Follistim or Gonal-F, or a combination of one of these drugs and a human menopausal gonadotropin (hMG), such as Menopur, the FSH made from the urine of menopausal women. Mixing pure FSH (made from recombinant DNA technology) with FSH/LH combinations (extracted from human menopausal urine) is done to gain the benefit of the LH in hMG preparations. With the advent of Luveris, a manufactured form of the luteinizing hormone, it is possible that patients may use Luveris instead of mixing drugs, but at the time of this writing this remains to be seen. Injectable FSH is started somewhere between the second and fourth day after your period, with day three being the average day on which to begin.

You will have a baseline ultrasound and a blood estradiol and progesterone test on day three to make sure that you have no large follicles in your ovaries and to be certain that your uterine lining is thin. It's not a bad idea to make sure you are not pregnant at the start of your treatment.

You will return for another ultrasound and more blood tests after having three to five days of medication to determine if you are getting ovarian activity. You and your doctor would like to see a rising estradiol level and evidence on your ultrasounds that your ovarian follicles are developing.

You will make frequent doctor visits over the course of the next five to ten days as your follicles get closer to the stage wherein they will contain mature eggs (oocytes). These visits could be daily or every other day, depending on how you are responding. At each visit, your doctor will get new information about the size of your follicles in comparison to your blood estradiol level. A mature follicle will produce an estradiol level of about 200 picograms. So, for example, if you have five follicles that appear to be mature and your estradiol level is 1,000, you are likely to truly have mature follicles. But if you have ten follicles that seem to be mature but your estradiol level was 1,000, you may have to continue your stimulation until your estradiol level gets closer to 2,000.

Problems can also occur at the stimulation phase of your cycle. You may be taking your drugs but they may not be working. This can happen if your medication has expired, if you left it in your car when the temperature rose, or if you are not mixing it correctly. These things happen. You are only human and probably under a great deal of stress.

It's also possible not to respond to medication. You should be concerned if you are somewhere between day three and day seven of your medication protocol and your estradiol level hasn't risen or your follicles aren't developing. If you don't respond to FSH within seven days, you are unlikely to respond at all. Your doctor may decide to review your injection techniques, order a fresh batch of medication, and even consider raising the dose a bit. Adjustments can be made, but you may not be able to overcome understimulation.

Step 3: You Take Your GnRH Antagonist and hCG Shot

When the biggest follicle (called the lead or dominant follicle) gets to be about 12 millimeters or greater in size, a GnRH antagonist (Antagon, Cetrotide) will be added to your protocol to prevent your natural LH surge from occurring and your eggs from being released before they are in the right stage of maturation. (See the box on page 208 for a more thorough explanation of this drug.) If you were using a GnRH *agonist*, such as Lupron or Synarel, you would have already been on this medication about a week before your stimulation.

Most IVF programs base their decision to conclude the stimulation phase when you have one or two 17- to 18-millimeter lead follicles. Generally, when you have lead follicles of this size, an appropriate estradiol level, and no problems with your LH or progesterone levels, you are ready to go to the next stage at which final follicular and ovarian maturation are triggered by a medication that acts like your natural LH surge—the hCG injection. The hormone hCG actually loosens the eggs and their surrounding cells from the walls of their follicles and primes the egg to resume meiosis (division). Approximately thirty-six hours after your hCG injection, your oocyte (egg) retrieval will take place. Because you may need to take your hCG injection late at night in order to time your retrieval during the day, many IVF programs will make special arrangements to provide hCG injections.

Here, too, problems can occur. Occasionally, women break through GnRH antagonists or agonists to have a small LH surge. This can also happen when a GnRH antagonist is started too late. If you are stimulating briskly, you should be checked earlier than day six, and if you are stimulating slowly, the GnRH antagonist may not be given until much later. Your doctor should watch your progress around day four or five of stimulation by checking your LH levels.

Step 4: Your Oocyte (Egg) Retrieval

Your egg retrieval (also called egg harvesting) will usually be done in an operative or semioperative setting. Most patients are given intravenous sedation. While you are under sedation, your vagina will be cleansed. A vaginal sonogram (ultrasound) will be performed. Under sterile conditions, a needle will be put through your vaginal wall into your ovary to aspirate (draw up) follicular fluid. The follicular fluid will be removed and inspected under a microscope to identify the oocytes (eggs).

The procedure takes about ten to thirty minutes. You will go to the recovery area for about an hour or two, after which you can go home and resume your usual activities.

It is possible to have your sonogram and find that you have already ovulated. This can happen if you take your hCG too early or if your egg retrieval is too late. If your retrieval happens forty hours after the hCG shot instead of thirty-six hours later, a good number of your follicles will

GnRH Analogs: Controlling Your LH Surge

IVF works most efficiently when your physician can control the timing of your LH surge and plan the retrieval of your eggs precisely according to that surge. (Remember, it is the hormone that stimulates ovulation.) Although necessary for natural reproduction, significant amounts of LH in your system can actually interfere with artificial reproduction. That's where the use of GnRH analogs comes into play. These agents turn off all or most of your own FSH and LH.

The first clinically available GnRH analog was a GnRH agonist, which initially causes ovarian stimulation before it shuts down FSH and LH. Newer analogs called GnRH antagonists work by a different mechanism but also shut down FSH and LH. Agonists can take up to two weeks to shut your hormones down, while antagonists have this effect almost immediately. Lupron is the most common GnRH agonist. It is also used to treat endometriosis by creating a low estrogen (hypoestrogenic) state. When used during IVF, Lupron is given subcutaneously and daily for three to four weeks in a row and causes some significant menopause-like symptoms, such as hot flashes, mood changes, and sleeping and memory problems. Lupron can also promote ovarian cysts, which will defer your cycle, because they must resolve before you can begin stimulation.

Today, many clinics are switching to GnRH antagonists, brand-named Antagon (ganirelix acetate) and Cetrotide (cetrorelix acetate). Clinically, there is little difference between these two antagonists. Again, antagonists quickly shut down your hormones. LH doesn't affect the follicle and egg in the early part of your cycle. It's only toward the second half of your cycle that you must be on guard against the premature emergence of LH. A subcutaneous (under the skin) injection of a GnRH antagonist can be given on the last three or four days of ovarian stimulation. Most people inject themselves without any problems. This type of GnRH analog, a GnRH antagonist, can shut off LH within two hours.

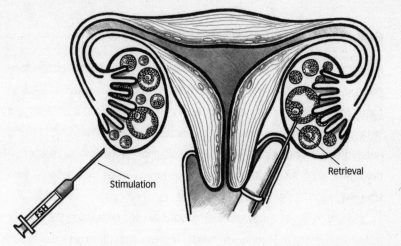

FIGURE 9. *Ovarian stimulation and egg retrieval*

already have ovulated. Once the egg has left the ovary, it isn't useful any-more, even if you could recover it. Women who are less stimulated or who have fewer follicles should be the most concerned about ovulating before retrieval.

> *You are in the post-retrieval area with other women under anesthesia and everybody is talking about how many eggs were retrieved from this person and that person. It's very upsetting. The only time they ever retrieved viable eggs from me, I had seven, and I was happy until I found out that the woman across from me had fourteen.* —SANDRA

Step 5: Your Eggs Are Fertilized

Your eggs will be put into a culture medium that contains water, buffers (substances that maintain acidity at a normal range), salts, sugars, proteins, and antibiotics, and then placed in incubators. About five to six hours after your retrieval, your eggs will either be inseminated—that is, placed in a dish with, say, something like 50,000 of your partner's or donor's sperm—or prepared for intracytoplasmic sperm injection (ICSI).

EMBRYO QUALITY IS EGG QUALITY

An egg is a three-dimensional sphere surrounded by a shell called the zona pellucida. That sphere remains the same size for five or six days as it transforms from a one-cell structure called a zygote to become a blastocyst, a structure that may have more than a hundred cells. Yet the total mass of the embryo does not change. Almost all of the material that's in the early embryo came from the egg. The male deposits twenty-three chromosomes and little else, so in fact embryo quality is really egg quality.

Identifying a good, day three embryo is an art. Embryologists look for good alignment of the pronuclei (genetic material from both parents) on day one, early cleavage (cell division), embryos that are relatively symmetrical, embryos that have seven or eight cells on day three, and a minimal amount of debris. (See "Assisted Hatching and Fragment Removal," page 211.) Cell movement inside the embryo is also a good sign.

Blastocyst (five to six day) embryos are often judged by the size of the blastocoele, a fluid structure inside the embryo; the definition of the membrane that forms the wall of the blastocyst, called the trophoblast; in the inner cell mass; and the number of cells in the blastocyst. The more cells, the better.

The inseminated eggs are then placed back into an incubator and approximately sixteen hours later removed and examined under a microscope to see if fertilization is taking place. These normally fertilized eggs are incubated for another two days (or four to five days in the case of blastocysts—see page 216) and then readied for embryo transfer.

Getting a fever can compromise fertilization. Over the years in our clinic, we have a seen a few cases where women who have had many previous cycles come in for retrieval. They have a smooth procedure and good eggs.

Everything looks fine until we get to the stage where we attempt to fertilize them and they don't fertilize at all. Backtracking some of these patients we found that they had a couple of days of fever during stimulation. If you have a bad viral illness or a fever early to midstimulation, you might consider deferring the cycle until you are better.

One of the most emotional and stressful events during an IVF cycle happens when a man is not able to produce sperm to be mixed with the newly retrieved eggs. If you know that your partner may have trouble producing the specimen, you can easily overcome this by freezing sperm before your procedure.

Some of the normally fertilized eggs seen on the day after your egg retrieval will not divide or progress over the next two to five days. These embryos are nonviable, but it would be uncommon for all of the embryos to arrest prior to transfer.

ASSISTED HATCHING AND FRAGMENT REMOVAL

Many IVF programs employ the technique known as assisted hatching. This involves making a hole in the shell (zona pellucida) surrounding a day three cleaved embryo. It is felt that since an embryo ultimately has to break through this shell in order to implant in the uterine wall, some removal of this obstacle might aid implantation. Assisted hatching should not be performed before the third day of embryo culture, because embryonic cells at that stage may break apart and cause monozygotic (identical) twinning. Assisted hatching is also not performed at the blastocyst stage, because many times the hatching has spontaneously begun by the fifth or sixth day of embryo culture. When assisted hatching is performed on day three embryos, there is an opportunity to remove fragments or debris from around or between the embryonic cells (called blastomeres).

The quality of cleaved (dividing) embryos is determined by the number of cells and the degree of fragmentation around those cells. Fewer cells as well as debris inside the embryo tend to lower quality. This debris may be called fragments, or "frags," which include cells that have died or collapsed. Embryos seem to grow better when they don't have a lot of debris at the cleavage stage. Clinics initially tried fragment removal with the hopes of improving an embryo's chance of implantation. As useful as fragmentation removal seems, it's probable that you cannot simply take bad embryos and make them as likely to implant in the uterus as good embryos just by removing the fragments. Whether fragment removal is really beneficial may depend upon in whose hands it's done.

When it comes to techniques of embryo cultures and transfer, clinics try different methods. There is no uniform way of achieving the best results. For example, some clinics would be comfortable abandoning the practice of assisted hatching while others do assisted hatching on every case. In the same way, embryologists are divided in their approach to handling embryos, with some people feeling that they achieve more success without manipulating the egg, and others cleaning up the egg to an incredibly pristine state. In either case, people are trying to achieve the best result possible. So when an embryologist is proficient at fragment removal it may be beneficial, whereas with another embryologist who isn't as good or as accustomed to removing fragments, the procedure may do more harm than good.

Whether you should consider fragment removal depends on the clinic and your IVF history. If you haven't gotten pregnant with the standard IVF techniques and you have embryos that don't look as good as they could, it's reasonable to try to modify as many aspects of IVF as you can. You may change drug protocols, lab techniques, and/or culture media. (We talk about this later in this chapter.) On the other hand, if you are under thirty-seven and you did one IVF cycle during which everything went well but it just didn't work, you might consider that you are simply facing the law of averages and that your next cycle, or the one after that, will be the one to succeed.

Step 6: You Have Your Embryo Transfer

Between two and six days after your oocyte retrieval, the embryos that appear to be the most viable are placed into your uterus under ultrasound guidance. The embryos are replaced into the uterus by a catheter (tube) introduced through the vagina and cervix, usually under transabdominal ultrasound guidance.

For this procedure, you will usually be required to have a full bladder. Your bladder sits in front of the uterus. A full bladder outlines the uterus so that your physician can more clearly see the embryo catheter as it moves through your cervix into your uterus. Sometimes it happens that you fill your bladder so much that the transfer is too uncomfortable to endure. A middle ground between not being full enough or being too full is best. If your uterus is retroflexed, or tilted backward, having a full bladder isn't helpful because the uterus does not lie against the bladder. About 15 percent of women have this condition wherein the uterus is tipped toward the spine. In some cases, transfer may be done along with transvaginal ultrasound to visualize the procedure.

It may seem like a simple procedure, but embryo transfer is the most crucial and difficult part of the entire IVF cycle. The skill, knowledge, experience, and ability of the physician you choose matters most here. The object for the physician is to introduce the embryos into the optimal part of the uterine lining with as little disturbance of the uterus and cervix as possible. Any doctor who tells you that every single embryo transfer he or she does is smooth is not telling you the truth. There is often a little glitch, and the skill and experience of the person doing the transfer can really determine the success or failure of the whole IVF procedure. Before your transfer, in the early stages of planning your cycle, ask your doctor who is going to actually do your transfer and whether there are any differences in skill level between the doctors proposed. Embryo transfer is the most "operator-dependent" aspect of the entire IVF cycle. Don't be afraid to ask for the best practitioner.

In our clinic, we do a trial transfer before the actual embryo transfer, passing an empty catheter that is very similar to the catheter loaded with embryos. We usually start doing this before the actual IVF cycle in the context of a saline sonohysterogram, gaining the advantage of looking into your uterus at the same time we are making sure that the catheter will pass through your cervix. There are times when the test catheter doesn't go in easily and the embryo catheter does and vice versa. The uterus is muscular and catheters are very soft, flexible, and delicate, making them tricky to use.

During the trial transfer, we will be able to determine if your uterus has a problem, such as being tipped away from the bladder, or if your cervix is very tight, which makes it difficult to pass the catheter through. If there is a problem, you and your doctor will know that you are going to have a tricky transfer. You can remind your doctor at the time of your transfer that it might be difficult. You can both take a deep breath and begin the procedure prepared.

Once the catheter is in, the embryo must be placed in the right part of the uterus. That is why all transfers should be done under ultrasound guidance to allow the doctor to actually see the embryo being placed.

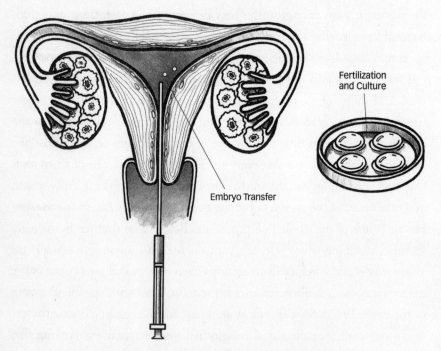

Fertilization and Culture

Embryo Transfer

FIGURE 10. *In vitro fertilization and embryo transfer*

Making Your Embryo Transfer Easier

Embryo transfer is the culmination of a great deal of effort on your part and the clinic's, and it's important that your physician be able concentrate and focus on the procedure. Although it seems a little odd to say to yourself, "This is important, so relax," you can help the procedure by doing just that. You may have had dozens of speculum exams during the course of your cycle or cycles, but that doesn't necessarily mean that you have gotten used to them. If you know you have trouble with speculum exams, talk to your doctor well before your transfer for solutions to problems caused by unease. Some people get through the procedure by bringing a squeeze ball, a religious icon, or using meditation. Use whatever feels right and natural to you. Some women choose sedation. This is preferable to tensing up and clamping down on the speculum or involuntarily rejecting it, which is counterproductive to completing this very delicate procedure. Some women have their partner or husband with them, and while some doctors are happy to have others in the room during the transfer, I personally prefer not to have any distractions, and so I ask that partners remain outside in the waiting room. Ask your doctor about this as well so that you and your doctor will know what to expect.

> When they were transferring the embryos. I tried to open my heart as wide as possible. I saw the embryos on the screen, and I just said to myself, "Receive." My body was open to heaven. I became emotional, and I know that everyone in the room could feel it. I was trying so hard not to cry because of the overwhelming reality of opening to my child. —KATHLEEN

Problems that Can Occur at the Embryo Transfer

Many women who are undergoing a lot of ovarian stimulation have copious cervical mucus. Sometimes the mucus can actually capture the embryos during the transfer. Embryos can also become stuck in the catheter. Because the doctor can only see the movement of the fluid entering the uterus on the ultrasound, it sometimes happens that when the embryo catheter is removed, flushed, and inspected, embryos are found remaining in the catheter. Although this is disappointing, it's actually a good sign because these embryos are sticky. Sticky embryos have a good chance of adhering to the uterine wall. The embryo catheter should always be checked immediately after transfer to make sure the embryos have been released. If they haven't been, the embryos can be reloaded into another catheter and the transfer can be repeated. This is done under controlled circumstances so the embryos are not overly exposed to the atmosphere.

The embryo catheter can cause bleeding or irritation of your uterine lining. That's why it's important that the catheter not touch the top of the uterus. This can induce contractions. Also, it is not uncommon for a woman's cervix to bleed, because the cervix is quite vascular and sometimes even washing the cervix causes it to bleed. Your doctor should be careful to avoid this, if possible.

After the embryo transfer, many people are concerned that the embryos are going to fall out if they do heavy lifting, hit a speed bump on the way home, or go to the bathroom. While these concerns are natural, the embryos do not fall out, because they are sticky and sandwiched in your uterus, which is in fact very much like a sandwich, because the uterine walls touch each other. There is not much you can do to dislodge the embryos. Even intercourse, which seems the most traumatic activity, has only been shown to be neutral or helpful to implantation.

Although many physicians prescribe hormonal supplementation, such as progesterone, baby aspirin, which increases uterine blood flow, or antibiotics, these additions may have only incremental benefits. So, as you move into the last phase of your IVF cycle—the wait—you should know that there is little you can do or not do to change the course of events.

Blastocyst Versus Day Three Embryo Transfer: Which Is Better?

If you are having or contemplating IVF, you may have heard a great deal about the pros and cons of transferring an embryo on the second or third day of its development, that is, an embryo at the cleavage stage known as a *day three embryo,* versus transferring an embryo at the fifth or sixth day of its development, called a *blastocyst.*

There are two ways of looking at an IVF cycle. One is to look at your chance of getting pregnant on your fresh cycle, which means that you receive ovarian stimulation and produce follicles from which eggs are then retrieved. The eggs are inseminated to create embryos and transferred into your uterus. An alternative to doing a fresh cycle only is to do a fresh and a frozen cycle. You can transfer some of your embryos and freeze the remaining embryos to be transferred later. If you don't get pregnant right away, you won't need to go through ovarian stimulation again, and the cost of frozen cycles is considerably lower than that of doing another fresh cycle. Day three embryos and blastocysts can be frozen.

You can look at the clinic's pregnancy rate for a fresh cycle, keeping in mind the clinic's rate for high-order multiple pregnancies, which can occur when more than two embryos are transferred at a time. Or, you can look at the total pregnancy rate achieved over time through the combination of fresh and frozen cycles. There is no doubt that on an individual basis a blastocyst has a higher chance of implantation than a cleaved, or day three, embryo (or a day two embryo, for that matter). But there is a chance that an embryo that survives until day two or three won't survive to day five. Yet these same embryos can be frozen at day two or three and transferred later on, giving you more embryos to try with over time. In addition, when you can afford to limit the number of embryos you transfer to your uterus at one time, you reduce your risk of multifetal pregnancy. Unfortunately, many programs that do blastocyst transfers do a substantial amount of transfers with more than two embryos at a time. If you are looking at the clinic's average transfer number and see the figure 2.5, that means that half of the time they are transferring three embryos.

Presently, there is no one right answer as to whether a blastocyst transfer is better than a day three transfer or visa vice versa, and much depends on the clinic's experience with day three embryos and blastocysts. Some programs can individualize the number of embryos they transfer based on your age and the number of embryos you have. For example, if you had twenty embryos, the clinic could freeze twelve to fifteen of those embryos on day three, allowing the remaining embryos to grow to the blastocyst stage, even freezing some blastocysts. On the other hand, if you have only two or three embryos, there is no point in waiting to see if they grow until day five, because you risk having no embryos if none survive.

It's important to note that some programs cannot tailor individual cases. If you are in such a program, you should know what is possible for you and should come to an understanding with your physician about whether you want to transfer day three or blastocyst embryos. You certainly should decide how many embryos you want transferred, as this is a major decision that could have a lasting effect in your life.

There is a growing concern about the use of blastocysts that is still being investigated at the time of this writing. There is worry that the longer we hold an embryo outside of the body in culture media, the more chance it might be affected by imprinting disorders such as Beckwith-Wiedemann syndrome, an overgrowth disorder that leads to the development of hemihypertrophy (one side of the body being bigger than the other). (See "The Risk of IVF Hurting Your Baby" on page 224.) We don't yet know if there is a difference in these disorders in people who were born from embryos transferred on day three and people born from embryos transferred on day five.

What we may learn is that we need to get the embryo back into the body sooner. In some countries, embryo transfers are still done at day two. In fact, there is a Swedish study in the *New England Journal of Medicine* that showed high birth rates for women with single embryo day-two transfers—not just pregnancy rates, but delivery rates—in addition to a lower risk of multifetal pregnancy. In this prospective randomized trial, one group of women got back two embryos while the other group got back one embryo. If the women in the second group failed with their first cycle of IVF, they got back their other frozen embryo for another cycle. The total birth rate of the people with two embryo transfers was 42.9 percent. The total birth rate of the group that got one fresh and one frozen embryo was 38.8 percent compared to the overall 50 percent success rate with IVF. While these are excellent delivery rates, it must be remembered that these outcomes were achieved in a very ideal population. Almost all of these women were young and going through their first IVF cycle.

Importantly, the twin rate for the group that received two embryos was 33 percent but only 0.8 percent in the group that got one embryo first and then another. We can see from this study that if we want to eliminate the risk of multiple pregnancies, putting back fewer embryos is the key.[1]

Make Sure Those Embryos Are Yours: Does Your Clinic Take Precautions?

A good IVF lab will be scrupulous in its attention to detail when it comes to embryo transfer. When you go to your embryo transfer, you want to know that you are getting your embryos and no one else's. Here are some precautions clinics should take to avoid mix-ups:

- Clinics should etch the patient's name into the embryo dish. Some clinics not only etch their embryo dishes, but also actually place a TV monitor on the microscope so the patient can read her name on the dish from which the embryos are removed.
- Before a patient's eggs are retrieved, the patient should sit up and state her name to the embryologist. The doctor should ask her name and double-check her hospital ID wristband to make sure it matches her spoken name.
- Only one patient should be scheduled for retrieval at a time.
- Every patient should have her own shelf in the incubator.
- Two patients' embryos should not be out in the laboratory at the same time so as to avoid any possibility of mix-up.

Step 7: The Hardest Part: You Wait

After the embryo transfer, most people will be given supplemental progesterone either with vaginal suppositories or through an intramuscular injection, if you prefer. Some women prefer intramuscular shots to suppositories. Others dislike the shots because they are deep, oily, and painful. Some doctors prefer to give the injections to be sure that the medication was administered. As a practical matter, there is no difference in the efficacy of either the injection or suppository delivery.

Once your transfer is complete, you must then wait two weeks to find out if you are pregnant or if you get your period. I often tell patients that this is going to be the hardest part of the entire IVF procedure. Up to this point, you've been engaged in a lot of activity, making frequent doctor's visits, having ultrasounds, blood tests, daily injections, and many interactions with doctor and staff. Now all that activity has stopped. You may be on medication, but it will be a relatively straightforward application. There is nothing to do but wait for fourteen days. During this difficult time, many have a tendency to think that what they do or don't do now will make a difference. Once again, there is really nothing you can do to change the course of the outcome. Some people are naturally optimistic in their style of thinking, and others need pessimism to handle possible disappointment. It's important to know what works best for you but to try to keep as neutral an attitude as you possibly can. It's very hard not to become obsessed thinking about the result, and there may be no remedy for this. Talking to someone can help. Keeping busy can help. Think about what might work for you, and try as many approaches as you can to help you cope.

IVF was stressful, because you think of the possible outcome. What if it doesn't work? How can we afford to do it again? Halfway through we knew we had some frozen embryos, but we didn't know what we were looking at. Then there's the heartache. You just don't want to have to go through it again. Our transfer went perfectly, and we were blessed not to have to go through more heartache. —JANIE

The days just go so slowly. You don't get your period. They test you on day thirteen and they don't tell you anything, which is excruciating. Days thirteen to fifteen were tortuous. —DINAH

In my head, I thought that it wasn't going to work. I'm by nature rather pessimistic, so I always have a plan B. People would say to me, "If this doesn't work, you can always adopt." But we didn't want to adopt. If infertility treatment didn't work, my husband and I were going to buy motorcycles and tour the country. —CYNTHIA

A SAMPLE IVF CALENDAR

Sunday	Monday	Tuesday	Wednesday	Thursday	Friday	Saturday
		Day 1 of your period	Start birth control pills day 2	→		
→						
→		Last day of birth control pills	No pill	No pill	Blood test and ultrasound @ 9 a.m. for 3–6 days	Begin stimulation medication
Continue	stimulation	medication			→	Possible hcG
	Possible egg retrieval	Fertilization call		Embryo transfer	Start progesterone caps	
	Pregnancy test 10–12 days after embryo transfer					

THE RISKS OF IVF

When people come to my office and say they want to get pregnant, we always discuss this desire a little further. Most people, it's safe to say, don't just want to be pregnant, they want a baby, and they don't just want a baby, they want a healthy baby, one who will grow into a healthy adult. Most people have questions about the safety of IVF, about the risks not only to themselves but to their offspring as well.

The Risk of Not Having a Baby

For some women or couples, IVF is the first step into fertility care. But for most, it's a procedure contemplated after a long struggle with other methods for conception that didn't work. By the time many reach the decision to undergo IVF, they are frustrated, disappointed, stressed, and exhausted. Regardless of your situation, the first question on your mind is probably, "Is this going to work?"

The best IVF programs in the world rarely exceed birth rates in over 50 percent in all patients. And although some clinics may have a success rate of over 50 percent in highly selected subsets of patients, this is not a reality for most people. This means that in the best of circumstances, you have a fifty-fifty chance of having a baby. IVF can be an attractive possibility, but in no sense is it guaranteed.

As always, your age matters. The older you are, the more likely it is that IVF won't succeed. Older eggs tend toward chromosomal and metabolic abnormalities that can result in no pregnancy, miscarriage, or a pregnancy that is abnormal. It's also possible that you won't produce enough eggs to do IVF. This doesn't mean you *won't* succeed, only that you must be realistic about this procedure. Otherwise, you may be profoundly disappointed.

Everyone comes to IVF with a distinct history and set of problems. Before embarking on IVF, ask your doctor, "For somebody of my age with my fertility problem and my history, what do you think my chances are of achieving a pregnancy and maintaining that pregnancy to delivery with

IVF?" It's very important that you consult directly with your doctor. While a staff professional can take you through a general overview of the procedure and provide you with a calendar or timeline for specific procedures, only your doctor can advise you about your individual chances and risks.

People kept saying to me, "How are you getting through this?" (Fourteen in vitro fertilizations.) And I would often say to myself, "Why am I not in a funny farm?" I got through the disappointments by staying in bed for two days each time I learned I wasn't pregnant. Think about what you are going to do if the doctor tells you that you aren't pregnant. You don't have to have the answer, but you've got to figure out what you need to get through it. If you don't want to talk to anybody, then don't talk to anybody and don't apologize for it. And plan what you will do if infertility treatment doesn't work. —JILL

The Risk of Carrying More Than One Fetus

Typically, IVF involves putting back more than one embryo into your uterus for implantation, giving you a higher statistical chance of having an embryo implant in your uterus. Putting back two embryos doubles your chance of success. Putting back more than two is an issue that should be thoroughly discussed with your doctor because of the risk of multiple pregnancy beyond twins. When multiple fetuses develop, couples confront the difficult topic of multifetal reduction in which some of the pregnancies are terminated to try to reduce complications to the remaining fetuses. In Chapter 11, we talk about this critical topic about which everyone considering IVF must be informed.

The Risk of Ovarian Hyperstimulation

In Chapter 7, we talked in detail about ovarian hyperstimulation. Younger women, women with PCOS, and women who don't ovulate regularly are most at risk for ovarian hyperstimulation. Hyperstimulation is rarely a surprise. If it is going to happen, hyperstimulation almost always happens in a first cycle, and if you are at risk, you should be monitored closely. While cancellation for this reason can be a disappointing setback, it is actually a good sign. You are someone who will make a lot of eggs and, hopefully, a lot of embryos. The goal is to get you through your cycle safely. At your next cycle, you can be stimulated much more gently with a much lower dose of medication.

The Risk of IVF Hurting Your Baby: Will IVF Do Harm?

Many couples are justly concerned about the risks of IVF and IVF/ICSI to their offspring. For all babies born in the United States, there is between 2 and 4 percent incidence of birth defects. From the most optimistic to the most pessimistic of studies concerning outcomes of IVF, it appears that there is somewhere between no increased incidence of birth defects from children born with IVF to two times the risk of birth defects. Some of the increased risk may be due to advanced maternal age in women using IVF, because advanced age in and of itself increases the risk of birth defects. But certainly we are concerned that some of that risk may be due to the actual technical aspects of IVF. This is one reason among many that people who don't need IVF should not have it.

There is an increase in abnormal findings at amniocentesis in women with pregnancies through ICSI. (See page 225.) In the general population, we would expect to see 0.5 percent chromosomal abnormalities on amniocentesis. The incidence is raised with ICSI pregnancies to 1.6 percent,[2] which you might interpret as a threefold increase. Most of these chromosomal abnormalities are inherited from the Y chromosome. Currently, the recommendation is that couples with ICSI pregnancies have amniocentesis to detect and address chromosomal abnormalities.

There are also certain very rare conditions called imprinting disorders that may be associated with IVF. These include Beckwith-Wiedemann, an overgrowth disorder, and Angelman syndrome, a rare syndrome characterized by speech impairment, balance and movement problems, an unusually happy or laughing demeanor, and retinoblastoma, retinal tumors.

Studies have looked at the incidence of cancer in children who are the result of IVF and found no increase in the risk of cancer in these children.

IVF WITH ICSI: NEW HOPE FOR MEN

IVF with *intracytoplasmic sperm injection* (ICSI; pronounced ick-see) revolutionized fertility treatment for men. In the past, donor sperm or adoption were the only options for parenthood for men with no or severely abnormal sperm counts. Today, a man with a very low sperm count—even a count as low as one sperm—may be able to father a child using a relatively new procedure that allows for the injection of a single sperm into an egg to promote fertilization. If you are having IVF and you have poor morphology on your semen analysis, then you should have IVF/ICSI. (See Chapter 3 for more about semen analysis.)

The first successful ICSI was described in 1992. Two years later, the procedure became widely available, and now, more than ten years later, almost all IVF labs offer ICSI. ICSI can be performed with sperm that has been either ejaculated or surgically removed.

ICSI is done in conjunction with the full IVF procedure described in this chapter. With ICSI, a single sperm is injected into the cytoplasm of an egg with a very tiny glass conduit called a micropipette. The embryo is placed into the uterus for implantation and, it is hoped, pregnancy ensues. You will need IVF/ICSI if:

- your partner has an extremely low sperm count;
- you and your partner have a history of not being able to fertilize an egg in vitro;
- your partner is using testicular or epididymal sperm for IVF. (We will talk about this later in this chapter.)

ICSI Half: When Your Partner Has a Borderline Sperm Count

It's not always simple to define who is a candidate for traditional IVF versus IVF with ICSI. There is always a small number of people (under 10 percent) for whom there can be a surprise fertilization failure with traditional IVF even with obvious, unrelated infertility factors, for example, tubal blockage and a normal semen analysis.

Couples with borderline sperm counts or unexplained infertility may choose to have half of their eggs used in ICSI procedures and the other half used in IVF without ICSI. ICSI can cost anywhere from $500 to $2,500 in addition to your IVF bill. Some larger labs have struggled for years attempting to sort out who can benefit from ICSI and who won't benefit, and often end up doing ICSI for every patient. This is not bad medicine, but it is a bit of overkill, not to mention a possible unnecessary financial expenditure.

Going Through IVF/ICSI as a Couple

Some physicians prefer to use fresh sperm for IVF/ICSI, although the medical literature repeatedly confirms the equal efficacy of frozen and fresh sperm in IVF/ICSI, except for TESE. (See "Microsurgical TESE," on page 229.) However, if you choose to use fresh sperm, you and your partner will be cycled together. This means coordinating his sperm retrieval and your oocyte (egg) retrieval with his urologist and your reproductive endocrinologist. The logistical and financial costs may make this feasible only in centers specifically geared toward doing these procedures.

When Your Partner Has No Sperm in His Ejaculate

In Chapter 6, we talked about some of the reasons men have azoospermia, or no sperm in their ejaculate. Obstructive azoospermia describes conditions in which a man produces sperm, but it simply can't get out of his body to fertilize his partner's eggs. This can happen when he was born without a vas deferens; if he had a vasectomy; or if he has scarring caused by infections, or an injury such as might have happened during a hernia operation. So what can he do to get sperm out for conception?

If he had a vasectomy, he may choose a vasectomy reversal. This is the best choice for a man whose vasectomy is less than three years old, or at the very most five years old, and whose partner is thirty or younger.

For other men with obstructive azoospermia who choose IVF/ICSI, sperm must be retrieved either in an open biopsy (surgery) or through in-office procedures in which a fine needle or other instrument is used to draw sperm from the epididymis or testicle. Recall that the epididymis is the place where sperm is stored after it is produced in the testicles (although it continues to mature even beyond the epididymis). For IVF/ICSI, it's preferable to have epididymal sperm rather than testicular sperm, because testicular sperm cells are less motile (they move less) than epididymal sperm and are harder to identify and evaluate as viable. Moreover, most studies show that epididymal sperm can be used effectively whether it is fresh or frozen.

Even though there are advantages to epididymal sperm, men who have questionable sperm production may need to use testicular sperm for IVF/ICSI. Later in this section, you will read about options for retrieving either testicular or epididymal sperm. When contemplating IVF/ICSI and sperm retrieval, there are a number of things to think about, including whether the male partner is a candidate, whether you are a candidate for and want to undergo IVF, as well as costs and insurance.

MESA: Getting Sperm from the Epididymis

MESA stands for *microsurgical epididymal sperm aspiration*. MESA is an "open" surgical procedure that can be used to take sperm from the epididymis. This is the place where the most mature sperm are likely to be found in someone without vas deferens or with a failed vasectomy reversal. An "open" procedure means surgery conducted through an incision rather than a needle puncture, in this case by a microsurgeon who is an expert at surgery using a microscope.

In this procedure, the testis and epididymis are surgically exposed as your doctor uses microscopic guidance to collect sperm from the tubules of the epididymis with care not to contaminate the specimen with blood. Sometimes, the surgeon can also retrieve sperm from efferent ductules connected to the testis. These are tiny ducts that convey sperm to the epididymis.

MESA has the advantage of enabling a surgeon to get a lot of sperm at a single surgical procedure. MESA is also the best option for a man who wants to freeze (cryopreserve) sperm for multiple IVF attempts. Other retrieval methods don't have the same IVF success rates with frozen sperm. Because sperm from MESA can be frozen, it's the most convenient retrieval before IVF. If sperm is found with MESA, a couple can schedule what's known as an "interval" procedure. The male partner can do his sperm retrieval and have the sperm frozen. His partner's retrieval can be scheduled later, for example, even two months later. Couples with children or other shared family and work responsibilities may prefer this option, if it's available, because both partners won't be recovering from a procedure at the same time.

MESA is best for men with obstructive azoospermia, that is, men with obstructions that prevent sperm from reaching the ejaculate, including:

- congenital bilateral absence of the vas deferens (CBAVD);
- ejaculatory duct obstruction;
- men with failed vasectomy reversals who opt for MESA and IVF over or a second vasectomy reversal;
- men who have had obstructions due to scarring caused by infection or injuries that occurred during surgery.

Although MESA has advantages of retrieving the most sperm, and allowing for freezing and coordination of egg and sperm retrievals, it has the disadvantage of requiring microsurgical expertise and of requiring surgery. There are somewhat simpler techniques that can be used to retrieve sperm for IVF procedures that require fresh sperm, such as percutaneous epididymal aspiration (PESA).

PESA and TESA: "No Surgery" Sperm Retrievals

Undoubtedly, most men would prefer to undergo a simple in-office procedure to retrieve sperm from the epididymis, rather than an open surgery in the hospital with general anesthesia. For some people this can work well. If your partner has obstructive azoospermia, he may be able to have his retrieval by aspiration.

Percutaneous (under the skin) *epididymal sperm aspiration* (PESA) is a procedure in which a urologist can draw sperm from the epididymis with a fine needle, biopsy gun, or other instrument. PESA can help men with obstructive azoospermia. Success rates for percutaneous aspiration are low for men with nonobstructive azoospermia and are not recommended.

Testicular sperm aspiration (TESA) is an in-office procedure that allows a urologist to draw sperm from a man's testis. Again, this technique is best when there is a good chance he has a testis full of sperm (obstructive azoospermia). Further, its diagnostic aspect is only useful when it is positive, that is, if sperm can be retrieved. If no sperm is found—and TESA is negative—it doesn't necessarily mean that a man has no sperm. Men with nonobstructive azoospermia may have mere islands or areas of sperm undetectable by needle biopsy methods, but that can be found by surgical methods.

The disadvantage of PESA, TESA, or of any "blind" procedure is the risk of causing bleeding and potentially causing long-term pain. This is particularly true with the epididymal procedures.

Microsurgical TESE: Advances for Men with No Sperm Production

While MESA, PESA, or TESA can help men with obstructions to sperm delivery, men with nonobstructive azoospermia cannot benefit from these methods of retrieval, because rather than merely having an obstruction to sperm production, men with nonobstructive azoospermia are not producing enough sperm to reach the ejaculate. For example, men with Klinefelter's syndrome have few seminiferous tubules containing sperm, and these tubules may be seen only within areas in the testes.

If you have nonobstructive azoospermia, you may still be able to find viable sperm by removing a sample of testicular tissue. Investigators have found that by actually opening the testis under a microscope, taking very small samples of the testicular tissue, which is replete with tiny seminiferous tubules that contain Sertoli cells and spermatogonia (immature sperm cells), and then carefully going through these tissue samples, sperm can be found for use in IVF/ICSI. This procedure is called *microsurgical TESE*, which stands for testicular sperm extraction. Clearly, this is a labor-intensive process. A microsurgeon conducts the surgery, during which an embryologist must be present to accept the small portions of tubules. The samples are placed immediately into a sperm-washing medium. In the lab, the embryologist or a team of embryologists must hunt through the samples for sperm with some degree of motility.

Even if only one sperm is found, it can be injected into a woman's egg during IVF/ICSI. It doesn't matter if the sperm is highly motile. To be combined with an egg, it must simply be living. Until fairly recently, there was no treatment for men who don't make sperm because of hormonal or other problems. This includes men with:

- Sertoli-cell-only (SCO) germ cell aplasia;
- maturation arrest;
- Klinefelter's syndrome;
- men who have undescended testes;
- men with other genetic anomalies that hinder sperm production.

Finding Sperm with Microsurgical TESE. When talking about success rates in these procedures, it's important to remember that we're talking about getting sperm, which is a first step toward conception, but not conception itself. Being able to find sperm is no indication of whether you and your partner will conceive with that sperm. Nonetheless, the startling news is that at least 30 to 50 percent of men whose biopsies show no sperm—not even early spermatogonia—will find sperm cells at retrieval that can be used with ICSI. These are figures for Sertoli-cell-only (SCO). When maturation arrest is the issue—when the problem is that sperm stop developing at some point in spermatogenesis—success rates jump to between 70 and 90 percent, meaning that most men with maturation arrest will be able to find sperm at microsurgical TESE. Even men with Klinefelter's syndrome, men with other karyotype-specific abnormalities, and 46XX men can find sperm. But as you can imagine, the procedure is not guaranteed. It also has the potential to damage blood supply to the testes, which can impair hormone production and may then necessitate testosterone supplementation. This may not be as much of a deterrent to men who already need supplementation—for example, men with hormonal deficiencies—or it may be a trade a man is willing to make if there is no other way to retrieve his sperm for reproduction.

What We Know About Testicular Sperm and the Health of Your Baby.
Although testicular sperm is in a more primitive state of development than mature sperm, the data on the offspring of testicular sperm is reassuring. While we have to bear in mind that the oldest child born from ICSI would be approximately fourteen years old in 2006, children conceived using testicular sperm and ICSI are healthy.

As we mentioned previously, there is an increase in abnormal findings at amniocentesis in women with pregnancies through ICSI. Most of these are chromosomal abnormalities inherited from the Y chromosome. Certainly, if a man uses ICSI because of a problem with his Y chromosome, his son will inherit the identical problem. There may be a slight increase in sex chromosome errors such as XXY (Klinefelter's syndrome), XYY syndrome (a chromosomal condition that affects males and can be associated with learning disabilities and behavioral problems), or Turner's syndrome (which describes girls and women with a missing X chromosome or defects in one of the two X chromosomes). Depending on the wishes of the couple, these disorders can be screened out through amniocentesis.

Will He Need More than One Retrieval Procedure? If your partner's sperm retrieval yields sperm, he may not need to have another procedure. More often than not, extra tissue and extra sperm can be frozen and used again, if you want to try for repeated IVF procedures. Sometimes a second retrieval may be offered, if the first attempt to retrieve sperm failed. About less than half the time, men will have to have this second procedure, but having a third is very unusual. The risk of having too much testicular tissue removed is that a man will have testicular failure and need testosterone replacement therapy. But again, some men may decide to tolerate this, if a retrieval procedure is the only means of having a genetically related child.

Choosing a Center for Microsurgical TESE. Choosing a center for microsurgical TESE means choosing an IVF program with an experienced microsurgeon who does at least ten of these procedures a year and embryologists who can devote time to the labor-intensive search for sperm. The best place to start your search is to look for an IVF program and ask questions of those programs. (See Chapter 4.) Microsurgical TESE clearly affects the cost of IVF/ICSI. The cost of a microsurgeon's fees, fees for the operating room, and anesthesia can increase the cost of your IVF procedure between 50 and 100 percent.

When to Think About Donor Insemination

IVF can either be done with fresh sperm—that is, sperm that is recently ejaculated or retrieved—or frozen sperm. If you and your partner are planning to do IVF with fresh sperm from a surgical procedure on the male, and there is a chance that no sperm will be found, you may want to consider having a backup of donor sperm for the IVF procedure.

Choosing donor sperm is a tough emotional issue for some people. If your partner's reaction to the possibility of recovering no sperm is, "Under no circumstances do I want a genetically unrelated pregnancy," you don't need donor backup. But if you are both uncertain of your feelings, it's good to start confronting this issue before your fertility treatment.

If he has azoospermia (no sperm) or he is considering a vasectomy reversal, you may want to talk about the prospect of using donor insemination if:

- You are doing a fresh IVF or IVF/ICSI cycle that is going to culminate with testicular sperm retrieval at the time of your egg retrieval. You may have retrieved eggs (oocytes) but find no sperm with which fertilize them to make embryos unless you have donor backup.
- You and your partner want to do IUI with donor insemination.
- He has a genetic anomaly that he doesn't want to pass on to his offspring.

If donor insemination is unacceptable to you, by all means you should not feel compelled to pursue it. If you do, however, want to consider donor sperm, your reproductive endocrinologist can coordinate this with you. You can choose a specimen from the sperm bank catalog, and either the doctor's office can arrange for the delivery of the sperm, or you or your partner can bring the sperm to the office, depending on your choice.

FROZEN EMBRYO TRANSFER

Most IVF labs can and do freeze embryos, because people may have more embryos that can be transferred at one time. Unfertilized eggs can be frozen, but as yet they don't freeze and thaw with the same high efficiency as embryos, and they don't produce nearly the same pregnancy rates. It seems that there is something about fertilization that appears to aid cryopreservation. However, successful egg banking and freezing is on the horizon.

Embryos can be frozen at any stage including the zygote stage, which is about sixteen to eighteen hours after fertilization. They can be frozen as cleaved embryos on day two or day three, or they can be frozen as blastocyst embryos on day five or day six. All of these variations have been done with approximately equivalent success rates. The stage at which a clinic freezes embryos is really a matter of lab experience and lab practices. In general, cryopreserved embryos account for about 5 to 50 percent of an IVF program's cases. Generally, success rates for pregnancy with frozen embryos are about 30 percent.

The rate at which a given clinic freezes embryos depends on the criteria used to select embryos for cryopreservation. Some will freeze embryos that look in relatively poor condition, as long they are clearly viable. Other programs will only freeze embryos that meet certain benchmarks, such as the number of cells they attain on a certain day or embryo grade, which is the way embryo quality is described.

Most embryos survive freezing and thawing, although the condition the embryo was in at freezing certainly makes a difference to its survival. The implantation rate of frozen embryos is somewhat lower than fresh embryos, so generally when doing a frozen cycle, clinics will put back one more embryo than they would on a fresh cycle. The total number of embryos you will put back depends on your age and other risk factors you have that lower your chance of success. So for example, if you were an older woman with a lot of embryos and chose to put back three embryos on a fresh cycle (not having the same risk for multiple pregnancy as a younger woman), you might put back four embryos on a frozen cycle.

It's important to recognize that you may not make a lot of eggs at an older age. Even more importantly, the number of embryos you put back will be determined by your age at the time the embryos were frozen and not your age at the time you wish to put them back. So if you are forty years old and you froze your embryos at forty years old, you can probably be aggressive about the number of embryos you want to put back. On the other hand, if you are forty years old and you froze your embryos when you were thirty-five, you should base the number of embryos you put back on the number suggested for a thirty-five-year-old woman.

The American Society for Reproductive Medicine (ASRM) offers guidelines for the numbers of embryos that should be put back on a fresh cycle depending on age and circumstances. Generally, you can add one frozen embryo to the number recommended by the ASRM for a fresh cycle. (Talk to your doctor about ASRM guidelines.) You may wish to be more conservative if you have already had a child from your embryos on a fresh cycle. This may be more evidence that the embryos were good and that you are at increased risk of multifetal pregnancy. Of course, these are discussions that you should have with your doctor well in advance of your embryos transfer.

Having a Frozen Embryo Transfer

Having a frozen embryo transfer differs from a fresh cycle protocol. In your fresh cycle, you most likely had stimulation to produce a number of follicles and eggs. With your frozen cycle, you transfer your eggs without having to go through ovarian stimulation. However, if you do not have regular cycles, you will need hormonal support.

There are two protocols for frozen embryos: a natural cycle and a hormone replacement cycle. If your cycles are regular, but you had IVF for a reason such as male factor infertility or tubal problems, you may be able to do a natural cycle, meaning you will have no medication. Your physician will follow you through your regular cycle with frequent ultrasound checkups until the day you ovulate, putting the embryos back into your uterus at the appropriate time. So, for instance, if you ovulate on day fifteen and you are putting back a day three embryo, you could probably put that embryo back three days later, that is, on day eighteen.

With a hormone replacement transfer, you will have estradiol supplementation either orally, transdermally, or by injection to develop a uterine lining. Once your lining is sufficient for implantation, as seen on an ultrasound, you will start progesterone, basing your transfer on the day of progesterone onset, which is analogous to the day of ovulation.

Some women who have regular cycles prefer to get their embryos back in a natural cycle, minimizing their use of medication. Other women prefer to use hormone replacement, because it requires fewer doctor visits and allows for a more controlled schedule. If you don't have your own cycle, you have no choice but to do a hormone replacement cycle. Rest assured that the pregnancy rates for natural and hormone replacement cycles are the same with frozen embryo transfers.

How Embryos Are Frozen

Embryos are made of cells, and cells are made primarily of water. Normally, when you freeze cells that contain water, ice will form. As you can imagine, ice formation will destroy a cell. That's why we must use a substance called a cryoprotectant to replace water in the cell. Cryoprotectants are substances that can be taken to extremely low temperatures without forming ice crystals. When an embryo is put into a dish with a high concentration of a cryoprotectant, water will go out of the cell and the cryoprotectant will go into the cell to replace the water.

Here again, many people worry whether this process will harm the health of the child produced from an embryo preserved in this manner. In the early 1980s, the first children were born from cryopreserved embryos. It's been over twenty years since the advent of this technology, and in this fairly lengthy period of time we know that these children are as normal as other children.

Problems to Watch Out for During Your Frozen Cycle

Just as with a fresh cycle, problems can occur with your frozen cycle. Your embryos may be stored for several years. Of course, your embryos should not be misplaced, but, depending on the length of time they've been stored, staff members may have come and gone from the lab, and changes may have been made that could conceivably lead to lost embryos.

Fifty to 90 percent of embryos survive thawing, which means that 10 to 50 percent of the time they don't. These are general survival rates. Uncommonly, embryos are not frozen according to strict protocols and are destroyed in the process. You may not discover this until your embryos are thawed. In Chapter 4, we list questions to ask when choosing a clinic, including questions about the way in which frozen embryos are stored.

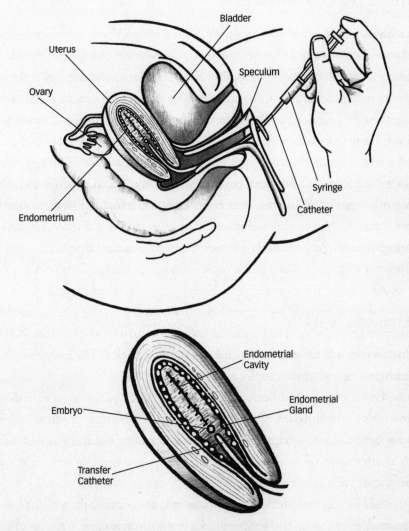

FIGURE II. *Embryo transfer*

Embryos are placed between the anterior (front) and posterior (back) uterine walls and are therefore "sandwiched," as opposed to floating free.

PREIMPLANTATION GENETIC DIAGNOSIS (PGD): TESTING YOUR EMBRYOS FOR GENETIC DISORDERS

Preimplantation genetic diagnosis (PGD) is a method by which doctors test chromosomes or the DNA of an embryo for evidence of a genetic disorder, giving a woman or couple the option to choose not to transfer that embryo and to instead select only those embryos that do not have genetic anomalies.

Most PGD is done on day three embryos on what's called a blastomere, a cell from a cleaved embryo. Sometimes it is also done on a day one polar body, a set of chromosomes ejected from a newly fertilized egg that does not become a functional part of the pregnancy. PGD is done to look for two types of problems. It is often done for structural chromosomal problems, such as having too many or too few chromosomes or chromosomes that might be broken or stuck together in unusual ways. It is also done for what are known as *single gene disorders,* wherein defects in a specific gene cause the disorder. Some single gene disorders are called recessive disorders because both members of a couple must be carriers of the disorder in order for it to be passed on, such as with cystic fibrosis. PGD can also be used to look for sex-linked disorders, such as Duchenne's muscular dystrophy, which usually affects only sons.

PGD is *absolutely* indicated for known carriers of single gene disorders and for certain chromosomal rearrangements, including a problem called translocation, where fragments of one chromosome break off and attach to another chromosome. This will be visible on a karyotype, which is a picture of your chromosomes.

PGD is frequently indicated when people are at particular risk for having an embryo with the wrong number of chromosomes. This is called *aneuploidy.* Down syndrome is a very common form of aneuploidy called trisomy. Down syndrome occurs when one has three chromosomes 21, called trisomy 21, instead of the normal two chromosomes 21. Couples with recurrent pregnancy loss and women at advanced maternal age, that is, thirty-seven or older, are most at risk for aneuploidy. A case could also be made for testing women thirty-five years old and up for aneuploidy. However, as you will learn momentarily, the number of embryos you make will influence whether to do PGD in this circumstance.

Do You Have Enough Embryos for PGD?

One of the key issues with regard to doing PGD in these instances is whether you have enough embryos to benefit. The more embryos you have to sample, the more useful PGD can be to you, in terms of both diagnosing your current embryos and telling you about the likelihood of problems for embryos you make at any future attempts to get pregnant. For example, if you make eight embryos, and, say, two can't be diagnosed because of technical problems, leaving you with six embryos, a percentage will likely be normal. That percentage could differ, depending on your age, with a greater percentage likely to be normal if you are young. But let's say half are normal. Now you have three embryos left to transfer. That's why the number of embryos you have and your risk for really having an embryo with serious chromosomal problems should be taken into account when considering PGD.

If you have few embryos, but are definitely at risk for a chromosomal translocation (where part of one chromosome breaks off and attaches to another), or you definitely are a carrier for a single gene disorder, such as cystic fibrosis, you should go ahead and do PGD. But if you have a small number of embryos from which to choose and are just at risk for chromosomal aneuploidy due to your age, but not necessarily going to have a pregnancy with an abnormality, you may decide to forgo PGD. Embryos that are not normal because of aneuploidy are likely to miscarry or fail to develop. Ideally, you should have at least six to eight embryos to sample for PGD.

As we learn more about genetic diseases, testing embryos for genetic problems will likely increase. It takes an expert to adequately counsel a couple about their specific risk for genetic disorders. While couples who are not undergoing IVF may not seek genetic counseling before trying to conceive, couples having IVF are spending so much time, effort, and money trying to get pregnant that an argument could be made that everyone undergoing IVF should be counseled about their genetic risks so that they can make choices about whether or not to have their embryos tested.

Once you have had genetic counseling, know your risks, and are contemplating PGD, the next question you want to ask yourself is whether you will transfer an embryo with a genetic disorder or an embryo that, if it develops into a pregnancy, will become a person who is a carrier for a genetic disorder, as can happen with cystic fibrosis.

Will PGD Harm Your Embryos?

The first PGD baby was born in Great Britain in 1989. Thousands of children have been born using this technology since, with no apparent detriment to their health. This may be because embryonic cells are "totipotent" cells, meaning that they have the potential to develop into any kind of cell. You may have heard of this with regard to stem-cell research. Embryos at this state are also resilient and can lose a cell or two without being harmed. But it must be said that we have not yet seen the first PGD baby reach full adulthood. We do not yet know if there are repercussions of PGD for these children later in life.

How PGD Is Done

Testing for structural chromosomal abnormalities is done with a technology called *fluorescent in situ hybridization* (FISH). In this technology, a cell is fixed to a microscope slide, and a series of DNA labels with fluorescent attachments are applied to that cell. For example, chromosome 21 may be assigned the color red so that when it is stained and viewed under a fluorescent microscope, it can be seen as a red dot. If two red dots appear, we know that the embryo has two chromosomes 21, but if three red dots appear, we know the embryo has three chromosomes 21. This is trisomy 21, better known as Down syndrome.

FISH is done with between nine and twelve pairs of chromosomes out of the possible twenty-three pairs in a human being. This is the limit of current technology. Ultimately, we may be able to identify all the chromosomes. There may be a specific DNA sequence unique to each chromosome and we may be able to amplify the DNA to make sure that each chromosome is represented and no chromosome is overrepresented. At this point, testing will become an almost automated process.

Single gene disorders are tested for with a technique called polymerase chain reaction (PCR). This is a way of measuring DNA by replicating, or amplifying, it dramatically and quickly and then using probes to detect the presence of a sought-after gene.

PGD and Gender Selection

Gender selection is one of the most controversial areas of IVF. We can now determine gender with PGD with 99 percent certainty. Clearly, this is very useful in detecting sex-specific disorders, such as hemophilia, but should it be used to help ordinary couples select the sex of their child? Should a woman who is otherwise fertile be given the option of going through the entire IVF procedure, including stimulation, egg retrieval, and transfer, for this reason?

Among practitioners, there are honest differences of opinion about this issue. Most reproductive endocrinologists do not advocate PGD for gender selection. Admittedly, those of us who are against doing IVF and PGD solely for gender selection are not logically consistent. Most reproductive endocrinologists are pro-choice, believing strongly in a patient's right to exercise her autonomy. Although sex selection is an exercise of patient autonomy, most REs see PGD techniques as having been designed to treat disorders and reason that since gender in and of itself is not a disorder, PGD should not be used to "treat" gender. Certainly, there are physicians who provide this service and patients who are grateful for its availability.

The ease with which PGD may become available is an issue for the future. When and if PGD becomes an inexpensive and noninvasive service, as might happen if sperm—which determine gender—could be processed for gender selection, then we may see the widespread availability of this service, which may develop past the point of being something that is rendered solely by physicians. It may become what we might term an "off the shelf" commodity, as available as readily as using donor sperm.

JUST BECAUSE IT CAN BE DONE, SHOULD IT BE DONE?

We don't have to wait until there are further advances in technology to confront issues on the slippery slope of reproductive medicine. If gender selection becomes normalized as an elective procedure to which couples are entitled, why not provide for selection of embryos according to height, hair color, and other characteristics when we have the tools to identify these features in embryos? Sperm banks, of course, already market donor features, with some companies advertising specimens from men of a certain ethnic or racial background, such as sperm banks that provide specimens from Scandinavian men only. Women who provide donor eggs may also be solicited for certain physical and other criteria.

Today, it is entirely possible for someone to get donor eggs from women in struggling economies, such as Ukraine or Romania. These women could undoubtedly be paid far less for their eggs than donors in the United States. Conceivably, these eggs could be combined with sperm frozen in the United States or abroad. Or donor embryos could be produced outside the United States and shipped back to this country without any barriers. You could make as many embryos as you like. You might even have the embryos placed into gestational carriers in states where there are no laws against being a gestational carrier. All this is entirely legal and possible right now. It concerns me that at the time of this writing there is nothing on the horizon to prevent this scenario from being realized.

As professionals, reproductive endocrinologists must begin to adopt some standards and guidelines about what we do and do not endorse, because in the long run if we don't apply these standards to our practices, they will be supplied to us by outside forces.

FALLOPIAN TUBE TRANSFERS

Gamete intrafallopian transfer (GIFT) allows sperm and egg to be directly introduced into the fallopian tube. Until the mid-1990s GIFT had a significantly higher success rate than IVF, but since then, developments in laboratory methods have closed that gap to the point where the less invasive procedure, IVF, is almost universally employed.

In order to introduce sperm and egg directly into the fallopian tube, it's necessary to have a laparoscopy, a relatively minor but invasive surgery. The upside of having to have a laparoscopy for GIFT is that the laparoscopy can also be used to check for any undetected problems, such as endometriosis. Another consideration for the use of GIFT may be religious in that it allows for fertilization inside the body as opposed to in the laboratory. Therefore, some Catholic institutions will condone GIFT.

Other tubal transfer procedures include zygote intrafallopian transfer (ZIFT), which involves transferring a day-one embryo into the fallopian tube, and tubal embryo transfer (TET), which refers to the transfer of a day two or day three embryo into the fallopian tube. These procedures may be used when a severe cervical obstruction might prevent normal embryo transfer.

WHAT TO DO WHEN IVF JUST ISN'T WORKING

One of the misconceptions about IVF is that if it fails, you must move on to other options, such as using donor eggs or adoption, and while this is certainly a realistic course for women who are thirty-seven or older, and is especially true for women over forty, it is not necessarily so for younger women. Before thinking about other options, ask yourself if your IVF cycle went well.

- Did you have a normal period of stimulation, meaning twelve days or less?
- Did you respond well to the fertility drugs, meaning you produced a good number of viable embryos?
- Do you have good ovarian reserve?
- Is your uterine lining good?

If you are under thirty-seven and you answered yes to these questions, and everything went well with your IVF cycle, it may just be a matter of time before you get pregnant with IVF. It may be reasonable to do another cycle, without changing anything.

On the other hand, if there were problems with your cycle, and age is not an issue, you and your doctor may then want to look more closely at the features of your cycle, considering whether some changes can be made to improve your chances the next time.

Should You Change Your IVF Protocol?

The most crucial elements of your IVF cycle are how well you stimulated and how viable your embryos are. If you are thirty-seven or younger, ask your doctor what went wrong. Inquire if your stimulation or embryo quality was poor. Or were both aspects of your IVF cycle unsatisfactory?

Some physicians are inclined to change one thing at a time. If you didn't stimulate well, the next step may be to change your stimulation protocol. If your embryos don't look good, changes may be made in the lab to try to improve their quality. Depending on how bad the situation is, some doctors would like to change as much as they can. The worse an IVF cycle is, the more I want to change as much as I can to try to improve it.

Changing Your Drug Protocol

In Chapter 7, we mentioned that raising the dose of injectable FSH beyond 600 units will rarely do anything but waste your money. Many physicians will not give over 450 units of injectable FSH for the good reason that this is the maximum dose for someone of an average body size. If you are already at the maximum dose, your doctor might consider dividing your doses, giving you 225 units twice a day in "spikes" rather than once daily. When you take an injection of FSH, you get a peak level about an hour after the injection and then the level starts to decline. With two shots a day rather than one, your "mean" daily FSH level will be higher. Sometimes doctors will consider changing the GnRH analog that you use to shut down your ovaries toward the end of your cycle, switching from an agonist like Lupron to an antagonist like Antagon or vice versa. Switching FSH preparations is sometimes done, but there is no evidence that a drug made by one company is any more potent than another. Adding clomiphene citrate (Clomid or Serophene) or letrozole (a drug that blocks estrogen) are other potential courses.

What if Your Embryo Quality Isn't Good?

When an embryo doesn't look good, it means it isn't growing in the laboratory. Doctors and embryologists would like to see an embryo grow to four cells on day two and eight cells on day three. Lower numbers can signal a poor embryo. Fragmentation (debris) is another sign that an embryo isn't as good as we would like it to be.

When your embryos aren't doing well, you might ask your doctor if there is something that can be done to improve their quality. In hopes of improving embryo viability, some laboratories may switch culture media, the substance in which embryos are placed to develop. There are a number of good culture media commercially available, but that doesn't mean one size fits all. Most labs will use one medium and change the medium if necessary; some labs use a variety of media. One IVF program I know uses two different types of media, dividing embryos into two different sets, putting one half in one medium and one half in the other.

Coculture is a technique sometimes employed but fading from use. With coculture, a woman's own endometrial cells are put into the culture along with the embryo, in accordance with the theory that cells grow better in the presence of other cells, either because they secrete growth factors into the culture medium or that the cells metabolize waste products from the embryo. Coculture might be something to consider in cases where embryos are consistently bad without any other explanation, such as age. If you are forty-two, for example, poor embryo quality is most likely due to your age, but if you are thirty, as another example, the reason your embryos are consistently bad may be far from clear.

In the Future: Media Showers?

Embryos sit in little dishes of culture media, as if in little baths. But instead of sitting in a dish of stagnant medium, the embryo may soon sit in a receptacle wherein media constantly circulates around it. Engineers are getting close to a developing a system in which the embryo will be continuously exposed to new media while the old medium is washed away, a bit like an embryo shower. Although still under development, this technique may be very beneficial and available in the near future.

IVF programs and laboratories do what works best for them, and no single approach is better than another. A good lab or IVF program is one that gets results. How a program gets there can differ from lab to lab. Some labs adopt a rigid and fixed method, and others make changes as they go along. And although in the best of circumstances, discussions about the culture media occur collaboratively between the doctor and the laboratory, this isn't always practical, especially in larger laboratories where cases may not be individualized. Still, if you are younger and your embryos don't look good, you may not necessarily be told about the possibility of changing the culture medium unless you ask.

If Your Embryos Don't Look Good and You Don't Stimulate Well

If you have had one or two IVF cycles, and you didn't stimulate well and you didn't produce good-looking embryos, you may really want to consider donor eggs or adoption as possible next steps, regardless of your age. If you are young, you still have the option of going to another IVF program. But if you are already at a highly regarded IVF program, there may not be much benefit in going to another such program. In Chapter 12, we will talk about third-party options in depth. It isn't always easy to adjust to the thought that you may have a child genetically unrelated to you, and this isn't a desired option for all couples or women, but it is something to think about sooner rather than later. Some women and couples reject these options initially, but find they are the best answer later. Some women or couples decide to remain child free. It is painful to have to face these choices. But the more information you have about your likelihood of succeeding in the future with your own eggs, and the steps involved in donor egg or adoption, the more certain you will be that you have examined all of your options for creating your family.

What Can You Do the Next Time? An Overview of Changes

- If you didn't stimulate well, your doctor might increase your FSH dose within limits or divide your FSH dose.
- If your embryos didn't develop well, you might ask about changing the embryo culture.
- You and your doctor may want to discuss growing your day three embryos to the blastocyst stage, if you have enough embryos to make this feasible
- If fewer than half of your eggs fertilized with traditional IVF, IVF with ICSI may be a consideration.
- You and your doctor may decide to transfer your embryos on day two rather than day three. No study has shown that day three transfers are better than day two transfers. If you have poor embryo quality and few embryos, this may be a reasonable course of action, because taking the embryos out of the laboratory and putting them back into the body sooner rather than later may be beneficial.
- If the transfer didn't go well, ask what went wrong. Your doctor will certainly want to take steps to prevent future problems.
- Although not available in all IVF programs, a transfer of your embryos directly into your fallopian tube may be another alternative. However, this alternative does involve laparoscopic surgery.
- If you have a high number of embryos and your cycles went well, you

and your doctor may want to discuss PGD to test the embryos for aneuploidy. If you have seven embryos, for example, and all are aneuploid, you will know why your cycles didn't work. On the other hand, if there is no evidence of aneuploidy, you are young, and your cycle went well, but it just didn't work this time, you may feel encouraged to do another IVF cycle with the thought that it may work the next time. If you have too few embryos for PGD, that is, fewer than five or six embryos, PGD may not be worth the cost.

• You may ask your doctor if a laparoscopy is a possible next step. Endometriosis or pelvic adhesions may be what's preventing conception. Treatment may enable you to get pregnant spontaneously without the intervention of IVF.

Although it's not common, a few people will get pregnant without intervention after a failed cycle of IVF. These are not patients who have blocked fallopian tubes or partners with severe male factor infertility, of course. They may just be people who have a certain amount of statistical luck. Or it may be that there is something about having IVF—the stimulation of your ovaries, the needle introduced into the ovary during retrieval, or undergoing prolonged periods of high estrogen and progesterone—that has a positive effect. If you are young, say, in your early thirties, with a fertility problem that isn't definitive, such as blocked tubes or male factor infertility, and you haven't succeeded with IVF yet, spacing out your IVF cycles might make some sense for you. You might try doing a cycle of IVF and taking off one or two cycles before planning your next cycle.

In the next chapter, we will look at another difficult aspect of infertility care: recurrent pregnancy loss. Even if you have not had a pregnancy loss, and especially if you are just starting or contemplating infertility treatment, you may want to look at this chapter in order to understand the risks of having a miscarriage—or more than one miscarriage—when undergoing treatment. Being prepared for the unexpected is one of the best things you can do to help yourself through the ups and downs of infertility care.

10 | Recurrent Pregnancy Loss and Ectopic Pregnancy

MISCARRIAGE IS ONE OF THE SADDEST, MOST DEVAS-
tating events for a woman and her partner. Finding out that you are pregnant and feeling the joy of anticipating a child, only to experience the
horrible disappointment of loss soon after, can be crushing. When you
have recurrent miscarriages, the repeated cycle of hope and loss, along
with the physical trauma of miscarriage, can be almost unbearable. Human beings can be expected to endure only so much grief, and many who
go through numerous losses feel their hope wane or cease altogether. Miscarrying during infertility treatment is especially difficult, because of the
tremendous effort, time, and money spent trying to get pregnant. Women
and their partners can begin to feel as if pregnancy is impossible. They
may strengthen their resolve and try again, or they may opt to stop trying.

Before you decide to stop trying, make sure that you have a complete pregnancy-loss workup to try to find out why you are miscarrying. You may be able to avoid or prepare for another loss.

Some women have what's called a biochemical pregnancy, a positive pregnancy test that goes away. All too often couples who endure this type of loss have few ways to mourn or express their sorrow. Other people may not understand what they are going through. Or a couple may not want to talk about it. Many women who aren't having infertility treatment may actually have a biochemical pregnancy and not know it if they don't have a pregnancy test. Were they to be tested, they would see a temporary rise in their beta hCG levels, suggesting a pregnancy. Without testing, they may bleed close to their periods, experiencing the miscarriage as part of their menstrual period. But when you are being treated for infertility, having a positive pregnancy and then suddenly not being pregnant can be excruciating, because you are so aware of your cycles and trying so hard to have a child.

WHAT CAUSES RECURRENT MISCARRIAGE?

Recurrent pregnancy loss is defined as having three miscarriages in a row. The vast majority of these losses take place in the first trimester. Miscarriage is fairly common, affecting 10 to 15 percent of pregnancies. Recurrent miscarriage is more unusual. About one in one hundred women will go through recurrent miscarriage, with the risk increasing for women thirty-seven and older.

Along with the heartbreak of consecutive losses is the troubling fact that while most women (about 60 percent) will be able to find out why they are having miscarriages, many others (about 40 percent) won't know why, despite testing. Fortunately, even when the cause is unknown, there is a very good chance that you can still go on to have a successful pregnancy, if you keep trying. In fact, about 75 percent of women with recurrent losses do. Unfortunately, the prognosis worsens for women as they age and as the number of losses increase. On the following pages, we will look at known causes of pregnancy loss.

Hormonal Problems (Luteal Phase Defect)

A lack of progesterone or progesterone effect on the uterine lining, sometimes termed *luteal phase defect*, can cause the uterine lining to be in the wrong phase of development at the time the embryo is available to implant.

A blood test (serum progesterone) is the least invasive way to find out if you have an adequate amount of progesterone for implantation. Ten nanograms is an adequate level of progesterone, but to some degree that's a judgment call. The higher your progesterone level, the more likely it is that progesterone is not the problem. The lower the numbers, the more likely progesterone is a problem. When there is doubt, your doctor may suggest an endometrial biopsy, in which a small piece of your uterine lining is removed. The endometrial biopsy can help determine whether you need progesterone supplementation. (See Chapter 3.)

Uterine Septums

When you have a uterine septum, the inside of your uterus is shaped like a V, while the outside is formed like a triangle. (A uterus is normally shaped like a triangle on both the inside and the outside.) The septum, a wedge of tissue within the uterus, does not get blood supply, which flows from outside into the uterus. When a pregnancy attaches to the septum, it can't survive, because there is decreased blood supply to support it. Fortu-

TRYING AGAIN?

Most often couples can try again the month following a miscarriage. Each time you shed your uterine lining you are readied to build an entirely new uterine lining. What happened last month won't affect the next month. In effect, you are getting a clean slate from which to begin.

nately, treatment for a septate uterus is a same-day surgery done with a narrow telescope called a hysteroscope. The hysteroscope is inserted through the vagina into the cervix. Instruments can be put through the hysteroscope to cut away the septum. In the past, this operation used to be done abdominally, making the removal of a septum major surgery. Today, it can be done with minimal recovery time and no scars. You can probably try for another pregnancy in the next month after the procedure.

Cervical Problems

There is no hard-and-fast way to diagnose cervical weakness, medically termed *cervical incompetence*. Often, cervical problems are diagnosed when a woman has a history of having dilatation without pain. Unlike the uterus, the cervix is not a muscular structure. It is not resilient. Every time the cervix is dilated through the following ways, it gets a bit weaker:

- multiple surgical procedures through your cervix, such as a number of hysteroscopies and/or D&Cs;
- multiple surgeries on your cervix to treat dysplasia, such as cervical cone biopsies and LEEP procedures;
- cervical laceration such as during childbirth;
- premature delivery that was relatively painless;
- DES exposure;
- a congenital cervical anomaly, such as a unicornate uterus.

Cervical cerclage, a procedure in which a purse-string suture is put around the cervix once you are pregnant, effectively tying your cervix closed, is the treatment for cervical weakness, but whether it is effective is a controversial issue. It's not practical to test outcomes of this procedure by taking two groups of women who have precisely the same histories and cervixes and doing cerclages in half of these women and not doing this for the other half. It's hard to perfectly design two equivalent groups of these complex patients. Thus, the decision to do a cervical cerclage becomes a matter of the physician's clinical judgment. Like many such issues in medicine, clinical judgment is very much subject to a doctor's unique experience and training. Treating with a cervical cerclage is no trivial matter. The procedure can tear the cervix. When you don't have a history of pregnancy loss due to cervical weakness, the use of this technique to try to prevent a loss is even more controversial, because the physician is treating something that may or may not happen with the risk of actually damaging the cervix. When making this decision with your doctor, you must trust that your doctor has your best interests and those of your pregnancy at heart.

A cervical cerclage is not usually done until the eleventh week of pregnancy. Cervical incompetence is a very unusual cause of miscarriage in the first trimester when there is usually not much strain on the cervix. But many miscarriages in the first trimester are caused by chromosomal abnormalities, and most of these occur by the eleventh week. Therefore, doctors usually perform cervical cerclage after this point in order to avoid performing a surgical procedure unnecessarily.

If you have a cervical problem, it's key to have close monitoring of your cervix with ultrasound, which is a very good way of visualizing the cervix and tracking your pregnancy from week to week. There is no known risk of doing ultrasound.

Fibroids

You've just read that multiple instrumentations can contribute to the possibility of a pregnancy loss. If you were treated for fibroids (myomas), you may have had more than one hysteroscopy. You may be concerned about whether having these procedures puts you at risk for pregnancy loss. As you know, fibroids that distort the uterine cavity can sometimes cause pregnancy loss. Removing fibroids in order to avoid miscarriage is advisable, especially when you are being treated for infertility and undergoing IVF. The advantage of removing a fibroid that is protruding inside the uterine cavity far exceeds the danger of doing a hysteroscopy. Still, if you have had multiple hysteroscopies, your doctor should watch your cervix more closely, looking for any potential changes in the cervix as a routine precaution.

Chromosomal Problems

Chromosomes are structures in the nucleus of a cell that contain our genes. Normally, each human cell has forty-six chromosomes. We get our chromosomes from our mother and father, with each parent contributing twenty-three chromosomes when the egg and sperm fuse. Your mother contributes an X chromosome and your father an X or a Y. When you are born, you will have two sex chromosomes, XX if you are a woman and XY if you are a man, as well as twenty-two pairs of additional chromosomes.

If you and your partner have normal chromosomes, but you lost your pregnancy because the pregnancy had too few or too many chromosomes, the risk of this happening again is low, far less than 5 percent. Having more or less than the normal number of chromosomes is called aneuploidy. Down syndrome is the most well-known form of aneuploidy in which one has an extra number 21 chromosome. In other words, instead of having two number 21 chromosomes, there are three number 21 chromosomes. This form of aneuploidy is called trisomy. If you find out that you have had a miscarriage for this reason, know that it is an infrequent, sporadic event, which does not necessarily require intervention. While you might be worried that you will have another such pregnancy, you can try again, knowing that statistically you have a very good chance of having a normal pregnancy the next time.

More complex issues arise when you have or your partner has a chromosomal abnormality. To find out whether you have a chromosomal problem, you and your partner should have a karyotype, an actual picture of your chromosomes. Each of the twenty-three chromosomes contained in a sperm or egg cell are very well described and can actually be seen in a karyotype where a growing cell is fixed in a stain, making all of its chromosomes visible under a microscope for photography.

A translocation is the most common chromosomal problem. This is a structural abnormality wherein a piece of one chromosome is stuck to another chromosome. Either the male or female partner could have a translocation affecting the pregnancy. If you have a translocation, it's likely that you have all of your genes and are completely normal, except that half of your gametes (sperm or eggs) are not normal. When half of your gametes are imbalanced, a proportion of your embryos will be imbalanced—that is, they will not have the appropriate number of chromosomes in their genes—resulting in a miscarriage. If you have had two to three miscarriages and you carry a translocation, the odds it will happen again are 30 to 60 percent.

You could take a number of approaches to miscarriage because of chromosomal problems. You could take the "war of attrition" approach, trying again and hoping to have a normal pregnancy, which will probably happen over time. For some, the emotional pain of repeatedly trying may be too much to bear, and there is certainly a limit to how much difficulty and disappointment with which one should be expected to cope. You could also have IVF with preimplantation genetic diagnosis (PGD). With PGD, you can find out which of your embryos are affected by the chromosomal problem and choose to transfer only those embryos that are not affected. As the pregnancy develops, you could also choose to have chorionic villus sampling (CVS) to assure yourself that the pregnancy was normal. (This is a procedure done at ten to twelve weeks of pregnancy in which a small piece of placental tissue, chorionic villus, is sampled.) However, the vast majority of chromosomally imbalanced pregnancies miscarry before CVS or amniocentesis can be done.

A last alternative would be to try using donor eggs or donor sperm, depending on which member of the couple is affected, although the affected parent will lose a genetic connection to the child.

Thyroid Problems

Severe hyperthyroidism and hypothyroidism can cause recurrent miscarriage. There is a body of literature that suggests antithyroid antibodies can be associated with pregnancy loss, but the vast majority of women with antithyroid antibodies do not have pregnancy loss and in fact usually manifest their thyroid disease after delivery with what's called postpartum thyroiditis. Extreme hyperthyroidism and hypothyroidism may be associated with pregnancy loss. While mild hypothyroidism does not cause pregnancy loss, it should be treated, because the mildest form of hypothyroidism is associated with impaired mental development in offspring. Hypothyroidism can be treated with a thyroid hormone. Similarly, lack of diabetic control is tightly correlated to birth defects of the fetus.

Blood Clotting Disorders (Thrombophilia)

There are a number of blood clotting disorders, called thrombophilic, that are or may be related to pregnancy loss. If discovered, they can be treated fairly easily.

Blood doesn't just course through the blood vessels. It's dynamic, always clotting and unclotting at a microscopic level. There are mechanisms that cause the blood to clot and unclot, creating a balance between either state, but when that balance is off, either due to an immunological or genetic problem, you are more likely to clot or to bleed. Disorders that cause you to hypercoagulate (to clot more often) may be detrimental to pregnancy. The uterus and the pregnancy need a blood supply to grow. When blood flow is impeded in any way, there is less blood flow to the uterus and to the placenta. When the placenta can't grow, or the fetus can't get enough oxygen, the pregnancy may not continue.

Generally, tests for blood clotting disorders are not done to screen everyone attempting pregnancy but should be strongly considered in women who have a personal or family history of coagulation disorders (such as pulmonary embolism or stroke) or recurrent pregnancy loss. You and your doctor may also suspect a need for testing when you have a history of pregnancy loss, a history of autoimmune disease, such as lupus, or previous pregnancy with hypertensive (high blood pressure) disorders, such as preeclampsia, as well as other hypertensive disorders of pregnancy.

You should be tested for:

- *Antiphospholipid antibody syndrome.* This is the most common blood clotting disorder, affecting about a third of infertile women. There are two main types of antiphospholipid antibodies, anticardiolipin antibodies and lupus anticoagulant. You don't have to have lupus to have these clotting disorders. In fact, most people with these antibodies don't have lupus. These antibodies can cause platelets to stick together, decreasing uterine blood supply. The good news is that this and other blood clotting disorders can be treated with low-dose heparin, which is an anticoagulant medication, and low-dose (81 mg) aspirin. Antiphospholipid antibodies have been found to be associated with both early and late pregnancy loss.
- *Factor V (Five) Leiden* affects about 5 percent of the population. Although this gene mutation may make you more prone to coagulation, its high prevalence suggests that it may have had some evolutionary advantage. In fact, the overall fertility of carriers of Factor V Leiden mutation is equal if not superior to the normal population. However, in the setting of an otherwise negative workup for recurrent pregnancy loss, individuals with Factor V Leiden mutation may benefit from anticoagulation with low-dose aspirin and low-dose heparin.
- *Protein S deficiency, protein C deficiency, prothrombin gene mutation, and antithrombin III* are other blood clotting conditions that might be associated with pregnancy loss. These are much less common and should be checked only in the face of a positive personal or family history or in the setting of recurrent pregnancy loss.
- *Homocysteine.* There is an enzyme mutation called *MTHFR* that causes high levels of an amino acid, homocysteine. High homocysteine levels have been shown to damage blood vessels, predisposing a person to cardiovascular disease, atherosclerosis, and perhaps even dementia. Damage to the vessel walls makes one more likely to develop blood clots. There really isn't proof-positive literature that high homocysteine levels or MTHFR mutations cause recurrent pregnancy loss, but it can be treated with high-dose folic acid, which helps you to metabolize homocysteine.

Polycystic Ovarian Syndrome (PCOS) and Miscarriage

Some studies suggest that there may be an increased rate of pregnancy loss in women who have PCOS or isolated elevated levels of LH. Other studies suggest that women with PCOS who are insulin resistant may decrease their risk of pregnancy loss in the first trimester by taking metformin. Whether metformin should be continued beyond the first trimester is an open question.

WHAT TO DO IF YOU KNOW YOU ARE GOING TO HAVE A MISCARRIAGE

More than half of all women have some bleeding in their first trimester of pregnancy. Most of these women will not miscarry, but should be evaluated. If you have any bleeding or cramping and feel like you may be having a miscarriage, call your doctor. Your doctor will look at your progesterone and beta hCG levels and do an ultrasound to assess the progress of your pregnancy. When everything looks all right, but the bleeding is of some concern, your doctor may suggest that you return for a follow-up visit, if the bleeding continues or gets worse.

On the other hand, an ultrasound may show that the pregnancy is no longer viable or that it hasn't progressed and that you are going to have a miscarriage. At this point, you and your doctor will discuss whether or not you would want to have a D&C to end the process or wait and go through the miscarriage on your own. You should also make sure that you know your blood type. If you are Rh negative and your husband or partner is Rh positive, you are going to need a RhoGAM injection so that you do not become immune to a future Rh positive pregnancy. This is because when you are Rh negative and your fetus is Rh positive, there is a chance that some of the fetus's blood may enter your system, causing you to develop antibodies to it. The antibodies you make at this time can destroy a future fetus's red blood cells, causing severe harm to the fetus as it develops. If you are Rh negative, this can happen in any future pregnancy, if you are not given the RhoGAM shot.

Most women elect to go through the miscarriage on their own to avoid having an operation with all that it entails. If you choose to go through the miscarriage on your own, you should know that you will have major bleeding with a lot of cramping and clotting sometime in the coming weeks.

Going Through the Miscarriage

Miscarriage can be a terrifying and profoundly sad event. You needn't go through it alone. If you are partnered, it's very important to involve your significant other, because he or she is also experiencing a major loss. You and your partner can help each other through this very difficult time.

Although it may seem like a medical emergency, there is usually no reason to go to the ER unless you are bleeding excessively or you are in extreme discomfort. There is nothing to stop a miscarriage in progress. Putting your feet up or resting won't help stop the event, although it won't do any harm.

If you have never had a miscarriage, you may not know exactly what is happening in your body. It may make the experience a little less frightening to know what is going on. The uterus is a muscular organ designed to expel. When you menstruate, you expel tissue and blood. Having a miscarriage is like having a period exaggerated many times over. When the process is complete, the uterus clamps down and stops the bleeding. It does this when you menstruate, when you have a miscarriage, and when you have a delivery.

The most dramatic part of the miscarriage—the time when you are having extremely heavily bleeding—should last no longer than two to three days. If it does, call your doctor. The entire miscarriage should last no more than a week, but it can take up to two weeks to resolve. You will feel like you are having your period for this length of time. You also want to be aware of the signs of ectopic pregnancy, which can be dangerous. There can be similarities between symptoms of a miscarriage and those of an ectopic pregnancy, for example, pain and bleeding. (See the section on ectopic pregnancy in this chapter.)

Your doctor should see you within two to seven days after your miscarriage. You will need an ultrasound to make sure that your uterus has emptied. You and your doctor will also want to discuss your having a complete pregnancy loss workup (page 261) to try to assess why you had a miscarriage. A test for chromosomal problems, called a karyotype, should be done immediately, because it will take three to four weeks to get the results. Other tests should probably wait until the miscarriage is completely over or until your next menstrual cycle. Shortly, we will talk about what you need for a complete workup.

Having a D&C

A dilatation and curettage (D&C) is a procedure in which the contents of the uterus are gently removed. You will find a discussion of having a D&C in Chapter 5, in the section on polyps. But a word of warning: don't let anybody talk you into having a D&C without a short-acting general anesthesia. The uterus has a nerve supply, and scraping the uterus can be extraordinarily painful, such that having anesthesia is absolutely justified. It would be easier to have an egg retrieval without anesthesia than to have a D&C without it. The anesthesia can be done without intubation. Alternatively, you can have a spinal anesthetic or an epidural to completely anesthetize the area.

Your D&C should be done in an appropriate setting, such as an office where anesthesia is available, an ambulatory surgery center, or a hospital.

The procedure takes about fifteen to twenty minutes, although you should get to the facility early and allow some time to recover after anesthesia. Make sure that you have someone to drive you home. You should not drive after having anesthesia. Be aware of the signs of infection, such as foul discharge, a fever over 100.4°F, or chills.

GETTING TESTED AFTER RECURRENT PREGNANCY LOSS

If you have had only one miscarriage, you do not need a complete pregnancy loss workup. After your second or third miscarriage, it's time to take a closer look at the possible causes.

Some tests should be done once you have reestablished your cycle. The amount of time it can take to complete the array of tests differs from woman to woman, but most testing can be done within one to two months. You should have:

- *A profile of your chromosomes and your partner's chromosomes, called a karyotype,* to look for chromosomal problems that may have caused the miscarriages.
- *A complete blood count (CBC)* should be done once the miscarriage is completely over. This is done to detect anemia, because some anemias are associated with pregnancy loss. Pernicious anemia is a vitamin B_{12} deficiency that occurs when you can't absorb B_{12}. Injections of B_{12} can correct the problem. The most common cause of anemia, iron deficiency, is not associated with pregnancy loss.
- *An ultrasound and a hysterosalpingogram (HSG) or a saline hysterosonogram* to evaluate your uterus for an anomaly, such as a uterine septum. (See Chapter 3.)
- *Thrombophilia tests* for blood clotting disorders, which can be implicated in pregnancy loss. These should be done once your beta hCG levels are back to normal, indicating that you are no longer pregnant. Pregnancy can interfere with some of these studies.

- *Testing for luteal phase defect.* (See Chapter 3.)
- *A day three FSH/LH/estradiol test.* No matter how old you are, you should have this test if you are having recurrent miscarriages. Among those women for whom no cause of repeat miscarriage can be identified, some will ultimately find that their ovaries were failing. Luteinizing hormone (LH), the hormone that stimulates ovulation, is potentially important even for ovulatory women who have recurrent miscarriage, because a higher LH level is associated with an increased incidence of chromosomal mistakes, which can bring about miscarriage. Recurrent miscarriage can also be a sign of perimenopause.
- *Fasting blood glucose* (fasting blood sugar) to rule out diabetes.

Having a miscarriage ruins the excitement that you have when you find out that you are pregnant. The first time I found out that I was pregnant, I was completely excited. We went to the doctor, and there was no heartbeat. I couldn't believe how devastating it was. From that time on, when I got pregnant, which happened continually, they would draw the blood, and I knew right away that something was wrong. My numbers kept going up, but not the way they should go up. It became torturous. I had to choose between having a D&C and waiting to see if the pregnancy just stopped on its own. I think about it now, and my heart starts to ache. Everyone tells you, "You're just a little bit older. It's going to work. It's going to be okay." I was pregnant. I wasn't pregnant. This went on continuously. I could never tell my son what was going on, but he knew Mommy was crying and upset. It invades every aspect of your life. I had two bedrooms upstairs. Do I turn one into an office or a nursery? Every time I walked into that extra room, I would think, what am I doing? My oldest son had tons of clothes and toys. Do I throw them out or pack them away? It got to the point that every single closet in my house was completely filled with his clothes and his toys in preparation for this baby who was not coming. So every closet door you open, you ask, "Am I moving on, or am I not moving on?"

I pursued a miscarriage specialist who spent an hour and a half with me and basically told me it was bad luck and that there's no problem. To satisfy me, he did all the blood work, and lo and behold, they found two abnormalities in my blood that were clotting problems and so in all likelihood those were the reasons why I was having all these miscarriages. At that point, the infertility doctor who I was working with said, "Well, let's put you on heparin, which prevents your blood from clotting at the beginning of IVF. You can't just be on heparin indefinitely waiting to try to get pregnant naturally." The miscarriage specialist didn't want to do it, because academically my problem should cause a miscarriage at ten to twelve weeks, and I kept having a miscarriage at six to eight weeks. I said I don't care about the academics, if it's only a difference between being on heparin for six extra weeks. I don't want to keep going through this. If you are going to do it, you might as well go full force, and we did. We got pregnant with the twins. I was on heparin for the whole pregnancy, and I had two healthy babies.

—SARI

INTRAVENOUS IMMUNOGLOBULIN THERAPY (IVIG)

IVIG is a very controversial issue in infertility care. Immunoglobulin is a blood product that contains antibodies pooled from screened donors' plasma. Antibodies are proteins that help the body fight viruses, bacteria, and other pathogens. Much like any blood product, immunoglobulin is transfused into a vein. (Immunoglobulin is not associated with the same risks of red blood cell transfusions.) Doctors using IVIG theorize that pregnancy has a protected immunological status and that special blocking antibodies prevent a woman's body from attacking her developing embryo. Theoretically, if a woman doesn't have these blocking antibodies, she will reject her pregnancy. That's where the use of IVIG comes in to strengthen the immune system. Some studies suggest that the therapy may play a positive role in controlling miscarriage, but it has not been recommended by the American College of Obstetrics and Gynecology or England's Royal College of Obstetrics and Gynecology. At this point, it is still an experimental therapy.

IVIG is both extremely expensive, costing around $3,000 a treatment, and in short supply. It's used to treat people with diseases of immunosuppression. If you are considering IVIG, you may be wrestling with an ethical issue when you consider that its benefit is unproven and people with genuine immunosuppression need it to stay alive.

ECTOPIC PREGNANCY

Normally, a fertilized egg, or embryo, should pass through the fallopian tube into the uterus, where it implants and develops. With ectopic pregnancy, the embryo begins to grow outside the uterus. Although the most common place for ectopic pregnancy to develop is within the fallopian tube, ectopic pregnancies can rarely occur in the abdomen, in an ovary, or in cervical tissue.

Undetected, ectopic pregnancies are potentially life threatening. As the pregnancy develops and gets bigger, it expands the walls of the tube (if present in a fallopian tube), causing the fallopian tube to rupture. If the tube bursts, severe hemorrhaging, shock, and even death can result. Complications of a nontubal ectopic pregnancy usually involve surface bleeding rather than tubal rupture. In the end, any ectopic pregnancy can result in hemorrhagic shock from blood loss.

Although ectopic pregnancies are not usually counted as recurrent pregnancy loss, they do, of course, cause pregnancy loss and are more common not only in women with tubal problems but in women who have had multiple uterine miscarriages. Infertility doctors often underestimate the frequency of ectopic pregnancies in their patients. It's my own bias that if somebody has had a number of pregnancy losses, it's more likely that one or two of those losses will be an ectopic pregnancy. The pregnancy losses will have caused multiple traumas to that woman's uterus, making her uterus less hospitable than her fallopian tubes and raising the chance of an implantation in the tube rather than in the uterus. People at risk for ectopic pregnancies include with women with:

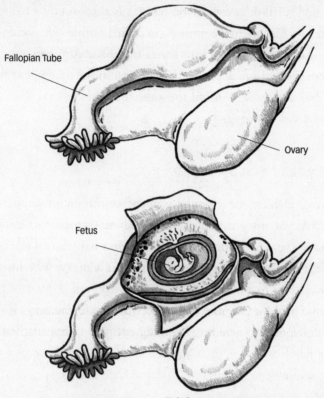

Fallopian Tube

Ovary

Fetus

FIGURE 12. *Tubal ectopic pregnancy*

- History of PID;
- Tubal blockage or damage;
- Previous tubal procedures;
- Reversal of tubal ligation;
- Congenital abnormalities in the tube caused by DES exposure;
- IUD use (Technically, an IUD can put you at risk of an ectopic pregnancy because IUD use increases your risk of tubal disease. You are also much more likely to have an ectopic pregnancy with IUD use if you get pregnant with the IUD in place.);
- Recurrent pregnancy loss.

If you have had tubal disease and you have IVF, there is still a risk of ectopic pregnancy. Although the embryo is placed within the uterus, it is possible for it to move upward into the fallopian tube. When your tube isn't damaged, the embryo will move back down in the uterus, but with a damaged tube, it may stay inside the tube, developing into an ectopic pregnancy, if not detected early.

Warning Signs of Ectopic Pregnancy

Before you can identify the warning signs of an ectopic pregnancy, you must know that you are pregnant, which, with an ectopic, isn't always as easy as it seems, even if you have been trying. You might have some bleeding around the time of your expected period, but it may not be like your normal period. Two to three weeks later, you may notice onset of pelvic pain, especially pain that is more one-sided than usual. You may also have signs of early pregnancy, including being more tired or premenstrual than

WARNING SIGNS OF AN ECTOPIC PREGNANCY

- You had some bleeding around the time you would have had your period, but not normal bleeding.
- When your beta hCG or progesterone levels are checked, they are low for your stage of pregnancy or not rising appropriately. For instance, a progesterone level of less than 20 nanograms is sometimes associated with an ectopic pregnancy. Beta hCG levels that are not doubling at least every two to three days can be another sign of an abnormal pregnancy.
- Bleeding or spotting through the early weeks of pregnancy.
- Pain, especially on one side or the other.
- Dizziness.
- Shoulder pain.

usual, or having nausea. Soon you may develop pelvic pain. In the late stages of an ectopic, you may notice shoulder pain, which is caused by bleeding into the peritoneal cavity. The bleeding actually irritates your diaphragm (the muscle system that helps you breathe), but you will perceive it as shoulder pain. As you lose blood internally, you may feel as though you are going to pass out whenever you get up suddenly.

If recognized early, ectopic pregnancy can be resolved. If you think you may be pregnant and you are at risk for an ectopic pregnancy, or you have a period that is not normal, see your doctor. Today, ultrasound and very sensitive pregnancy tests allow your doctor to detect a developing pregnancy through transvaginal ultrasound. When a measurement known as your beta hCG level is over 2,000, your doctor should be able to see a cystic structure (the developing pregnancy) in your uterus. When no such structure is visible at these levels, an ectopic pregnancy may be the reason.

Treating Ectopic Pregnancy

If caught early, ectopic pregnancies can be treated with methotrexate. Although methotrexate is excellent for treating ectopic pregnancies, you must not be exposed to this drug when you have a viable pregnancy. It will not end a uterine pregnancy with any certainty, and it will cause birth defects. Therefore you and your doctor should be absolutely sure that your pregnancy is *outside of the uterus* before using methotrexate. This is why many physicians strongly believe that before being treated with methotrexate, a woman with a pregnancy outside the uterus should have a D&C to evacuate her uterus and to make sure the pregnancy is extrauterine (outside the uterus), that is, ectopic.

Many doctors make the mistake of considering pregnancy as if it were an infectious disease and methotrexate as if it were an antibiotic. It cannot be overemphasized that methotrexate is a terrible drug for intrauterine as opposed to extrauterine pregnancy. It's ineffective and it causes birth defects. The use of methotrexate in the setting of "Maybe it's an ectopic or maybe it's a bad intrauterine pregnancy" is inappropriate, sloppy, and generally bad medicine. If your doctor cannot assure you that you have an extrauterine pregnancy, then do not take methotrexate.

Once an ectopic is confirmed, you can be treated with methotrexate, which is effective in one dose about 80 percent of the time. The dose can be repeated if your beta hCG level is not cut in half within a week's time.

Very rarely, a woman can develop a pregnancy in the fallopian tube and in the uterus. This is known as heterotopic pregnancy. Normally, it is so rare that it is not even entertained when resolving a diagnosis of ectopic pregnancy, but whenever a woman has taken fertility drugs or has had IVF, a pregnancy of this kind must be considered, because fertility drugs cause multiple ovulations. Certainly, a woman with a heterotopic pregnancy is not a candidate for methotrexate and should instead have surgery to remove the pregnancy in her fallopian tube. Often, a surgeon will remove the entire tube (salpingectomy), because methotrexate can't be used in the event that there is residual pregnancy in the tube after a less aggressive surgery.

Unfortunately, there is nothing than can be done to save an ectopic pregnancy, except in the case of heterotopic pregnancy. Removing the fallopian tube with the ectopic pregnancy will not usually impair the pregnancy in the uterus.

Surgery is another way to treat an ectopic pregnancy—either by removing the entire tube with a salpingectomy or by removing the pregnancy through an incision in the tube in a procedure called salpingostomy. Most ectopic pregnancies are treated with a minimally invasive surgery called laparoscopy, although a laparotomy (a major operation) may become necessary, depending on the complexity of the surgery.

If your fallopian tube has ruptured, it may have to be removed. While it would be rare to have residual pregnancy after the total removal of the fallopian tube, it's not uncommon after the more conservative approach of salpingostomy, because the idea of the surgery is to remove the ectopic pregnancy with minimal trauma to the tube. Often residual tissue resolves by itself, or it can be treated with methotrexate. Rarely, a second operation is performed to remove the residual tissue.

Getting Pregnant after an Ectopic Pregnancy

If your other tube is in good condition, your chances are still better than fifty-fifty that you will get pregnant again after an ectopic pregnancy and that you will have an intrauterine pregnancy. About 85 percent of women having conservative surgery—that is, surgery wherein the pregnancy but not the tube is removed—have open tubes after surgery, and about 70 percent have a pregnancy thereafter. Eighty percent of these pregnancies are in the uterus. The risk of a second ectopic after conservative surgery is about 20 percent. One study found that resolving a pregnancy with methotrexate is also associated with an approximately 85 percent rate of open tubes and an 89 percent rate of conception after surgery. Ten percent of those pregnancies were ectopic.[1]

As you can see, the risk of a second ectopic pregnancy still remains, because the problems that led to the ectopic, such as damage to or a defect in the tube, may have also affected your other tube. You should be monitored for another ectopic pregnancy, but you can start trying again as soon as you ovulate.

Your Emotions After an Ectopic Pregnancy

Ectopic pregnancy loss often gets overlooked as a source of emotional pain and grief. If you experienced a medical crisis as a result of your ectopic pregnancy, you and the important people in your life may have initially focused on your medical crisis and treatments. Your loved ones may have experienced a mixture of emotions, including fear and relief. At first, the potential threat to your life may overshadow the loss of your pregnancy. Doctors don't always provide the same support to women who have lost ectopic pregnancies as they do to couples who go through miscarriage, because they tend to get so caught up in treating this potentially life-threatening condition that they overlook the disappointment of losing an expected child. As with family members, doctors too may be relieved that you will recover.

The disconnection between your own feelings and the feelings of those around you may lead you to experience a certain amount of emotional confusion. The loss of anticipated pregnancy often brings grief, anger, and disappointment. Not only do you lose a potential child when you have an ectopic pregnancy, you experience an abrupt loss of all of the excitement, hopes, and dreams that surround the news of a pregnancy. Adding to your pain may be the knowledge that once you've had an ectopic pregnancy, you are more likely to have a second ectopic, a fact that can make the prospect of getting pregnant again troubling, if not actually frightening. Thinking that you may not be able to get pregnant again can also be devastating.

Some women wonder why they had an ectopic pregnancy and if there was anything that they could have done to prevent it. Most ectopic pregnancies are spontaneous and happen as complete surprises. Often there isn't any known preexisting tubal disease or even any tubal disease seen at the time of treatment. Even if there is tubal disease, it is a disease, not something that you caused or asked for. You may have some or none of these feelings, or you may experience them later on. There is no one right way to feel after an ectopic pregnancy, and each person must approach her loss in her own way.

Others may not understand what you are feeling. Your partner may feel differently than you. He or she may have seemed to have "moved on" more quickly than you. Sometimes it happens that partners hide their emotion, either because it's not comfortable for your partner to express feelings or because your partner wants to help you by shielding you from his or her feelings.

Just as everyone responds to pregnancy loss in his or her own unique way, each person may choose a different method of dealing with grief. You may want to speak with a grief counselor, talk with a supportive friend or clergyperson, talk with a therapist, read about ectopic pregnancy or miscarriage, or visit a bereavement group or an online support group. Make sure that you treat yourself well, giving yourself what you need to help you heal physically and emotionally.

There are few words to describe the traumatic nature of repeated miscarriage or loss due to an ectopic pregnancy. Each woman, and each couple, must decide whether or not to keep trying to get pregnant after recurrent losses. But if this is happening to you, make sure that you have had a thorough evaluation before making your decision. There may be a discernible cause of your losses, and it may be possible to treat that cause and succeed. It's always important to make sure that everything that could be done was done to treat your infertility. Talk to your doctor about tests and treatments that may be right for you and persist until you are satisfied that you can make your decision without regret.

11 | Multiple Pregnancy and Multifetal Reduction

OFTEN, THE RISK OF HAVING A MULTIPLE PREGNANCY—
that is, a pregnancy with many fetuses—is the last thing a woman or couple thinks about at the outset of infertility treatment. This chapter is intended for people facing this situation, but should be read by anyone considering IVF or ovarian stimulation, as there is a relationship between multiple pregnancy and stimulating multiple ovulations and transferring more than one embryo for implantation during IVF.

In the past, when IVF was just coming into use and pregnancy rates with IVF were very low, it was not uncommon for doctors to put back as many embryos as they could in the hopes of achieving a pregnancy and, frankly, building up a clientele for an IVF program. Fortunately, these days are coming to an end, and IVF programs are becoming more responsible about the number of embryos they transfer at one time for a given patient. Still, many women and couples pregnant with higher-order multiples, including quintuplets, quadruplets, triplets, and even twins, continue to need information about the risks and realities of multiple pregnancy.

FEELINGS ABOUT MULTIPLE PREGNANCY AND MULTIFETAL REDUCTION

Multifetal reduction (also called fetal reduction) is one of the most difficult issues in infertility treatment. It's not possible to underestimate the tragedy of a situation in which after having gone through so much to get pregnant, you find yourself pregnant with multiple fetuses, having to choose between two very difficult options to help improve the chance that your children will be born healthy: terminating some of the pregnancies to give the others an opportunity to develop to term or carrying the pregnancy with the best possible obstetrical care in hopes of getting far enough along to have healthy deliveries. Undoubtedly, neither you nor your partner ever wanted to have to make these painfully difficult choices.

A decision about multifetal reduction can never be made solely on the basis of facts. This is truly a decision of the heart, one that is made out of love and concern. Women and couples facing this situation must weigh their emotions, intuition, and knowledge with their religious, spiritual, and/or ethical beliefs to choose the path that is right for them.

Mixed emotions about carrying more than one fetus are very normal. These can be tentative pregnancies. As time goes on, a woman may lose the pregnancy or find out that some of the pregnancies have spontaneously reabsorbed. Fear, anxiety, guilt, and grief are all natural reactions to knowing that you are carrying multiples and certainly to losing a much-wanted pregnancy. The grief one feels at pregnancy loss is intensely private and profound. No one can tell you how to feel or what is wrong or right, because this is your experience, your life. Many people with multiple pregnancies call on or reconnect with their sources of spiritual support or support from loved ones. You may also want to reach out to groups that can connect you with people who have had to face a similar decision. (See Resources.) Be kind to yourself and remember that you are a human being, given to complex and varied emotions. You are doing the best you can to cope with an intensely painful life challenge.

FACING THE RISKS OF MULTIPLE PREGNANCY

In multiple pregnancies, called higher order multiples, there are both risks to the fetuses and to the women carrying them. The more fetuses you are carrying, the more risks there are.

Risks to the Infants

Prematurity and low birth weights are the most significant risks to a fetus in a higher-order multiple pregnancy. The greater the number of fetuses in the pregnancy, the greater chance there is of premature delivery. A child who is born prematurely isn't as fully developed as an infant born at term and faces a number of health challenges that can have lifelong repercussions. Babies who are born prematurely have a greater risk of getting sick and dying than other babies. After delivery, they may have to spend time in the neonatal intensive care unit (NICU). They may develop breathing problems, such as respiratory distress syndrome, lower respiratory tract infection, bleeding into the brain (intraventricular hemorrhage), retinopathy (blindness), hearing loss, or feeding intolerance, which can prevent them from getting adequate nutrition. Premature infants are more likely to have cerebral palsy and cognitive development issues, including mental retardation. Aside from the emotional anguish of having a child in the NICU, the financial costs can be devastating, even if you have insurance.

The average birth weight of a twin is 5.2 pounds, of a triplet, 3.7 pounds, and of a quadruplet, 2.9 pounds. Their average length of stay in neonatal intensive care is eighteen, thirty, and fifty-eight days, respectively. Twins have a fourfold increased risk of cerebral palsy, and the risk of a major disability for triplets is 20 percent and for quadruplets 50 percent.[1]

Fortunately, there have been improvements in care for premature infants in recent years. One of the most important is the introduction of surfactant to help premature infants breathe. Surfactant is a natural substance composed of proteins and fats that help prevent the small air sacs in the lungs, called alveoli, from collapsing during exhalation. Because premature infants don't have enough of their own surfactant, replacing surfactant can help newborns breathe more easily.

Risks to the Mother

Physical risks to the mother carrying multiples can include premature labor and delivery, pregnancy-induced hypertension or preeclampsia (toxemia), and diabetes. Hypertensive disorders in pregnancy are associated with blood clotting disorders as well.

Vaginal or uterine hemorrhages are also possibilities, because a uterus that is overly expanded with multiple pregnancies is less likely to contract after delivery than a uterus carrying a single pregnancy. The more placentas you have, the more likely one of them will be over the cervix. This is called *placenta previa*. When you have complete placenta previa, you must have a cesarean delivery. When the placenta covers the cervix only partially, a fetus can slip by, but a lot of caution must be taken. Another potential problem with placenta previa is that placentas that implant low in the uterus are more likely to implant deeply in the uterine wall. Because the uterine wall is thinner at the bottom than at the top, you are more at risk for what's known as *placenta accreta*, in which a placenta invades the wall of the uterus. These types of placentas often necessitate a hysterectomy after delivery and are sometimes associated with severe problems in pregnancy, such as severe blood pressure problems or blood clotting disorders of pregnancy.

Generally, cesarean section is likely with higher-order multiples such as triplets and quadruplets, and certainly breast-feeding can be an additional challenge, although it can be done. The care of a good maternal fetal medicine specialist (MFM), either alone or in consultation with your ob-gyn, can reduce or even eliminate some of these problems (see page 276).

The Risk of Losing Your Pregnancy

When you are carrying multiple fetuses, there is a risk that you could lose the entire pregnancy. It doesn't make the decision any easier to know that multifetal reduction itself can cause the loss of the entire pregnancy, with the risk being about 9 to 18 percent. This means that, generally speaking, if there were ten women with multifetal pregnancies in precisely the same situation, between one and two of them would lose their entire pregnancy after multifetal reduction. If you choose to have a multifetal reduction, it's imperative that you choose a doctor with extensive experience doing multifetal reduction. Such a doctor may have better statistics, but we will talk about this later in the chapter.

IF YOU ARE EXPECTING MULTIPLES: WHAT TO DO

It can take time to absorb the news that you are carrying more than one fetus. Sometimes, you may receive this information gradually at successive sonograms (ultrasounds). If you think you may be carrying more than one child, you can begin to gather information by talking to specialists who help couples with high-risk pregnancies with multifetal reduction and who care for infants born prematurely. Your reproductive endocrinologist should refer you to a *maternal fetal medicine specialist* (MFM), also called a perinatologist. An MFM is a board-certified obstetrician-gynecologist with two to three additional years of education and clinical experience in the obstetrical medical, surgical, and genetic complications of pregnancy. These additional years of training beyond medical school, internship, and residency are called a fellowship. An MFM should always be fellowship trained. Board-certified obstetricians and gynecologists are very well qualified to take care of single births (called singletons) and even twins. But when it comes to high-risk pregnancies, ob-gyns should consult with maternal fetal medicine specialists. Indeed, there are not enough maternal and fetal specialists to treat everyone on a one-to-one basis, but even if you cannot be treated individually, your ob-gyn can still consult with an MFM to develop a plan of care.

Unfortunately, many ob-gyns advertise themselves as high-risk obstetricians without having had fellowship training. One of the reasons doctors can do this with relative impunity is that the risks of a bad outcome are already high. Within these risks, the doctor's failure may go undetected. But in fact, a true specialist can make a major difference in the outcome of your pregnancy. At the end of this section, you will find a list of questions to ask when selecting an MFM.

You will also want to see a neonatologist. These are fellowship-trained pediatricians who care for sick or premature newborns. The neonatologist can tell you more about the effect of prematurity from a multiple pregnancy and the outcomes of those pregnancies. You may want to ask to tour the neonatal intensive care unit (NICU).

When seeking opinions about whether to carry a multifetal pregnancy or to reduce the pregnancy, you may need to consult two different MFMs. It is certainly fair to ask them what percentage of the patients they counsel go on to reduce or carry their pregnancies.

Considering Multifetal Reduction

Very accomplished physicians can differ in their opinions about when multifetal reduction is advisable. Most agree that, from a medical perspective, reduction is advisable when a woman is carrying quintuplets or more. Having a multifetal reduction from five fetuses to two will unquestionably improve the chance that you will get further along in your pregnancy and deliver healthy children. Most recommend reduction with quadruplets, but even some noted physicians reserve judgment here.

If You Are Pregnant with Quadruplets

It can be painful to read, but quadruplets and other higher-order multifetal pregnancies fare less well than other multiple births, such as triplets and twins. The risk of losing the entire pregnancy without reduction is greater with quadruplets. Quadruplets also are more likely to be premature, to need neonatal intensive care, to have disabilities, and to die before one year of age. Because of the potential risks, couples may elect to reduce the number of quadruplets to twins in the hopes of giving two of the fetuses a chance at a better outcome. Experienced MFMs have had success bringing quadruplets to thirty-four or thirty-five weeks. (A term delivery is anywhere from thirty-seven to forty weeks.) If you are pregnant with quadruplets, it is imperative that you see an MFM with long, demonstrable experience in caring for quadruplets, someone who will see you often and act quickly if problems arise.

If You Are Pregnant with Triplets

The use of multifetal reduction to improve outcomes for triplets is controversial. Citing the risks of prematurity and disabilities, as well as the potential risk of losing the pregnancy because you are carrying multiples, some physicians recommend reduction. On the other hand, physicians who specialize in obstetrical care of triplets do not broadly recommend reduction, adding that these recommendations are individualized for each person's medical and other needs. Within this controversy, some physicians feel that reduction does not necessarily eliminate the risk of prematurity or of losing the entire pregnancy. As we discuss below, even with multifetal reduction, there is still a risk of losing the pregnancy. Here again, the best thing to do is to gather resources from reputable specialists and consider your individual medical needs, your personal, religious, and spiritual beliefs, your desires, and your intuition about what is best for you.

If You Are Pregnant with Twins

Even more controversial than multifetal reduction for triplets is the recent extension of fetal reduction to twins, who are statistically more at risk for negative outcomes than single babies. This approach is indeed highly controversial, with some physicians citing the need to minimize risks of long-term health consequences to infants and others seeing no medical necessity for multifetal reduction with twins. As with every decision concerning multifetal reduction, you and your partner are the only people who can make this intensely personal choice. Personally, if both pregnancies appear to be normal, and there is no unusual maternal risk factor, I discourage the reduction of twins.

The Daily Challenge of Raising Multiples

Certainly, everyone facing the prospect of delivering multiples thinks seriously about what life will be like raising more than one child at a time.

No one can say exactly what your life will be like raising multiple children. One of the best things you can do to imagine what life might be like is to meet parents of multiples and find out how they manage day to day. Fortunately, there are good support groups for parents of multiples. Mothers of Supertwins (MOST) can put you in touch with people who are raising multiples. They can also put you in touch with people who have had children with a range of medical needs, from no or very minimal medical issues to ongoing challenges. If this or other organizations appeal to you, it may be worth your while to become a member.

There are a lot of myths about raising multiples. Many people have the misconception that raising higher-order multiples will be easier than having one child after the other because parents can get everything done at the same time. Some people are told that parents of multiples receive free products from companies. These are indeed misconceptions. Raising a number of same-age children all together can be very tough, and community resources for parents differ widely, with some people finding a tremendous amount of support and care from their communities and religious organizations and others finding little or no support.

Having a single child changes the dynamics of your entire life and your marriage or relationship. Having multiples can change your life even more profoundly and may put an excessive strain on couples. Almost every woman will need outside help, even during pregnancy when bed rest may be recommended. You may need more physical support from your partner than usual. Women and men often differ in their fears, anxieties, hopes, and concerns about the pregnancy. It can help to air your thoughts in a nonjudgmental way so that everyone's feelings can be heard and understood. Couples may want to talk with a therapist or counselor experienced in working with couples with infertility and multifetal pregnancies. (You can find more information about choosing a therapist in Chapter 14.)

Finances can be a major issue. In addition to the costs of having a child in the NICU and possible complications associated with a high-risk pregnancy, parents of multiples find themselves facing the enormous costs of raising more than one child into adulthood. There are costs of food, clothing, education, and children's usual needs. When a child has a disability, there may be additional costs of medical care and support. Children who are born prematurely may have educational needs that should be addressed early in life. Someone with cerebral palsy and other lifelong disabilities will face different issues as a teen and as an adult than someone without disabilities.

Many couples being treated for infertility and indeed many expecting multiples are not aware of the long-term repercussions of having twins, triplets, quadruplets, or more. This is not to say that everyone will have a difficult time. There are many, many people who are proud and happy parents of multiples. Again, try to touch base with people who can talk to you honestly about what to expect. Look for an organization that meets your needs and can put you in touch with people with a range of experiences. (See Resources for more information.)

As a professional, I know the morbidity and mortality with multiples. It's what I do. I'm a neonatal nurse practitioner, and I know the risks are enormous. If multifetal reduction is going to lower maternal or fetal risk, as a professional, I feel strongly about it in higher-order multiples. As a mother of quadruplets, an individual, and as someone with my own moral issues, I'm conflicted. It's very easy for me to give advice as a professional. But on a personal level, I want to tell people what the risk factors are, what might happen. I want people to be educated, to be able to let them make their own choice.

Visit a NICU, and take a tour. In my twenty-year career as a practitioner, I've seen at least ten sets of quads. Two of them of have been perfectly "normal" sets, and one of them is mine. The biggest problems with multiples are prematurity and low birth weight. The more fetuses you are carrying, the lower the birth weight of the children you are going to have and the more problems they are going to have. Then there are the financial costs. I had resources. I had an educational background that allowed me to find the best doctors. There are a lot of people who don't have these resources.

Everybody thinks the children are cute, and initially people are there to help you, but then everybody gets tired and goes home. You don't sleep. I didn't for three years. Women face anxiety and depression disorders.

This is a lifelong process. You don't think about safety issues. You don't think about how you are going to get them to the doctor's when there are three and four and five of them. How are you going to take a walk with a stroller? How are you going to feed them? Even after all of the physical tests and normal things that you go through with baby diapers and feedings, you have preschool issues, you have elementary school issues, and psychosocial issues related to their sense of individuality. Every single task of daily living is multiplied. Because everything is task driven, I think it impacts on them emotionally.

The pregnancy did a lot of damage to my body. I was very sick afterward. I was rehospitalized after I had them. I had to have surgery two years after I had them. Even after a hernia repair and a tummy tuck, I still have unbelievable stretch marks. I have not been a healthy person since. Much of this has to do with stress levels and lack of sleep and going in too many places at one time. I'm really blessed to have my kids. They're my miracles. I just think that people are very naive when they think that this is going to be easy.
— TRICIA

CHOOSING A MATERNAL FETAL MEDICINE SPECIALIST

It's absolutely mandatory that you trust the doctor who will help you. If you are considering carrying your pregnancy, choose someone who has a good reputation and long experience caring for multiples. You don't want to be your doctor's second or third patient with triplets or quadruplets. As mentioned, an MFM will often serve as consultant to your regular ob-gyn rather than as your primary doctor. But if you are planning to carry your pregnancy, find out if there is any possibility that the MFM can be your primary care physician and whether that physician will accept your insurance. When choosing an MFM, ask:

- How many of these procedures have you done?
- How many patients do you see yearly?
- How many of your patients have elected to carry their multiple pregnancies?
- How many sets of quadruplets, triplets (or the number of fetuses you are carrying) have you personally delivered in your career?
- What are your statistics? In other words, ask, What are your average gestational outcomes? That is, on average, how many weeks' gestation do you usually achieve for the number of fetuses I am carrying? Don't settle for a percentage. Ask for a numerator and a denominator. That is, how many pregnancies did the doctor care for? Out of that number, how many achieved the gestational age you are being quoted? For example, one out of two may be 50 percent, but it's a lot less impressive than one hundred out of two hundred cases seen.
- What is my long-term goal in weeks? When is my exact due date?
- At what point in my pregnancy will you be proactive in sustaining my pregnancy? What are some of the things I can do to help sustain my pregnancy?
- How many multifetal reductions have you done that resulted in healthy

live births? How many of the pregnancies you have reduced were lost entirely? Here, the number should be commensurate with the overall rate of loss, which is 9 to 18 percent. If a doctor gives you better odds, you should be suspicious unless the physician is able to give you specific numbers, such as the number of multifetal reductions performed and the exact number of losses. Physicians who are truly expert may be able to do this.

- Do you accept my insurance?
- At which hospital do you have privileges?
- What will happen if I have to go to the hospital on an emergency basis? Will you or my ob-gyn be able to provide care?
- What would you do in my position?
- What would you do if this happened in your family?

HAVING A MULTIFETAL REDUCTION

Generally, it's not possible to know if your fetuses will be affected by the problems that we have discussed. There are sonographic (ultrasound) markers for Down syndrome that may be seen at eleven weeks. Doctors who do multifetal reductions should also do prenatal testing beforehand, with chorionic villus sampling (CVS), in an effort to determine if one or more of the fetuses has a chromosomal problem. Your doctor will do CVS in conjunction with FISH (fluorescent in situ hybridization), a molecular test to look for problems like Down syndrome. You should know the next day if you have a fetus with chromosomal problems. This may then be the fetus that you choose to reduce.

How the Procedure Is Done

Multifetal reduction is done at eleven weeks of pregnancy. Under sonographic guidance (ultrasound), a needle is passed through the fetus's gestational sac either through your abdomen or vagina. A small amount of potassium chloride is then injected into the chest cavity of the fetus or fetuses. Potassium chloride is a chemical that stops the heartbeat.

Maternal fetal medicine specialists are trained to do the procedure and also to care for high-risk pregnancies. Reproductive endocrinologists are trained to help couples conceive. For many reasons, not the least of which is emotional, the reproductive endocrinologist does not usually do this procedure. This procedure is profoundly difficult for the woman and couple, and the reproductive endocrinologist is acutely aware of this. Everything in medicine has a complication rate, and even when complications are unavoidable, doctors feel bad, although they may not show it. Having to do the procedure may be very hard on the doctor as well, and so a referral to someone who is experienced in the procedure and uninvolved in your fertility care is best.

In this chapter, we looked at one of the most difficult issues in infertility and obstetrical care. Ironically, the problem of higher-order multiple pregnancy more frequently arises in patients who have been unable to conceive. As always, the best treatment is prevention, and the future holds great promise for the development of single-embryo transfer. In the Conclusion, we will talk about improvements in fertility care on the horizon. In Chapter 12, we will talk about third-party reproduction. This can also be a difficult issue for many women and couples to face, as it may involve changes in the course of your care and contemplating letting go of the idea of having children in the manner that you may have initially hoped. Although it's an emotional topic, it's one about which you should be informed so that, should it become an option, you will have had time to consider all of the factors involved in making this decision, which will have lifelong repercussions for you and your prospective family.

12 | Find Out About Alternatives

THERE ARE TIMES WHEN COUPLES NEED HELP FROM outside parties (third parties) to have children. This can happen when a couple lacks a critical factor in reproduction, such as eggs or sperm, when a member of a couple carries a genetic disorder that he or she does not want to pass on to children, or when a woman does not have a uterus or when there is a severe medical risk in her carrying a child to term. In this chapter, we will talk about issues of third-party reproduction. When we talk about third-party reproduction, we are simply talking about those instances in which you must work with another to achieve your goal of having a child. We will start with the most common issue that arises for people undergoing IVF, and that is the difficult consideration of using donor eggs to get pregnant and carry a child.

DONOR EGGS (OOCYTE DONATION)

As the use of assisted reproduction increases, and women continue to delay having children until later in life, myths about having children after thirty-seven abound. Many, if not most, people have come to believe that it's very possible for a healthy woman to have children in her late thirties and even in her early forties. Truly, more women are choosing to have their families later, but the number of women who can get pregnant with their own eggs and carry to term later in life is much smaller than the percentage of younger women who get pregnant and carry to term. Women are also done a tremendous disservice by stories of celebrities who appear to be having their own biological children past forty. It's likely that most of these people are in fact using donor eggs. Stories of ordinary women who have children well into or even beyond their forties don't help dispel the myths of prolonged fertility either, unless you consider, once again, that these women received donor eggs. If you have delayed parenthood until you were really ready, only to learn that you can't have your own biologically related children, you are by no means alone. Many women who wisely made the choice to grow and mature, develop their careers, look for a loving, responsible mate, or simply work hard to provide security for themselves and their future children are devastated to find out that when the time is finally right, it's too late. On top of this, women are sometimes made to feel guilty for having waited. Unlike men, women often find themselves having to choose between their careers, even their economic survival, and having children during their most fertile years, and as of yet there is little sensitivity to this issue in the workplace. Remember that you did the best you could. You made the choices that were right for you, and you may still have options for creating the family you want. In the near future, it may be possible for a woman to bank and store her eggs, but at the time of this writing this is not yet possible.

After having gradually accepted that they were not going to have children with their own eggs, many women who chose to use donor eggs or adopt have said that they look back on their fertility struggles as part of the process of coming to meet the children with whom they were ultimately meant to be. Some people choose to remain child free, knowing that it is more than possible to have a full and meaningful life without children.

Whatever path you take, it's important that you take time to make a decision. Often, couples tired and desperate from numerous IVF cycles are inclined, through their stress and vulnerability, to move quickly to the donor option. The same may be true for women who find out they have extremely high FSH levels. On the other hand, you may have always known that donor eggs would be an option for you, for example, if you have known that you have premature ovarian failure. Donor eggs may be the right choice for you, but you must be sure, because this decision will affect you for the rest of your life. There are lots of issues to consider, including whether you can come to terms with the loss of a genetic bond with your child, as well as the many other emotional, psychological, spiritual, and financial challenges that choosing to use donor eggs brings.

No Regrets: Making Sure That Everything That Could Be Done Was Done

Before choosing alternatives, many women and couples want to be absolutely certain that they have done everything they could to have a child with their own eggs. They don't want to look back on their decision to move on to other options with doubt or regret.

If your FSH level is very high, say, 25, it's very unlikely that you can have a child with your own eggs. It does not make sense in this instance to attempt IVF. On the other hand, if your levels are borderline, say, 15 or 16, or just beyond borderline, it's not unreasonable to try IVF and prove to yourself that either it will not work or you were one of the handful of people who did succeed with a very high FSH level. If you don't stimulate well enough to produce eggs for IVF, it can be very helpful to you psychologically to have experienced this for yourself by going through ovarian stimulation and literally seeing the result of your stimulation on your ultrasound.

When to stop multiple IVF procedures and move on to donor eggs can be a tricky question. Many people have heard of or known of someone who gave up on IVF and conceived on her own years later. It is true that about 30 percent of those with unexplained infertility will ultimately get pregnant on their own. But as with everything else concerning fertility, age matters. You are much more likely to get pregnant spontaneously with unexplained infertility if you are younger, say, under thirty-five, than if you are older, especially if you are in your forties.

Go Back to Basics: Do You Know if You Have Endometriosis?

If you have blocked or absent fallopian tubes or your partner has a zero sperm count, you cannot get pregnant spontaneously. The decision to quit IVF depends on your age and how your IVF cycles are going. Ask yourself, have you and your doctor looked at all options to allow you to get pregnant? Technology is attractive, and some clinics and doctors focus so tightly on IVF they may overlook basic issues, such as the possibility of endometriosis. I had a patient who was thirty-six. She did a number of cycles of IVF on high doses of fertility medication at a world-famous center,

HAVE YOU HAD ENOUGH?

Deciding to stop treatment depends very much on your personal, emotional, and financial struggles with the procedures you are having. But from a purely medical perspective, you may want to consider the following general rule of thumb, assuming that you have had a basic medical workup and you know that your progesterone levels are good and your fallopian tubes are open.

If you have had three to six cycles of IUI, a laparoscopy to check for endometriosis or pelvic adhesions, then three cycles of IVF at a good program, and things are not looking good, this is the time to think about other options for creating your family or remaining child free.

but her eggs were few and her embryos didn't look good. Yet her tubes were open, and her partner's sperm didn't look too bad. There was no apparent reason why she should not get pregnant, even with this discouraging set of circumstances. I suggested to her that we do a laparoscopy to find out if she had endometriosis. If she did have endometriosis, we could remove it and see if she got pregnant without IVF. It turned out that she did have endometriosis, and once it was removed, she did get pregnant without IVF. Of course, if she had already been treated for endometriosis, and she still had problems with IVF, doing another laparoscopy wouldn't have helped. But the point is that sometimes doctors skip this basic step. If you are doing IVF and not getting pregnant, ask your doctor whether there is anything else you and your doctor can do to find the cause of your unexplained infertility. It may be endometriosis.

Are You Ready to Quit? A Checklist

Before going on to another option, ask yourself:

- Do you really understand the reason for your infertility? Does it make sense to you? Even if your diagnosis is unexplained fertility, you should have done all the necessary fertility tests (see Chapter 3) and should have a clear sense that every diagnosis has been considered. Have you talked to your doctor in depth? If the answer is no, ask your doctor to detail the reasons for your infertility.
- Is the treatment you are receiving competent, sufficient, and thorough? In other words, has your doctor exercised care and skill, and given you all of the testing you need? Have you tried IVF enough times with this doctor to give it a chance to work? Do your doctors think it's a good idea for you to move on at this point, given all the tests and treatments you have had?
- Do you feel that you have no alternative but to quit? Sometimes the emotional, physical, psychological, and financial strain of doing numerous IVF treatments makes it impossible for someone to continue without peril to her mental and financial health, her relationships, and

even her job. If this is you, consider what impact continued IVF treatment is having on your life and whether you won't hurt yourself by going on.

Should You Go to Another IVF Program?

It's not unusual for someone who didn't get pregnant with IVF at one clinic to go to another clinic for treatment. Sometimes, this is a good idea, especially when you don't think you are getting thorough and competent care. But you have to be careful. Some doctors may take advantage of patients who have left one IVF program for another. You must realize from a clinic's point of view, you can be a very lucrative patient. It may hurt to hear this, but it's a reality. Some clinics may see you as vulnerable and as someone who may be willing to gamble against the odds. You may end up having repeated IVF cycles to no avail after your first doctor advised you that you are unlikely to get pregnant with your own eggs. Undoubtedly, you must follow your own inner dictates, and you have a right to choose to follow or not to follow your doctor's advice, but it's best to base your decision on a balanced examination of the facts, something that can be very hard to do when you want a child and are willing to do almost anything to have that child.

Before moving on to another clinic, review our checklist. Make sure you have a clear sense of your fertility status and why going to another clinic could make a difference.

Also, ask yourself whether you have given your doctor enough time to make IVF work for you. Remember, doing IVF is truly like gambling with at best fifty-fifty odds. Some women just need time. This is especially true for younger women who have open fallopian tubes and partners with healthy sperm.

Becoming Informed About Donor Eggs

The cost of donor eggs may be one reason why it's so hard to accept the news that an alternative may be necessary. Donor egg procedures are always costly, running between $20,000 and $25,000, and are not covered by most insurers, making this an option only for those who are either affluent or who are willing to go into debt. This is, of course, very unfair, because infertility is no more voluntary than heart disease or cancer. Unfortunately, these costs are fixed, and there is no way to get around them, because they include the cost of putting the donor through ovarian stimulation and compensating that person for her time and effort. On the other hand, the cost can match that of a domestic infant adoption, but not all adoptions by any means.

Your child will not be genetically related to you, if you are the mother. If you will be using your partner's sperm, then, of course, the child will be genetically related to your partner. For some people, this is a very big issue that requires an open and honest discussion of feelings. We'll talk more about this later in this chapter.

As with any IVF procedure, there is about a fifty-fifty chance that the donor eggs will work. This is why it's important to freeze donor embryos for later transfer should the first IVF cycle with donor eggs fail. The donor will not have to be stimulated again to produce more eggs, and the cost of using frozen embryos will be tremendously lower than your first cycle with donor eggs.

If you do get pregnant with donor eggs, you will be able to experience pregnancy and delivery, and your child will be a newborn. Adoption does not allow you to carry your child or experience childbirth, and you may not always be able to see the child right at delivery, depending on circumstances and the type of adoption you choose. When you use donor eggs, you are able to control all aspects of your pregnancy—the food you eat, your general health care, and the environment you're in. You can't do this with adoption.

Unless you seek a donor on your own or through an egg broker, the donor will likely be completely anonymous. Your child will not be able to meet the donor in later years. Adoption may be anonymous, open, or semi-open, meaning that there are various degrees of contact between the child and the birth mother. Depending on the arrangements you choose, your child may seek out his or her birth mother later in life.

Using donor eggs can be a very stressful experience, perhaps the most stressful event in your adult life. Ask yourself whether you have a good support system, including a good counselor or supportive friends or relatives. You and your partner will need people with whom you can talk and a place to air feelings and concerns.

> *Using donor eggs wasn't as difficult as I thought it would be. My husband had a vasectomy, so we knew we would use donor sperm. My husband was fine with that, and I was fine with that, so I had to ask myself why I wanted to have a child who was genetically my own when I'm telling my husband to use donor sperm, that it's no big deal. And then I thought about the fact that I was planning to adopt, if it didn't work. My adopted child wouldn't be genetically mine, but would still be my child, no matter what. I knew from the day the eggs were implanted that they were mine. There wasn't a day that I said, "Well, you know they don't look like me or they don't have my personality." You could raise six kids and they would all be different.*
>
> —MAXINE

Making a Decision About Donor Eggs

If you have been going through IVF, using donor eggs may seem like a logical extension of IVF, and in some ways it is, but, as suggested, the biggest and most obvious difference is that one parent, namely the mother, will not have a genetic connection to her child. Everyone must confront this issue before agreeing to use donor eggs.

Think about your own family. What characteristics do you cherish in your family members? Of what other features are you less fond? How many of these things are nature (genetics) and how many are nurture (environment)? Are there genetic disorders or illness in your family? Were there fertility issues? Was anyone adopted in your family? How does or did your family handle secrets? Are there cultural issues that make you uncomfortable with the idea of using donor eggs?

Thinking about your own background can help you imagine how you will handle questions that will inevitably arise after you decide to use donor eggs. Whether or not you and your partner will tell anyone that your child was conceived through the use of donor eggs is another difficult question that each member of the couple must confront. Thinking about this is a process. You won't know the answer right away. But ask yourself:

- Will you tell your ob-gyn? Why or why not?
- Have you thought about having amniocentesis? If you are over thirty-five, you may think you need amniocentesis, but it's the age of the egg contributing to the embryo that matters. If your egg donor is young, as she is likely to be, you won't need amniocentesis.
- Will you tell your child's pediatrician? Remember that the pediatric records are your child's records to which he or she could have access later in life.
- Do you and your partner agree on whether or not to disclose this information to anyone?
- If you decide not to tell anyone about your child's genetic origins, you must realize that if one other person knows—your parent, your best friend—there is a chance that your child could find out about his or her genetic origins. This is especially possible when you are using donor eggs from a known donor, whether the donor is a friend or relative or you have an open or semi-open donor relationship. Whether or not to tell is your decision, but you must look at the realities surrounding this decision and remember that your child's well-being should stand at the center of that decision. What will you do if you decide not to tell your child, but your child finds out from someone else? Again, think about how your family has handled secrecy in the past. Was your family open about these types of issues? How did your family's behavior hurt or harm your development?
- Will you tell your child? This, of course, is the big question. For some, it's easily answered. For others, it's not. When deciding when and how to tell your child, you may find talking to an appropriately trained counselor to be very enlightening and useful.

Being Honest with Yourself: How Do You Really Feel About Using Donor Eggs?

Be honest with yourself about your feelings. Don't try to force yourself to accept this alternative, if it's not for you. For some people, the loss of a genetic connection to their child is unacceptable, and that is okay. What matters is your comfort level. Ask yourself:

- How do you really feel about having a child who will be genetically related to your partner but not to you? Sometimes it's helpful to remember that the donor is only providing genetic material. Only when combined with your partner's (or a donor's) sperm does the egg become an embryo. The embryo depends on your body to grow into a baby. You will be the child's mother, raising the child into adulthood.
- How does your partner feel about donor eggs?
- Are you doing this for your partner more than for yourself? It's not unusual for a male partner to drive the decision to use donor eggs (and vice versa). For example, a woman with children who marries a man without children may find he wants a baby more than she does, and it's not unusual for someone in this situation to feel she must please her partner by giving him a child. Women in relationships with women who are using one partner's eggs may have to confront similar issues. Without a doubt, the decision to have a child should be a mutual decision, and these feelings should be brought to the surface and discussed.
- Are there hidden issues, such as blame or guilt, affecting your decision? The emotional issues that arise when the use of donor eggs is an option can sometimes create disagreements in couples. One member of the couple may be angry or blame the other for having to use this option. Like all emotional issues, feelings of anger, resentment, guilt, or blame should be resolved before going forward.
- What do you want in a donor? Someone who looks like you? Someone with a similar racial and ethnic background? Or is a healthy medical and genetic history more or equally important? You and your partner

may want to make separate lists of what's important to you so that you can compare and discuss them in depth.

Getting Counseling

Everyone affected by the decision to use donor eggs should receive counseling to fully understand the long-term psychological, emotional, legal, and financial implications of this decision. This includes you, your partner, and any others who will be directly involved, such as the donor's partner.

When you are vulnerable, as you may be, it's easy not to see all of the ramifications of this difficult decision. Donors should think about what it means to give up a parental relationship with the child and consider what might happen down the line if the child created with her egg is the only child she has. If she has children, will she tell them?

If the donor is a close friend or relative, how will she feel when she is in contact with the child? What are the terms guiding the relationship? If the donor is a stranger, and you are choosing an open or semi-open arrangement, have you given thought to the type of structured relationship you want to have with the donor and that the donor will have with the child? A donor who is a very young woman, for example, in her early twenties, may not fully appreciate the possibility that her feelings toward the child may change over time. As of yet, there is not a lot of data on the success of open and semi-open arrangements.

Your spouse or partner, and the donor's spouse or partner, if applicable, should also be counseled. Your clinic should either have a counselor on site or be able to refer you to one. You can also seek referrals from a good support organization, such as RESOLVE or the American Fertility Association. (See Resources.) Any therapist you choose should be a member of a support organization. In order to counsel you appropriately, the therapist must have a current knowledge of technological advances and the law surrounding these choices. (For more information on questions to ask when choosing a therapist, see Chapter 14.)

Because using door eggs is a step after IVF with your own eggs and because your donor should be a young woman with younger eggs, it's hard to remember that the odds of getting pregnant with donor eggs are the same with IVF under any circumstance, about fifty-fifty. You may have already done many cycles of IVF, or you may just be starting out. Either way, think about how many cycles of IVF with donor eggs you want or can do before you will try another option like adoption.

If you are overwhelmed, that's understandable. You are being given a lot of information and choices that can be very hard to make. Knowing your bottom line can make a difficult process easier. As pointed out earlier, it is easy to become obsessed with getting pregnant and, frankly, for some women, it can be addictive. Always remember the intrinsic inefficiency of reproduction. Even in the best of circumstances, a couple has only a 20 percent chance of getting pregnant each month. Donor eggs are an option, but they are no guarantee. Will you try one cycle with donor eggs before moving to adoption or before thinking about not having children? Will you try additional cycles with frozen embryos? How many frozen cycles will you do before moving on?

The Egg Donor

You may have an image in your mind of the donor as a college student seeking funds for tuition. Although many are students, donors can be any women under thirty-four. Your donor should be of legal age, preferably twenty-one and over. If you do work with a donor in her thirties, you should talk to a genetic counselor about the need for amniocentesis and the effect of the donor's age on your ability to get pregnant with her eggs.

People choose to become donors for various reasons. Usually, the donor is inspired by altruistic reasons. Some are adoptees who want to help couples have children of their own. Some are women who loved their experiences with motherhood, but don't want any more children and don't want their eggs to go to waste; and some are women who don't want children, but don't want to waste their eggs. I've met donors who had friends who suffered from infertility and wanted to help others with the same problem as well as women who have donated organs, too. The reasons for wanting to donate eggs differ, and although women are compensated, they rarely mention money as the chief reason for wanting to do this.

There are two schools of thought about whether women who donate eggs should have had a child previously. Those who see this as a desirable characteristic reason that having had a child proves the donor's fertility. The other school of thought feels that since natural fertility doesn't necessarily equate with a good response to fertility drugs, this prerequisite is not only unnecessary, it prevents a lot of women from becoming donors simply because they haven't had their families yet.

Finding and Choosing a Donor

Many IVF programs have their own in-house donor egg programs. There are advantages of using an in-house program. You know the doctor or doctors who run the program and have had a chance to form an opinion about them based on experience. If you work with a doctor you like, you've already established a kind of comfort level and trust that you may not have with a broker.

Egg brokers are middlemen who recruit and connect egg donors and recipients and collect a fee for that service. They are not the providers of the medical service but rather assume the role of agent. This activity has no requirements or qualifications, is not subject to licensure, and is usually significantly more expensive than dealing directly with an IVF center with a donor egg program.

A broker's motivations are not necessarily questionable, but you have to remember that a broker is a salesperson and a middleman. Because the broker takes a fee, it can be more costly to use a broker than an in-house program. Moreover, you don't know this person any better than anyone else, and while you might be comfortable buying something small from someone you don't know, this is a transaction that will affect the rest of your life. As mentioned, there are no criteria that one must meet to become an egg broker. You will have to rely on trust to determine whether egg brokers screen donors. Many times they don't. You have no way of really knowing who the donor is. An advantage may be that the broker program is much more likely to provide videotapes and photographs of the donor, which will make the arrangement less than anonymous. Varied structured degrees of contact between the egg donor and the recipient family can be arranged through semi-open and open egg donation, although most IVF donor programs are anonymous or "closed" with no contact between the donor and recipient. Egg brokers are easy to find on the Internet. But again, the best donor egg programs tend not to use brokers, but have their own donors.

Sometimes couples want to use eggs from someone they know, perhaps a sister or a cousin. This can work out very well provided that all are clear on the level of disclosure desired, keeping in mind that it may be very hard to keep this a secret. Everyone, including the spouse or partner of the donor, should be counseled so that any issues that may impair relationships can be discussed. Coercion is another vital part of this equation. A younger relative, such as a niece, for example, may not feel able to say no to her aunt. Age is important, but power relations are even more important. Someone who is not your peer may not feel comfortable turning you down and should not be put in the position of having to do that. If you ask someone you know to donate her eggs, you must delineate the limits of each person's relationship to the child or risk having social and legal problems in the future. Even in cases where the donor is a friend or relative, there must be a clear written agreement specifying the terms of the arrangement.

In my practice, unless there are special circumstances, we are committed to using anonymous donors, the reason being that we feel that there are a lot of potential problems between people who contract to create a child. It is possible that a donor may want to have more to do with the child than she initially thought or that the child or even the recipients of the donor eggs may want to have more to do with the donor than they originally thought. To be a donor with our program, a woman must fully

BEFORE CHOOSING A DONOR EGG PROGRAM, ASK:

- How long have you been in business?
- How do you recruit donors?
- What screening processes do you employ? How do you screen donors medically, genetically, and psychologically?
- How is drug testing done?
- How much are donors paid?
- Will I be able to see information about the donor written in her own handwriting? Why or why not?
- Will I be able to choose the donor for myself or will the agency make the match?
- Do you provide counseling for all parties involved?
- Are anonymous, semi-open, and open arrangements available?

understand that there is no future relationship with the child or the recipient and that once her eggs are retrieved, her involvement ends. We are not even enthusiastic about telling donors whether or not the recipient conceived with their eggs, and we do not share photographs of donors with recipient families.

What You Should Know About the Donor

You should know the age of your donor, her ethnic background, her height, her hair and eye color, and her educational level. You should know her family history, although this is something virtually impossible to verify for an unknown donor. You should know that the donor has been screened for genetic diseases, and for communicable and infectious diseases, including HIV, hepatitis B, hepatitis C, syphilis, gonorrhea, and chlamydia. The donor should also be tested for drug use and evaluated by a mental health professional. Her personal and sexual history should be known, to screen out people at risk for HIV/AIDS. If she has donated before, you have the right to know how many eggs she produced and whether the other recipients got pregnant.

Later on in this chapter, we discuss sperm donation. Sperm donors are tested; their sperm is frozen and quarantined; and they are retested to make sure that they don't have communicable diseases. You may wonder whether the same procedure is possible for donor eggs. At this point in time, eggs cannot be successfully frozen. Some have suggested that it is possible to test an egg donor, create embryos from the eggs, freeze the embryos, and retest the donor in six months, as well. You should know that the risk of transmission of a communicable or infectious disease via human eggs (oocytes) is very low and that the embryo will not be affected. The real disadvantage of freezing embryos for this purpose is that you miss having a fresh embryo transfer, which is associated with a statistically higher pregnancy rate than frozen embryo transfers. This is not to say that you can't get pregnant with frozen embryos, but you don't want to miss your best chance with fresh embryos. The likelihood of success improves over time, that is, with each transfer you have.

Drug testing is a very important aspect of screening that can directly affect the baby's health. At our clinic, we do drug testing with hair samples rather than with urine specimens, because hair samples are more reliable. There are products on the market people can take to flush drugs out of their systems before urine testing, but these are ineffective with the hair-testing methods we use, where the interior and not just the surface of the follicle is examined. We also follow up on our donors with numerous contacts and may even use a private investigator to pursue any red flags that come up during the selection process.

Couples and women using donor eggs will receive a multiple-paged document in the donor's own handwriting in which she describes her medical history, likes and dislikes, experiences with her family, and other information that will help you make a selection. Some feel that having such an unedited document is important, because you can tell quite a lot about someone from the way she expresses herself. Some clinics type the donor's history, which may create the possibility, intended or not, that the clinic will enhance her profile.

We like to have patients choose their donors. Some clinics will provide matches, but we think that this unnecessarily takes control away from the recipient parents. Having infertility entails so much loss of control that it is nice to be able to regain an aspect of control over the process.

Unfortunately, some clinics and programs that match donors may have too much of a financial incentive to be entirely honest about the criteria used in the match. If a donor program tells you that they found a perfect match, be wary. It may be more of a sales pitch than the truth. It's not easy to read yet another reminder of how perilous these types of trans-actions can be, particularly because this is a time at which you are so vulnerable, but it's best to use caution when making a decision as signifi-cant as this one.

HIGH SAT SCORES AND BLUE EYES: DO THEY REALLY MATTER?

You've probably heard stories of couples searching for the perfect genes, willing to pay exorbitant fees for an egg donor with an Ivy League pedigree, high SAT scores, blond hair and blue eyes, or other prized features. If you are looking for a sperm donor, no doubt you have seen advertisements for sperm from men who have taken on certain professions or achieved an edu-cational feat, such as getting a Ph.D.

When faced with a seeming array of possibilities for choosing a sperm or egg donor, it's tempting to add criteria such as these to your list of needs. Parents tend to want the best for their children, and trying to increase the odds of having a child who will perhaps be more intelligent makes a certain kind of sense, but you must remember that there is no guarantee that you'll have a child with characteristics you hope for. Genetics are not absolute. We all know tall parents with short children or dark-haired parents with fair children. And we all know that SAT scores don't always indicate one's likelihood of success later in life. What really matters is one's ability to learn and to pursue a goal.

While some couples may seek out young women with great achievements, sperm banks directly advertise to women and couples, featuring special specimens from people who might be termed elite donors. So why shouldn't you get "Ph.D. sperm," or sperm from an attorney or doctor for that matter? To my mind, these kinds of marketing ploys are egregious for a number of reasons. In the first place, acquired skills, such as becoming an architect or learning to lift weights, are not passed on genetically. Second, why one might ask, is a doctor or a person who has earned a Ph.D. more valuable than, say, a teacher without a graduate degree? And if we really do agree that certain specimens are more valuable than others, why would sperm banks sell ordinary sperm from ordinary men? It makes a certain amount of genetic and perhaps common sense to want to choose a donor who will give you the best chance of having a child who looks like you, but to try to cultivate characteristics beyond your control does not. Further, it's unfair to place unrealistic expectations on a child because of a supposed genetic endowment.

If you are like most people, you didn't choose your partner for his or her ability to produce a superior child. Like most, you probably just want a healthy child. The purpose of using donor eggs or donor sperm is not to increase the chance of creating an ideal child, if there is such a thing. Using donor eggs does not reduce the overall rate of birth defects, for example, which affect 2 to 4 percent of all children. At our clinic, we no longer provide SAT scores, because we feel that we are in the business of helping people overcome infertility and not of creating specific types of children.

The Donor's Fees

Depending on where she lives, a donor may get anywhere from $5,000 to $8,000 for her eggs. Once upon a time in New York City, the fee used to be $2,500, until a competitor raised the price, and all other IVF programs had to follow suit. Surely, a woman has a right to earn what she can in this process, and no one has a right to say that she should not get the highest price she can for going through ovarian stimulation, ultrasounds, and egg retrieval. On the other hand, when and if the compensation gets higher, one worries about coercion as an element in these arrangements. For instance, could the fees get so high that a woman might feel it is irresponsible of her not to become a donor in order to provide for her family?

Once a donor is selected, the patient will pay the IVF clinic, which will pay the egg donor. Make sure that you know who will pay for medical expenses, including those that may occur beyond what is normally expected. The donor should have her own medical insurance, or she can have payments for temporary insurance deducted from her fee to cover any extra expenses associated with providing donor eggs. Insurance issues become even more important when working with a surrogate or gestational carrier, which we will talk about later in this chapter. Get these agreements in writing.

When You Are Having Trouble Choosing a Donor

Using donor eggs is not for everyone, and it doesn't have to be right for you. Sometimes women and couples find themselves rejecting donor after donor, unable to make a decision. No one seems right. No one is good enough. You may wonder how many donors you should review before you choose the right one.

There will always be some uncertainty. This is the nature of the process. If you find yourself struggling with these issues, you may be wondering if you will come to the conclusion that using donor eggs is the wrong answer for you. It can help to go to another clinic for another view of how using donor eggs works. See how they do things at that clinic. Broaden your perspective so that you can get a feel for whether this option is one you really want to use. You may want to talk to your counselor again to shed light on problems that are keeping you from going forward. There is a balance between doing all you can to find the right person and letting go of what you cannot totally control. You may come to the realization that adoption or living without children is the best course for you. You have every right to take the time that you need to make this decision.

The Donor Egg Procedure

Your cycle and the donor's cycle must be synchronized. So while she is undergoing superovulation, you will be preparing your uterine lining for transfer of the egg to your uterus. If you are ovulating, you will take Lupron or Synarel to turn off your ovarian function. Taking this medication ensures that your hormones won't interfere with the timed development of your uterine lining. When or just before your donor starts ovarian stimulation, you will be given estradiol, usually by injection or suppository, to prepare your lining to receive the embryo. If you are in menopause, if your ovaries have failed, or you don't have ovaries, you only need to take estradiol. You won't need Lupron.

The day your donor's eggs are retrieved you will start on progesterone by pill, suppository, or injection. Meanwhile, the donor's eggs will be combined in the laboratory with your partner's sperm to become cleavage-stage embryos or blastocyst embryos. Between your fourth and sixth day of progesterone, you will have your embryo transfer.

You will continue on estradiol and progesterone to support your uterine lining until your pregnancy test, which usually is done two weeks after the transfer. If you are pregnant, you will stay on estradiol and progesterone for seven more weeks. If you are not pregnant, you will stop those medications. You will start your period in a couple of days.

If You Don't Succeed Right Away with Donor Eggs

You can try again, if you have frozen embryos. Using frozen embryos is considerably less expensive than your first effort with donor eggs when the donor undergoes ovulation induction, falling somewhere between $2,500 and $4,500 a cycle.

SPERM BANKS

In the days before IVF/ICSI, sperm donation was an extremely common way of helping couples overcome severe male factor infertility, which was treatable in no other way. Today, sperm donation is still occasionally used to help couples with severe male factor infertility, usually when a couple cannot undergo IVF or when a couple has had unsuccessful IVF attempts. Increasingly, single women and lesbian couples are turning to sperm donation to start their families. Whether you are using an anonymous donor or someone who is known to you, you should go through a sperm bank. The donor is screened prior to donation, the sperm is then frozen and quarantined until six months later, when the donor is retested, and the sperm is released only if the donor and specimen are free of communicable and infectious diseases, including HIV.

Choosing a Sperm Bank

Licensing for sperm banks varies from state to state, and some states do not require licensing. One of the most important things you should know about choosing a sperm bank is that you can have sperm shipped from a licensed and accredited cryobank (sperm bank) anywhere in the United States to your doctor's office without compromising the quality of the sperm. Accreditation by the American Association of Tissue Banks (AATB) is the best indication of quality. It may be slightly more expensive to use sperm from an accredited bank, but you will have the peace of mind of knowing that there are guidelines the sperm bank must follow in order to remain accredited. If the bank is not licensed and accredited, you have no way of knowing that any guidelines are being followed.

To help ensure your safety, the sperm bank should screen the donor for genetic, infectious, and communicable diseases prior to donation. These include:

- HIV;
- hepatitis B and C;
- HTLV-I and HTLV-II (human T-cell lymphotropic virus);
- syphilis;
- gonorrhea;

- chlamydia;
- CMV (cytomegalovirus);
- herpes simplex virus 1 and 2.

Prospective donors should be given a psychological assessment, medical and sexual history, and genetic screening. Some sperm banks do a full chromosomal analysis on each donor before accepting him.

The precautions for testing date back to the early days of the AIDS epidemic when, in the mid-1980s, a sperm donor infected four women in Australia. In those days, sperm was generally used fresh, and donors were sometimes on call to produce the sperm. As more became known about HIV and AIDS, it was apparent that there was an incubation period during which time a person infected with HIV could have HIV but test negative. An HIV test may not become positive until three to six months after infection. In order to protect against transmission of HIV, sperm banks freeze their specimens to retest the donors six months later to make sure they are HIV negative at the time of donation.

It takes a certain infrastructure and a certain number of years in business to maintain screening standards, to accrue a pool of donors who are geographically stable so they can be retested in six months, and to keep track of their outcomes. These are additional reasons to use a sperm bank with a rigorous method of oversight.

In addition to AATB accreditation, a good sperm bank should have access to a genetic counselor who can alert recipients to any problems discovered with a donor's sperm, for example, if another recipient gives birth to a child with a genetic disorder or the donor himself has such a child. As progress in identifying genes for recessive traits continues, new genes will be identified. Sperm banks should keep count of the children a donor produces so that future parents can be contacted if there are problems. It's also important to understand that not every disorder can be detected in routine screening. If this seems disconcerting, you must remember that reproduction does entail some basic risks that most couples—who don't usually undergo genetic screening before partnering—are willing to take.

The American Association of Tissue Banks provides a rigorous accreditation for sperm banks in the United States. For a list of sperm banks accredited by the AATB, visit its Web site at http://www.aatb.org/ or call 703-827-9582.

These should be balanced against risks that can be screened. During the difficult period of finding and choosing a donor to have a much wanted child, it's good to remember that no child is perfect, and no child should be rejected in any way for not being so.

Using a Friend as a Sperm Donor: What You Should Know

Some people want to ask a friend to donate. Even when your donor is a friend, you are strongly encouraged to use a sperm bank to do a semen analysis and screen the donor to protect against transmission of disease. In other words, your friend will be treated like any other sperm donor, the only difference being that his sperm is only designated for you.

You could certainly argue that if you chose to have sex with your donor, you would not be required to go through screening, and it's certainly easier and cheaper than processing the sperm through a sperm bank. This is true, but you are still exposing yourself to any diseases that person has—whether or not he knows he has them. You are only relying on your friend's account of his medical and genetic history, which may be inaccurate or not entirely known to him. In the end, there is no absolute way to know someone's family and medical history, but screening can provide some additional protections. When you are putting so much effort into having a baby, taking this important step is worth the cost.

Regulations that bar men who have had homosexual sex from becoming anonymous sperm donors have been a recent source of controversy. The regulations were enacted with the belief that such men have a high rate of exposure to HIV/AIDS. Other people considered at high risk for HIV/AIDS are also not accepted as anonymous donors. These include people who within a year of donation have undergone acupuncture, body piercing, or tattooing where sterile procedures weren't used or where it was unclear if they were used, and people who use IV drugs or who might have been exposed to the virus in other ways. People with a family history of encephalopathy, Creutzfeldt-Jakob disease (the human form of mad cow disease), or who have had had a tissue transplant are also prevented from donating.

Couples who want to use a friend may be concerned about these regulations. This issue has been of concern for people who would like to ask a gay friend to donate. Any man can be what is called a directed donor—that is, someone who is specifically asked to donate sperm—but this person, like any donor, should still be tested, have his sperm quarantined, and be retested before the sperm is released.

Anyone who uses a friend as a donor should also be aware that claims for parental rights may be made by sperm donors who consider themselves fathers. Even when the claim is unsuccessful, it is stressful to undergo such a contest. While it's always necessary to have a contract specifying each party's relationship to the intended child, you are far less likely to face such a claim with an anonymous donor.

Make Sure You Have Quality Sperm and That It Is Yours

When choosing a sperm donor, you will be able to choose the race, ethnicity, height, hair and eye color, hair type, and blood type of the donor. Sperm banks should not accept donors who don't have good semen analyses. Some sperm banks list the criteria they use for accepting specimens on their Web sites. When sperm is prepared for insemination, it gets recounted, and your doctor should know the sperm count and motility. In Chapter 8, we talk about the importance of identifying the specimen before having your IUI. You should know the number of your specimen and that the specimen brought into the room for you during your insemination is indeed the sperm that has been prepared for you. At our clinic, we have the patient who is receiving donor sperm go to the lab on our premises and physically take the specimen to carry it with her to her insemination. When the practitioner enters the room, he or she looks at the documents that accompany the specimen and verbally confirms that the patient has the right specimen.

The Cost of Sperm Donation

Costs for sperm can run from around $200 to $400 a vial (almost never covered by insurance), plus shipping costs, which can range in the hundreds. Added costs can include information about the donor and other items like baby pictures of the donor. The donor is typically paid about $100 for a specimen, and each specimen yields three vials. Often, people buy enough sperm from a particular donor so that they can have one or two inseminations per month. If you are successful with a particular donor, you might consider buying several of this donor's specimens for the future, especially if you want genetically related siblings. Otherwise, it's possible that when and if you decide to have another child, that donor's specimens will no longer be available.

You Must Also Be Tested

Before you use donor sperm, you should be tested for everything for which the donor is tested. This is necessary for two reasons. You want to be sure that you don't have any of these diseases so that you can address your health and protect the health of your child. For medical and legal reasons, it's important to know the status of both the recipient and the donor, because if you test positive for an illness after you received the sperm, all parties, including you and the sperm bank, need to know whether the disease is attributable to you or the donor. If you are not being tested for genetic and medical diseases, that's a warning sign that you are not being given optimal care.

Be Prepared for at Least Six Cycles of IUI with Donor Sperm

Using donor sperm is a lot like trying to get pregnant with a male partner, with the same one-in-five chance of success each month. It's vital that you understand the intrinsic inefficiency of natural reproduction, because essentially that's what you are doing. Because you are using excellent sperm and IUIs, it may seem that the insemination will work without a hitch and you will get pregnant right away. The truth is, it probably won't. You have to be willing to repeat attempts, giving yourself ample opportunities to get pregnant. Plan on six attempts and buy enough sperm to do this.

SURROGATES AND GESTATIONAL CARRIERS

There is much that could be written about choosing a surrogate or gestational carrier, far too much for a single chapter. While we can't provide complete coverage of this complicated subject, we can give you an overview of the key issues.

First, it's important to know the distinction between a traditional surrogate and a woman called a gestational carrier. A surrogate uses her own eggs and uterus. Her egg is combined with your partner's sperm and she carries the child until delivery. A gestational carrier uses her uterus and carries an embryo created with your egg or, alternatively, a donor embryo. (We will talk about donor embryos later on in this chapter.)

When You Might Need a Gestational Carrier or Surrogate

A woman who has had a hysterectomy or who was born without a uterus may choose to use a gestational carrier to carry her child. Similarly, a person with no cervix or an amputated cervix may choose to ask someone to carry her child. Another reason you might choose a gestational carrier is if you have a condition that might be significantly worsened by a pregnancy, such as cardiomyopathy (a very weak heart), potentially severe diabetes, or severe vascular disease.

Very often, people who have had multiple IVF failures with good embryos and a normal uterus will ask if it's possible to put the embryos in another person and have a child that way. No studies suggest that using a host uterus can improve the outcomes for people who have good embryos but who are struggling with repeated IVF procedures. In my personal experience, most people who ask this question themselves get pregnant in time. Perhaps this is an indication of their persistence or willingness to explore any avenue.

WHEN YOU MIGHT CONSIDER A TRADITIONAL SURROGATE

Traditional surrogacy is really insemination of a woman who can provide her eggs and also serve as a gestational carrier. Before the advent of IVF, surrogacy, where legal, allowed couples who couldn't have a child any other way to become parents. Today, the use of gestational carriers—women who only carry the child and who are not genetically related to the child—is more common than traditional surrogacy. However, there may be instances when it is more economical to have a surrogate, especially when the surrogate is both an ideal egg donor and an ideal carrier. A young woman who has already had her family might be a good candidate, although it is critical that she understand the implications of having a child who will be genetically related to her children as a half-sibling.

FINDING AND CHOOSING A SURROGATE OR GESTATIONAL CARRIER

Before using either the surrogacy or gestational carrier option, the first and most important thing to do is to find out if your arrangement is legal in your state and what limits are placed on the arrangement. In some states, these arrangements are illegal; in other states, it might not be illegal, but the exchange of money to secure the arrangement is against the law. If unpaid surrogacy or gestational carrier arrangements are permitted, find out whether the contract you make with your surrogate or carrier is enforceable. You want to know who will be considered the legal mother of the child under your state law and/or if you will have to adopt the child during pregnancy or after delivery. Your IVF clinic should know the laws in your state. You can and should also talk to an attorney.

Some people will choose to use a surrogate or carrier who is known to them, and others will contact an agency or attorney to find a gestational carrier. When choosing an agency or family law or adoption attorney, you want to know that that organization has been in business for a while and has many good recommendations. Ask:

- How long have you been in business? There is no substitute for experience.
- What is your philosophy and approach?
- What are the fees? What's included in those fees? Fees can be enormously expensive. Some agencies or attorneys charge higher fees than others, but that doesn't necessarily indicate a difference in quality. Fees should be negotiated up front.
- How does the agency or attorney screen carriers for medical and genetic problems? Does the agency or attorney have access to ob-gyn records? Many may not adequately screen prospective carriers. Not only do you want to know about any medical and genetic issues that may affect your

WHY YOU NEED TO KNOW HER OBSTETRICAL HISTORY

Protect your child and your carrier/surrogate by making sure that your carrier/surrogate is someone who is likely to carry your child to term without complications, such as diabetes and hypertension, which can not only put the carrier at high risk but also unnecessarily expose your child to conditions that may be detrimental to his or her development.

child if you are using the carrier's eggs in surrogacy, you also want to know that the carrier is someone who has had an uneventful pregnancy before and has an excellent chance of carrying your child to term.

- What happens if the gestational carrier or surrogate changes her mind?

The surrogate or carrier doesn't have to be a good friend, but she has to be someone you trust and with whom you can communicate well. Nine months can be a very long time, if you are not sure of the person you choose. When considering a surrogate or carrier, ask yourself whether you are able to communicate well together. Do you get complete and satisfactory answers to your questions? Do you trust this person?

You may or may not want an ongoing relationship with the carrier or surrogate. Many couples feel that a distant but cordial relationship works best. Or, you may find that you develop a bond with the woman you choose. You may have to learn to respect cultural and economic differences. There may be class differences, even if you consider yourself middle class or "ordinary." It's important to recognize these differences and to take the time to get to know the person you are choosing. If it is legal in your state to exchange money for this service, be aware that money can influence your relationship. If you get the sense that the person is doing this just for the money, you may want to move on, because when money is the goal, you don't have a lot of room to negotiate any problems that arise and work together to resolve them.

Everyone Involved Must Receive Counseling

Undoubtedly, choosing to use a surrogate or carrier is not something that a couple does lightly. There are many emotional, medical, financial, legal, psychological, and spiritual issues to be faced by both partners. Connecting with an experienced counselor or others who have chosen gestational carriers or surrogates is a great way to identify and cope with issues that come up as you move along this path. There are Web site communities for people considering these options. (See Resources.) The downside is that these sites can be dominated by a few people, and what you hear on the sites may not reflect typical experiences. The upside is they can be terrific sources of support.

If you have chosen someone you know to be the carrier, that relationship must be free of coercion. A younger relative may not be in a good position to turn you down and may not be able to voice her concerns, or she may not have fully realized all of her concerns at the beginning of this process. That's why it's important to take the time to have a third party help you find out what's at stake for everyone. Your surrogate/carrier's partner or husband should also be counseled. A man may not realize it at the time of the initial decision, but it is possible to develop feelings of jealousy and discomfort living with a partner who is pregnant with a child that is not his. He may understand the situation intellectually, but coping with it emotionally may be a different thing altogether. How will he get through the pregnancy with her? Will he support her? If you are using her eggs, how will both families cope with having genetically related siblings whom they may or may not see again?

Another very important and often overlooked issue is the degree of control you will have over your carrier's body. She is carrying your child, but her body is her own. What will you do if you want her to have amniocentesis, but she doesn't want to have this test? How will you and she monitor her diet and habits? Crucially, how many embryos will you have her put back and what will you do about the question of having to reduce the pregnancy should she be carrying more than one child? Who will breast-feed? What will happen if she suffers from postpartum depression? How will she get through having to give the baby up? All of these issues should be discussed up front with all parties, and everyone should have sufficient information to make an educated decision about their future.

If the person carrying the child is a stranger, someone whom you met through an agency or attorney, what relationship will you have with her before, during, and after the pregnancy? What relationship will she have, if any, with the child? This is a crucial issue to designate in writing with an attorney, whether or not the surrogate/carrier is someone you know.

Always Consult an Attorney and Check Your Insurance!

It is vital that the surrogate/carrier and the intended parents have separate attorneys to create a contract that fully designates each party's rights and responsibilities. Having a clear contract can help you avoid any disputes that may arise in the future.

If fees are allowed in your state, they should be written into the contract. It is customary for the intended parents to pay for the carrier's legal fees, but again, always check the laws in your state. Payment for medical expenses, including unforeseen medical expenses, should also be detailed in writing. Be sure to check your health insurance to find out whether it will cover medical expenses for the surrogate/carrier and/or for your child, if need be. You may need to register your intended child with your insurer. If there are problems with the pregnancy, affecting either the child or the surrogate/carrier, you will want to know that you have insurance and to what extent the insurance will cover these expenses. This can be vital in cases where, for instance, a child needs neonatal care. In one such case, a dispute with insurers occurred over coverage for newborn and pregnancy complications in a gestational carrier arrangement between sisters, when the child had to spend its first two months in the hospital.[2]

Deciding to Tell Others

When using a surrogate/carrier, most people tell others because they are having a child without having a pregnancy. Telling your family you are planning to do this may be difficult at first, because people are likely to have strong feelings about using gestational carriers or surrogates. But often when the baby comes, the family is content. Family members can be excellent sources of support for both the intended parents and the carrier/surrogate.

EMBRYO ADOPTION

There is still one last other option you may want to consider if you feel strongly that you want a newborn baby: embryo donation. Although embryos are not widely available at present, this can still be a very good solution for a couple who needs both donor eggs and donor sperm, but the woman's uterus is in good shape to carry a pregnancy to term. As with donor eggs, you eliminate worries about another mother's intrauterine environment or the possibility that the birth mother will change her mind about giving her child up to adoption. Similarly, you also get to go through the experience of pregnancy and delivery, which most people consider to be very rewarding.

Where the Embryos Come From

When a couple gets pregnant with IVF, they may have extra frozen embryos they don't need. In this case, they are often asked whether they would like to have their embryos discarded, donated to research, or given to another couple or woman. Although most people give their embryos to medical research, some donate them to others. This can be a boon to couples who can have children in no other way. While you might worry that embryos not chosen for IVF are inferior, remember that those embryos came from a couple that got pregnant.

You are most likely to find embryo donation programs in IVF clinics that do a large volume of cryopreservation (freezing) of embryos. In our program, we do much more cryopreservation than many programs three times our size, and we do have patients who use extra embryos. It is possible that the number of available embryos will decrease as IVF programs do less cryopreservation. One of the reasons for this is the increased use of embryos at the blastocyst stage, which are less amenable to freezing. (See Chapter 9.) Another reason is the financial gain clinics stand to make by doing fresh embryo transfers instead of frozen transfers, added to the fact that not every clinic does cryopreservation well.

It's also not unusual for two infertile couples to know each other. When one succeeds at IVF and the other doesn't, it sometimes happens that the successful couple donates their embryos to the other couple. This can be a good solution to a problem, providing no financial transaction takes place. However, the emotional and social consequences in the future are obvious, and should be broached with a counselor, as in all cases of third-party reproduction. A practical consideration for the donating couple is that they must return to the IVF program, have their blood drawn, and be screened for disease just as an unknown donor would. They will then sign a consent form relinquishing the embryos.

Some programs such as Nightlight Christian Adoption's Snowflakes Embryo Adoption Program in California (http://www.nightlight.org) match donors and recipients, giving the donors more control over the choice of recipients.

LOOKING AT ADOPTION

If you think adoption may ultimately be an option for you, do a little preliminary information gathering so that you will be prepared to enter the adoption process when and if you are ready. Consider that costs for adoptions can range from a very low cost to around $10,000 to $30,000 for international adoptions. The average cost for a private or agency adoption runs about $15,000 to $30,000. Adoptive parents can receive a federal adoption expense tax credit.

Some adoption agencies and some foreign countries have age cutoffs for adoptive parents. In private adoption, there is no age cutoff. Private, or independent, adoptions are adoptions in which an attorney facilitates the legal process of adoption. Although agency adoptions are legal in every state, private adoption is not legal in some states. Check for current laws in your state.

If you are single or lesbian or gay, find out if there are any barriers to adoption in your state or in agency adoptions. Does your state bar adoptions by lesbian and gay parents? May only one lesbian or single parent adopt, with the other parent applying for coparent status? Will an agency treat you differently than married adoptive parents?

Time is a factor in adoption, but not to the degree that most people imagine. The average wait for an adopted child is nine months to a year.

Many are concerned that they will not be able to find a child who blends into their family's ethnic heritage. Others are not concerned about this. One of the myths of adoption surrounds the desire for Caucasian infants. It is possible to adopt a Caucasian baby, although there are fewer available infants than there are waiting adoptive parents. Nonetheless, the wait is typically the same as for any child, about one year.

Some attorneys and agencies will ask that you close the door on infertility treatment before exploring adoption, but there is no reason why you should not gather information or start your investigations at some point during infertility treatment, if you are financially able. I once had a patient whose adoption came through between her egg retrieval and embryo transfer for IVF. The IVF worked and she wound up with two children nine months apart. Both adoption and infertility care are emotionally challenging and stressful. Choose a pace that you can manage and that feels right.

There are still many unfounded myths about adoption, including the notion that there are too few infants available, that adoptive parents pay exorbitant amounts to "buy" babies, and that birth parents can reclaim the child at any time. Organizations for adoptive parents are great sources of information about the adoption process, about myths and misconceptions about adoption, and about choosing private, agency, or international adoption. (See Resources for more information.)

Third-party reproduction can be a wonderful option. Without it, many couples would not be able to have children. But special precautions must be taken to make sure that everyone is protected. Once you've made the decision to use a third party to have your child, there is no turning back. As you make your decision, remember the child's best interests should always be, as they undoubtedly are, foremost in your mind.

Acupuncture and Traditional
Chinese Medicine for Infertility

LIKE MANY PEOPLE WITH INFERTILITY, YOU MAY WON-
der if complementary treatments can really help you become pregnant. Undoubtedly, health practices like eating a balanced diet, exercising, practicing
yoga, meditation, visualization, and prayer are all good things that can enhance your health and quality of life, but whether they will help you get
pregnant is unknown, at least from a Western scientific perspective. On the
other hand, treating your body well, preparing for pregnancy by eliminating
harmful substances from your diet and environment, taking prenatal vitamins, and thinking positively about your body and your ability to get pregnant can help you focus on your goal, reduce stress, and support you during
infertility treatment, which can be frustrating and emotionally painful.

With the exception of acupuncture, there are few good studies to support or negate the use of most complementary and alternative treatments. Complementary fields are not regulated as doctors' practices are, nor are they subject to the restrictions of managed care. The Food and Drug Administration (FDA) does not require testing of dietary supplements, including herbs and vitamins, whereas it requires rigorous testing for drugs. In the end, consumers have fewer ways to find out whether a proposed treatment is really effective.

You may well benefit from complementary approaches, but you are encouraged to be as discerning when choosing a complementary practitioner as you are when selecting a medical specialist, remembering that just as medical practices and clinics are businesses subject to profit motives, so too are alternative and complementary practices. In this chapter we will take a look at acupuncture, one of the most popular forms of complementary treatment for fertility.

ACUPUNCTURE AND TRADITIONAL CHINESE MEDICINE

More than 3,000 years old, acupuncture is a healing system that involves placing thin, solid needles into various points on the body to stimulate energy called qi (pronounced "chee") to produce healing effects. There are various styles of acupuncture, ranging from the practice developed in China to styles that took hold in Korea, Japan, and Vietnam. Although the first book about it was written around 500 BC, acupuncture is just beginning to be studied through Western scientific methods. A 2002 German study, which suggested that acupuncture performed for twenty-five minutes before and after embryo transfer improved pregnancy rates for women with good embryos,[1] sparked enormous interest in the use of acupuncture in conjunction with Western medical fertility treatment. Well designed and impressive, the study legitimized the use of acupuncture and gave Western doctors information that they could relate to and use in their practices.

One of the reasons the study made so much sense to Western doctors is that there are very good studies from all over the world that show that increased uterine blood flow is associated with better IVF stimulation and

IVF outcomes. If acupuncture can increase uterine blood flow or relax the uterus, which after all is a muscle that can contract and release, it is plausible that acupuncture could make the uterus more receptive to implantation. After the German study, reproductive endocrinologists began offering acupuncture services within their practices, and many patients have used this adjunct therapy to help them through treatment.

You may have heard of traditional Chinese medicine, called TCM for short. TCM is a blend of acupuncture, herbs, qi gong (pronounced "chee-gong"), a form of energy exercise that includes tai chi, massage (tui-na, pronounced "twee-na"), and diet according to the principles of Chinese medicine.

Underlying treatment in acupuncture and TCM are the principles of ying and yang, which represent the shifting, opposing forces of the natural world. Chinese medicine views health problems as arising from imbalances in interrelating systems of the whole body. When making a diagnosis, a practitioner of TCM or acupuncture will study relations between conditions, including opposites of excesses and deficiencies, heat and cold, and disturbances in the internal or external (surface or deep) organs. Your diet, lifestyle, exposure to toxins, energy, and emotional state are all considered when planning treatment with traditional Chinese medicine.

Qi is energy or life force. When qi is not flowing properly in the body, disharmony and disorder can result. According to practitioners of acupuncture and TCM, qi has its own intelligence, rising and falling, as different energies that do different jobs within the body. Qi, blood, and body fluids travel through the body within a network of channels or pathways called meridians, which are not channels that can be found on dissection of the human body. Chinese medicine is based on philosophies very different from Western medicine and uses different terminology. For example, when an acupuncturist speaks about "liver qi," he or she is not talking about the anatomical liver but about conditions associated with it. Liver qi is associated with emotion, and both the liver and kidney are said to be important to women with infertility. In TCM, the liver also directs blood flow to the uterus. The kidneys affect your hormones and menstruation, as well as other body systems. In TCM, stress, excessive work, and poor self-care and nutrition can block emotional energy and cause liver qi and blood stagnation. Stress can also affect kidney qi and your hormone production.

Some TCM practitioners treat with herbs as well as acupuncture. Herbology is extremely complex. It takes a long time to master the study of the use of herbs in TCM. The complexity of the preparations in and of themselves is one of the reasons why herbs haven't been researched in depth in the West. It's difficult, if not nearly impossible, to separate components of these preparations to understand how they work.

Moxibustion is another important TCM technique. In this practice, an herb called mugwort is burned in the form of a stick or cone to warm points on the body to stimulate qi and strengthen the blood. In the direct form of moxibustion, the herb cone is placed on the body, where there is the possibility of a burn, but in the indirect form, the stick is near the skin, not on it. Among its many properties, mugwort is said to increase circulation and effect menstruation.

To try to neatly summarize principles behind Chinese medicine is as difficult as trying to run through a quick history of Western medicine. There are great differences between these two disciplines, which are sometimes discussed as being opposed, one taking a "mechanistic" approach and the other a "holistic" approach to treatment. Some see Western medicine as focused on the machinery of the body's organs and systems, fixing problems when they go wrong, while viewing complementary practices as attempting to sustain health by looking at the patient's condition in the context of a spectrum of life issues, including diet, emotional heath, lifestyle, and habits. These are oversimplifications, but certainly complementary practitioners do aim to look at myriad aspects of a person's health and functioning in relationship to symptoms in order to diagnosis and treat.

> *I started going to a nearby acupuncturist. He did a medical history and asked about my cycles. He explained that we would first work to regulate my cycles and then relax for the IVF. I was in the office for about an hour and always left feeling very relaxed. It's very tranquil. If I had to do IVF again, I would definitely start acupuncture beforehand.* —LINDA

TCM and Infertility

When it comes to infertility, TCM practitioners often recommend a judicious synthesis of Eastern and Western approaches. See your doctor and make sure you understand your diagnosis before attempting to treat it with complementary therapies. You want to know what to expect from a complementary therapy, how it can help, and how you can tell if it's working.

Practitioners suggest that TCM and acupuncture can help with emotional balance and stress. Chronic stress, depression and anxiety, and grief can clearly affect your health. When you have infertility, stress is almost inevitable. Acupuncture may help to calm you before and during treatment. You may also want to consider yoga, meditation, massage, exercise, or other modalities to help relieve stress, improve your energy, and help you attain the peace of mind necessary to put life's challenges in perspective and to cope with the many emotional challenges of fertility treatment.

As a doctor, I view acupuncture as offering more of a potential benefit when treating what are termed functional problems as opposed to organic problems. Organic problems stem from a disorder in an organ or system. They are more absolute than functional problems. Organic problems include:

- a blocked fallopian tube/s;
- a large fibroid;
- no sperm count.

These are examples of problems that are much better served by Western medicine. Your physician can isolate sperm for treatments like IVF/ICSI or open blocked tubes through relatively noninvasive techniques such as catheterization. (See Chapter 5.)

Functional problems are those that occur when it seems as though you should be fertile, but you have infertility. Unexplained infertility is a prime example of a functional problem, as are repeated IVF failures in someone who is young. Mild endometriosis can be another example of a functional problem. Medical treatment of mild endometriosis can improve fertility, but some people with mild endometriosis get pregnant even when untreated. Conceivably, a synthesis of Western medicine and TCM could help in such a situation.

When your fertility diagnosis is unexplained or you are young and failing with IVF for no obvious reason, acupuncture may have a role in helping. Yet it's important to know where you stand with your medical treatment while having complementary care. If you did one cycle of IVF and you stimulated well, but you didn't get pregnant on your first try, it doesn't mean that you will fail again. It may only be a matter of time before you get pregnant, particularly if you are under thirty-five. Still, you may want to try acupuncture to reduce stress and potentially improve the chance of implantation at your next cycle. The same is true if you are not stimulating well for IVF. Acupuncture may, at least in theory, improve your chances next time.

Repeated miscarriage may be another place for acupuncture as an adjunct to traditional treatment after a complete pregnancy loss workup that includes an examination of the structure of your uterus, investigation of the possibility of chromosomal abnormalities and blood clotting disorders. Still, about 40 percent of the time, doctors find no clear cause for repeated miscarriage after a complete pregnancy-loss workup, leaving many women to simply try again. Trying again with acupuncture may help.

I always advise patients to fit their fertility treatment into their lives rather than restructuring their lives around their fertility treatment. Because physicians are starting to work with complementary practitioners, even offering treatment through their offices, it's getting easier to get acupuncture without having to book yet another set of appointments into an already tight schedule. But if this isn't available to you and you find yourself having to work hard to get to these appointments, consider whether you aren't creating even more stress for yourself. Complementary approaches should make you feel better, not worse. Try not to impose demands on yourself past what you can reasonably handle.

Do Not Mix Herbs and Fertility Drugs

Many doctors and TCM practitioners do not mix herbs and fertility drugs, as a precaution against any potential adverse effects. After checking with your reproductive endocrinologist, the practitioner who uses herbs may treat only in a cycle when you are not undergoing ovarian stimulation, such as during a rest between cycles.

As we pointed out, acupuncture and herbs may help with mood. Clomiphene is notorious for causing mood swings in some people, and some may want to try acupuncture and herbs to calm their moods. Unlike injectable FSH, clomiphene is relatively inexpensive. Were herbs to have any negative effect on clomiphene, the risk of interference with your cycle is lower, at least from a financial standpoint, than with injectable FSH, which can cost thousands of dollars in drug and monitoring expenses. It's inadvisable to do anything that may tamper with an IVF cycle.

Choosing a Provider: What You Should Expect

As with medical doctors, a practitioner should be licensed (if provided for in your state), certified, skilled, and competent. Before choosing a practitioner, educate yourself about the style of acupuncture you are choosing, the aims of that treatment, and the likelihood of attaining these goals. There are many good books about acupuncture that you can read to get a sense of how fertility is treated. Just as in any field, there are good practitioners and those who are less knowledgeable and skilled. When acupuncture is practiced poorly, you can have temporary adverse symptoms, the risk of which should be discussed beforehand with the practitioner. At best, you may get no result from treatment. So choose your practitioner wisely.

Tell your doctor that you are considering complementary treatment. Your reproductive endocrinologist may work with a practitioner or be able to refer you. You will also want to talk about the way in which your complementary treatment will fit into your medical care. Your doctor needs to know as much about your reproductive health as possible and should know if and when you are being treated with herbs. As mentioned, herbs should not be combined with fertility drugs until more is known about the possible side effects.

If your doctor cannot refer you, ask friends, support group members, or others who have recently had infertility treatment, for recommendations. When speaking to the practitioner over the phone or in person, ask the same questions as you would a doctor, including questions about licenses and certification and seven-day-a-week availability.

When choosing a practitioner of TCM or an acupuncturist, make sure that person is certified by the National Certification Commission for Acupuncture and Oriental Medicine. If your practitioner uses acupuncture and herbs, he or she should be certified in both acupuncture and herbology. Some states license acupuncturists, and some do not. You can check with your state department of health, listed in the phone book. You can verify that your provider is certified, through this site:

The Directory of Health Organizations onLine (DIRLINE; http://dirline.nlm.nih.gov/) offers information about professional health organizations, including complementary and alternative practice organizations. Using the site, you can search professional organizations for almost any field, including fields of holistic medicine. Professional sites often detail the standards to which they hold their members. Looking at these standards should give you a good idea about what to expect from your practitioner.

At Your First Visit

Every practitioner is different, using a different style of acupuncture in combination with his or her own personal style. Because the practitioner will seek to investigate the root causes of your symptoms through various means, she or he may ask you about your sleep patterns, digestion, lifestyle, energy levels, and stressors, placing your condition in the larger context of your daily life. Your practitioner should spend a good amount of time with you, trying to understand your treatment needs. It's not unusual for someone to meet with you for one to one and a half hours. The practitioner should have a treatment strategy; and you should understand the rationale behind that strategy. Importantly, you should feel comfortable with your practitioner. As with any other complementary practice, you want to know your practitioner is skilled and knowledgeable, and you want to feel as though you have a good connection. After all, you are going to spend time with this person, who will be working with you on a number of levels, so trust and confidence are important.

Although timelines for results differ in medical and complementary practices, you should begin to see results within two to three months. Some practitioners aim to treat with a minimum number of weekly visits. This can really help when you are juggling numerous appointments. If you aren't feeling better or seeing results within two to three months, consider reevaluating your care. This is similar to my "three-month rule" for Western infertility techniques, such as ovulation induction or intrauterine insemination.

Consider, too, whether you are being overtreated. If your practitioner wants to see you week after week for many months, find out whether this is truly necessary. Consult with another practitioner. Overtreating someone or extending their treatment beyond what is necessary is called "churning," and at the very least this practice can cost you a lot of time and money. Again, as with any practitioner, you should feel that he or she has your best interests at heart.

You should always feel comfortable asking questions, and your provider should readily supply you with answers. If you are not getting the information you need, go elsewhere, just as you would when selecting a medical doctor. And again, remember that complementary care should make you feel good—not frustrated or hurried. If you can't get to a practitioner because of traffic, tight scheduling, or emotional overload, don't beat yourself up. You are doing everything you can to get pregnant. There is no need to try to push yourself beyond your limits.

14 | Make Sure You Have Emotional Support

MANY PEOPLE IN THE FIELD OF MENTAL HEALTH CARE are trained to help people through stressful life experiences, but there are some therapists who focus their practices specifically on helping people who have infertility. The issues connected to the experience of infertility are often so technical and complex, and different from most other life issues, that when you do seek help, it's a good idea to choose someone who understands the varied challenges that you face. Harriette Rovner Ferguson, LCSW, is such a therapist. A licensed social worker who has been helping people with infertility for fifteen years, she is the coauthor of *Experiencing Infertility: An Essential Resource,* published by W.W. Norton in 2000. She was a support group leader for RESOLVE for twelve years and is a member of the mental health professional group at the American Society for Reproductive Medicine. Many of the insights in this chapter have come from conversations with Ms. Rovner Ferguson, who was kind enough to share her experiences working with thousands of infertility patients and with other professionals in her field.

> *I was very, very depressed. The only way I could cope was to find out what we were doing next. I couldn't stand being without a plan. We never stopped. I mourned and replanned, but not without terrible depression.*
>
> —FRANCIS

INFERTILITY IS A CRISIS

If you are feeling anxious, depressed, and scared, you're very normal. According to research by Alice Domar, one of the leading experts on psychology and women's health, women with infertility have levels for depression and anxiety that are as high as women who are facing life-threatening illness.[1]

As soon as women find out that they are having trouble getting pregnant, they typically respond by getting busy, doing research, educating themselves about infertility, and making medical appointments with a specialist. Once you start making frequent doctor visits, the goal of getting pregnant begins to become concrete and seemingly within grasp. Of necessity, you may start to organize your life around trying to get pregnant. And as your life becomes increasingly directed toward your goal, pursing pregnancy can even feel like an obsession. In order to deal with this overwhelming feeling, you may want to talk to a therapist or meet with a support group, or read about infertility online or in books such as this. Taking control can be an important step toward coping with the inevitable stress of infertility.

Differences Between the General Reactions of Men and Women

While women often react to an infertility diagnosis with justifiable alarm, thinking, "What are we going to do?" men may not see infertility as a crisis at all. Instead, men usually take a kind of wait-and-see attitude, thinking that their partners are overreacting or being unduly negative. They try to reassure their partners that everything will turn out fine, given time. Right from the beginning of infertility treatment, women and men are in two different emotional places. Even if the fertility problem is due to male infertility, it is the female partner who will undergo most of the tests and treatment. She is the one who will have to redo her entire schedule. Her partner may accompany her to doctor visits, but she may soon start to feel alone in her struggle. It may take time for a man to catch up with his partner's reactions and consider infertility to be a crisis. For a woman, infertility is not only a physical or medical crisis; it's a crisis that affects her entire life, emotionally, spiritually, financially, as well as in her relationships.

Part of the gap in attitude between women and men may be due to the strong differences in the way men and women are socialized. As girls, many women practiced for motherhood by playing with dolls and role-playing in a variety of nurturing activities, developing a sense of the inevitability of parenthood. For many women, motherhood is at the core of their identity. Not so for many men, who are more focused on career as a source of their identity. They may want to become dads or see themselves as the person who supports the family financially, but they are not as motivated as their partners are to make pregnancy happen.

When men take a backseat role in infertility treatment, as they very often do, they can unintentionally frustrate or hurt their partners. When a woman first comes to a support group, she learns by listening to other women's stories that her partner's reaction is typical.

The truth is that although men don't share the same identity-based crisis around infertility, they often feel other difficult emotions that they tend not to express. Many men feel inadequate when it comes to helping their partners. Even if a man feels bad about what he and his partner are going through, he may not communicate this, thinking it will burden her. Unable to talk openly, some men may get angry with their partners. Men may complain that they "want their wives back." Sometimes they say they don't know what to do to help and that it's difficult to live at such a high emotional pitch. Some women don't realize that their partners may have to endure insensitive comments from other men and experience feeling left out when other men exchange pictures or stories about their children. When men begin to open up about their feelings, they may express feelings of sadness at not being able to have children easily, much to their partners' amazement and relief.

> *My wife and I always shared stuff. We worked it out. We had to. There's no choice in the matter. She needs me. I need her. I wanted this to work. I tried to make her comfortable. I would say things like, "You know, maybe this is the month. Maybe this is the time. Don't give up. We came this far already." But there were some nights when we were both stressed out. I'm a construction worker. I work a lot of hours. I can work all night, so there was a lot of concern with trying to fit in sexual contact. If I was working overtime on a certain day at a certain time, it got to be very stressful. You were basically going to blow the whole month if you didn't come home.* —BILL

> *Whether you have children or not, you are still going to be with each other, and it's important to remember that, especially nowadays when people are much more "me" oriented than "we" oriented. Stress is always easier to manage when you have somebody in your corner. But I think, as individuals we tend to lash out when we're hurting like wounded animals. It's hard to admit your vulnerability. "Will they still love me if they know I'm such a wimp about this?" It's a hard thing to get through. Every couple has to find their own way of doing that.* —JERI

FOR COUPLES: WHAT TO DO

Most couples are not prepared for the crisis of infertility. When you are married or partnered, you may never have imagined that infertility could have stopped you from reaching the next seemingly natural step of pregnancy and childbirth. This may be the first crisis you have faced together, and it can be frightening. However, the way you handle this crisis can be a template for the way in which you handle future difficulties together. If you are having problems, know that being patient with each other's style of communication and acknowledging the differences in your coping skills may increase your ability to love and respect one another. Be assured that couples rarely split because of this. Think of this as an opportunity to grow together.

Many women want to talk about the problems of infertility all the time. This can make their partners feel as if their relationship revolves solely around trying to have a baby. Some therapists believe that partners should plan a time each day when they can review information about their infertility care. Fifteen to twenty minutes is usually enough time to express feelings and discuss details of treatment. Turn the TV off, let the answering machine pick up phone messages, and concentrate on these few minutes. Don't let the conversation drift from subject to subject. Focus on what must be discussed and remember that you can pick up the discussion tomorrow. Having this time to talk may make you feel less anxious.

Most of the women in my support group were having relationship problems. My husband and I had dual infertility, so there was no feeling of culpability. We were very supportive of each other. We shared the burden. He went with me to as many appointments as he could. I didn't have to do it alone. It's hard for men. It's hard to see the woman they love go through this, especially when conceiving a child is supposed to be so simple. —CINDY

It's hard to speak for others because everyone copes differently. Some people cope by distancing themselves. I thought it would help us cope better if I was involved and aware of what of we were doing. But it's hard to tell people that they should get more involved, because it may be that in certain situations the husband's involvement creates more tension. —BOB

WHAT YOU MAY NOT KNOW ABOUT HIM

Women are relentlessly marketed the idea that men look at females as potential sex partners or mothers. When a woman is infertile, she may feel undesirable and that her body has let her down. She may not feel attractive or sexual, and she may believe that her husband or partner is thinking the same thing. This is rarely true. Men find their partners desirable even when they are going through infertility treatment together. Some women think that sexy, skinny blond women are ideals of beauty, but most men don't actually share these ideals.

Most likely, you and your partner are committed to one another because you are friends and because you like and respect one another. Your partner wanted to spend the rest of his life with you not because he expected you to be a "breeder," but because he loves you. Imagine if he became ill. Would you love him any the less? Probably not. If not, why would he leave you or love you any less because of this crisis? Infertility is a couple's problem. It's something that you can work on together. This is a perfect opportunity for you to deepen your trust of one another. One of the hardest but most rewarding things that you can do is to begin to trust that your partner cares. It may amaze you how communication opens up when you approach him with that foundation.

DEALING WITH FERTILITY DRUGS

Doctors may not acknowledge it as much as they should, but fertility drugs can wreak havoc with a woman's emotions. Most women report that when they are taking fertility medications, they feel as though they are in a chronic state of PMS. Some women say that they don't feel like themselves on these hormones. They may cry or get angry or irritated when they wouldn't normally. Empathy and understanding can go a long way. Both partners should resist taking these emotional surges too personally and remember that the woman is taking very serious medication. It can be very difficult for a couple to get through this time, but keeping your ultimate goal of parenthood in mind can help.

SUPPORT GROUPS: WHY THEY WORK

One of the things you can do for yourself is to get support from other women who are experiencing infertility, and one of the ways to do this is to join a professionally monitored support group led by a psychotherapist who specializes in infertility. You can also ask your doctor's office for a referral to a group in your community or to a local therapist.

Women often say that they don't want to go to a support group because they fear that it will make them more depressed. Support groups that teach coping skills using mind/body techniques, such as guided imagery, meditation, and journal writing provide excellent means of relief for anxiety and depression. You can also be part of an online community, many of which are very helpful. However, some are not professionally monitored, and you may receive erroneous medical information from these groups.

Although support groups can be very helpful, they are not for everybody. If you are a very private person, competitive, or just a very busy person, going to a support group may increase your anxiety and stress levels. You may find a one-on-one relationship with a therapist to be more beneficial.

> *A friend who knew I was having infertility treatment called and asked me if I would mind speaking to her friend about infertility. And I said, "I would love to help anyone who needs to talk about infertility."* —ROXANNE

WHEN FRIENDS AND FAMILY DON'T UNDERSTAND

It's often said that unless you have experienced infertility, you don't get it. While many close friends and relatives are able to offer support, many don't understand and aren't able to give their loved ones the empathy and kindness they need. Someone you love may disappoint you. That is almost certain. But it is also very difficult for people to know how to help. Because each person's style of coping differs, families and friends are often in a bind, not sure what to do or what to say. A healing and helpful tactic for one person may be the wrong approach for another. Some people want to talk about infertility, others don't. Some people want to be questioned about their experience, and others will be offended if asked. Decide what works best for you and let people know. Sometimes we think others will know what we need without having to be told, but they don't.

When you don't get the help you need from family and friends, or when you need support to deal with loved ones' reactions and expectations, support from people who have experienced infertility can be very helpful. For example, friends may not understand why going to a baby shower may hurt too much or why you react when someone unthinkingly asks when you are going to have children. People who have been there know what it feels like, and can offer assistance, acknowledgment, and support.

Right from the beginning, infertility treatment becomes a group activity. There were so many hopes pinned on my uterus. I was going to have the first grandchild on both sides. Everybody was waiting for the results. I wear my heart on my sleeve. That's me. So I wasn't quiet about it. Do I wish I could have done it differently? Yes. Do I think I have that capability? No. You have to go with your style. Personally, I don't know how you could bear this burden without anybody knowing. —SHERI

I think we made the right decision in keeping it a private matter. I think if we had gotten our parents involved there would be more questions. If we ended up failing, the frustration would be greater for all the other people who would have been privy to what we were going through. —DAVID

I work as a psychologist in an elementary school. Most of the teachers are in their twenties. For the last three years, we have had no less than seven

pregnant teachers a year. There are ten psychologists who work in my school district. In one meeting I found out that four of them were pregnant. It's been hard. It's been tough to deal with. —MAUREEN

It's normal for a person with infertility to have ambivalent or angry feelings toward people who are pregnant or who have children, even if they are close friends or relatives. It's part of human nature. You're not a bad person. You are not unusually selfish. You are dealing with a major life crisis that can affect your sense of identity and future. Think about ways in which you can remain close to your friends or relatives but protect your emotions. You don't have to do things that cause you pain, such as going to baby showers or children's birthday parties. There will be times when you will feel more open to such invitations and times when it will hurt too much. For instance, if you have just learned that your infertility treatment failed, perhaps you can acknowledge your friend or relative by sending a gift. As each situation arises, think about what you can do to preserve your well-being and the relationships you value.

Baby envy. The first time around, it was unbearable. I couldn't go to a park in the spring because everybody was out with their new babies. I couldn't go to baby namings or bris celebrations, and I especially couldn't deal with people calling me to tell me they were pregnant. —CINDY

WHEN YOU HAVE SECONDARY INFERTILITY

Secondary infertility can be a lonely experience. Women who have one child and who are struggling to have a second may not get support. If this is you, you may have heard comments like, "You should feel lucky that you already have one. Why do you want another?" No reasonable person would ever say such a thing to a couple without infertility who are planning to have a second or third child. Even women with primary infertility can't offer support, a fact that can make having secondary infertility an even lonelier experience.

Many women with or without infertility say that they don't feel complete until they are finished creating their families. This has nothing to do with their love for their first child. But going through infertility treatment while trying to raise a young child can bring about unique challenges. Some people report feeling guilty that their attention is not wholly directed to the first child. Some women are concerned that while their bodies once "worked," they are not working now. This can be a frightening experience. Questions like, "Should we adopt? Is one child enough?" arise for people with secondary infertility and should be addressed in a supportive environment. Finding support is a bit more difficult when you have secondary infertility, but there are groups out there. Check Web sites related to infertility and look for links about secondary infertility.

Secondary infertility is a completely different beast. My secondary infertility was worse than my primary infertility. With primary infertility, you are desperate to have a child and everybody feels for you. The first time I conceived more quickly than the second time. The second time, I went through six procedures. I spoke to doctors all over the country, and I was told I would never have another baby. It was really lonely. Nobody in primary infertility understands because they justifiably want their first child. How can they relate to somebody who already has a child? —SHARON

After I had my son, I didn't want people to know I had to do this (IVF) again, because I didn't want them involved in the process. People's constant comments are very draining. "Just be lucky you have one." You don't want to hear that. —RAMONA

We brought my son into the infertility specialist's office a couple of times and there were people looking at us like, "Okay, why are you here?" I felt very uncomfortable with that. It almost made me mad. We considered our first one as a gift from God, you know. We are all in this together. We are all trying to accomplish the same goal. I would ask people not to put others down. —MARC

CHOOSING A THERAPIST

There are many good therapists practicing today, but you are looking for someone who has experience working with people who have infertility. There are medical, financial, insurance, legal, relationship, and family issues that are particular to having infertility. Many kind and empathic people don't understand these issues and don't have the background to integrate knowledge of these issues into therapy. You may not want to spend precious time in therapy explaining to your therapist what an endometrial biopsy is, for example, when you could be working on your concerns.

Your doctor or clinic may have a therapist on staff or provide recommendations to therapists who work with infertility patients.

When interviewing therapists over the phone or in person, ask:

- How long have you been in practice?
- What licenses and certifications do you hold?
- How much experience do you have working with people with infertility?
- Are you a member of ASRM, RESOLVE, INCIID, the American Fertility Association, or any other fertility organizations? (See Resources for descriptions of these organizations.)
- What is your approach to therapy?
- Are you familiar with mind/body solutions such as guided imagery, meditation, and cognitive/behavioral therapy?
- Are you knowledgeable and comfortable with my religious, sexual, or cultural orientation?
- Can you refer me to a good local support group?
- Where are you located? (Driving to yet another appointment can be stressful. You may want to consider if you can really make it to appointments easily.)
- Can you be reached in an emergency? (If you have a miscarriage and you need to talk to someone, this can be vital.)
- Can I bring my partner in for therapy?

- Can I bring in a family member who doesn't understand what I'm going through?
- How many times a week may I see you? How long are sessions?
- What is the cost of services? Do you accept my insurance? Do you have sliding-scale fees?
- What is your policy on canceling a session?

As with any relationship, you and your therapist should be a good match. You should feel comfortable with your therapist's approach. You want to feel as though you are being listened to and that your concerns are being met in a way that makes sense and feels productive to you. Know that you can change therapists, if need be. You do not have to go to the first therapist you interview. Professionals understand that not every client-therapist match is a fit. You deserve good care that is right for you. Keep looking until you find someone who can help.

INFERTILITY MAY BE A CRISIS, BUT IT'S TEMPORARY

Sooner or later, life will return to normal. This is important to remember. You will find a resolution. You can have a family. There are options. Fortunately, we live in a time when third-party reproduction, such as using donor eggs or donor sperm, is available and acceptable to most people. Although the decision to create your family in a way that you did not envision can be difficult emotionally, it is important to remember that you can have a family, if you wish. Child-free living is also an option for some couples who want to redesign their family of two, and many times can bring unforeseen wonderful experiences. It is important to always remember that there will be resolutions. Keeping your eye on the light at the end of the tunnel can help you keep your life and your relationships in perspective. At the same time, trying to live in the moment and enjoy what you have in the present is key to coping with the emotional ups and downs of the infertility crisis.

15 | Plan Your Finances

MANY PEOPLE START INFERTILITY TREATMENT WITHOUT a true understanding of just how much infertility treatment can cost and how little insurance may cover. Unless you live in a state where insurance coverage is mandated for infertility care by law, be prepared to pay for many, if not most, services out of pocket and to advocate for yourself whenever possible. Among the most important things you can do for yourself before or during care is to know what your insurance really does and does not cover, persist in getting reliable answers from your insurance company, and use all resources available to you to help you cover the costs of treatment.

Learning to advocate for yourself, if you don't already, is great preparation for parenthood, where you are often called upon to stand up for your child. And while you may not have control over whether you get pregnant at each cycle, you can take charge of the decisions you make about insurance and finances. Think about what you will and will not spend—*before* you enter treatment. Learn as much as you can about your insurance coverage and other options so that you can make objective decisions about your financial health. In this chapter, we will outline key areas that will help you get the most out of your insurance and help you avoid losses.

FIRST, PARTNER WITH YOUR DOCTOR'S OFFICE

A good IVF program should have someone on staff who can review your insurance, tell you what coverage you have and what you don't have, and whether the office participates in your plan so that you will know where you stand even before you sit down with your doctor for a consultation. Not every program does this. Even if there is no one designated as an insurance counselor or insurance coordinator in your doctor's office or clinic, find out if you can talk to the head of the billing department. While this person may not officially be given the responsibility of helping you understand your insurance, you may be able to develop a working relationship with the department head, who can give you some very helpful information about handling your claim.

Ask your clinic or doctor's office about any available programs that can help with costs of care. Drug companies may have trial studies. Some states may have demonstration projects that help cover part of the costs of care for people who meet certain criteria. Such programs may or may not be available to you, but asking may provide you with new information and resources.

FIND OUT: ARE YOU COVERED?

Your insurance coverage can range from nothing at all to full coverage for diagnostic tests and treatments, including IUIs and IVF. Unfortunately, no coverage is much more common than complete coverage. And when coverage is offered, specific restrictions and limitations usually apply.

Unless you are fully covered for infertility treatment, your diagnosis will be key to determining whether or not your insurance will help you pay for the procedures you need. Each diagnosis is given an insurance code, as is each procedure. The insurer determines whether you are covered by linking the code for the procedure to the code for the diagnosis. For example, an ultrasound done for someone who is pregnant will be linked to a different code than an ultrasound done for someone who has been diagnosed with infertility. If you have an ultrasound for an IUI, but your plan doesn't cover infertility, your ultrasound won't be covered. If you're pregnant and your plan covers maternity benefits, the ultrasound will be covered.

When infertility treatment is covered, ultrasounds, tests, and other procedures connected to treatment are usually covered. When treatment is not covered, you must generally pay for these procedures out of pocket, unless there is a possibility that you can document that the tests and procedures you need are being done for a reason unrelated to infertility. Endometriosis, polyps, and fibroids are excellent examples of medical issues that may or may not be associated with treatment for infertility. Your doctor can help you by documenting your care in detail, including documenting what was found at your procedures.

Having more than one diagnostic code may allow your insurer to repay your claim rather than denying you flatly for infertility care. You may have to work with your insurance company to make them see this. Most employees of insurance companies are not trained to understand the fine details of various medical diagnoses and treatment. The person to whom you are speaking may not understand the difference in the diagnoses, but it is possible to make a good case that the treatment was not done to treat infertility but for other medical reasons.

While it sounds like your doctor's office should be able to fudge the codes or lie to help you get insurance, a reputable clinic will not do this. But you should ask your doctor's office for the insurance code for your diagnosis or diagnoses. When you supply the insurer with the codes, you, your insurer, and your doctor's office will all be on the same page, talking about and referring to the same procedure. Ultimately, your goal is to make sure that there are no surprises. There is no advantage to being misled by having an insurer tell you that you are covered for a procedure when you aren't, because down the line you may get a bill for that procedure, which may be quite expensive.

You should also be aware that if your insurance excludes coverage for infertility and you seek treatment from a reproductive endocrinologist—who, of course, focuses on the treatment of infertility—any test or procedure that you have done through that office may be construed as infertility treatment and therefore be denied. If you have not yet started treatment, you may want to factor in the possibility of seeing your ob-gyn for some services when strategizing your plan for care.

> *Money is always well spent on initial evaluations, because you can get an answer. Then your question is, how do you solve the problem? What's involved? If it's IVF and more intricate infertility techniques, services that are in the thousands of dollars, you and your partner should discuss this upfront and decide what you are going to do. Feelings about incurring debt add to the emotional stress and the grief of not conceiving.* —ANN

Consider Whether Your Regular Ob-Gyn Can Help

If you live in a state that mandates coverage for medically correctable causes of infertility (see page 348), it certainly behooves you to go to a specialist for treatment, but when you don't live in such a state, and when your healthcare plan excludes infertility, you may want to be selective about when you actually see the RE. Your general ob-gyn may be able to stretch your coverage further prior to or in conjunction with your RE visits. For example, could you save money by getting a regular sonogram through your ob-gyn? Can your husband do a semen analysis at his regular doctor? Asking these questions may save you some money, if your insurer covers these routine tests when done outside the context of infertility treatment.

Know What Type of Plan You Have

Most people are insured through their employers. In many cases, employers offer a variety of plan options. Before starting care, find out:

- The type of health insurance plan you have. Are you in an HMO, a PPO, or a fee-for-service (indemnity) plan? (See below.)
- If your infertility doctor accepts your insurance. This is crucial. Some offices may accept only very limited types of insurance.
- If there is an enrollment period when you can change plans. Normally, the open enrollment periods are annual. Keep up to date on them so that you can switch plans if necessary.

HMO (Health Maintenance Organization)

If you are in an HMO, find out if there is a board-certified reproductive endocrinologist within the network. Do you have to be referred to the doctor through your primary care provider? Most likely you will. If you will need special services, such as the care of perinatologist (a doctor who takes care of high-risk pregnancies), find out whether you will have access to this physician. (This may be necessary if you get pregnant with more than twins. We talked about this important risk factor in Chapter 11.) If there isn't a reproductive endocrinologist within a certain mile radius of your home, your plan may have a clause that allows you to go out of the network. Find out if this is available. If your insurance doesn't provide for this, there is no coverage for infertility, and you can no longer work with your ob-gyn, you may consider opting out of your HMO, if possible.

PPO (Preferred Provider Organizations)

With a PPO, you may have more flexibility in choosing your provider, paying less to see doctors who are within your network, but retaining the option to go out of the network by paying more.

Fee-for-Service Plans (also called Indemnity Plans)

These are traditional arrangements where the patient pays the provider for each service and then submits a claim, or the provider submits the claim, for reimbursement. You can choose any hospital or physician you like.

Self-Insured Plans

Many people are in self-insured plans in which the employer owns and manages its insurance company. The company gives the insurer a certain amount of money each month out of which claims are paid. If you are in such a plan, you should know that these plans are *exempt* from state mandates to cover or offer infertility services. (See page 348.) There may be an upside to self-insured plans, however. Your company can tell the insurer to cover services even when they are not designated, because the company has the power to determine what will or won't be covered. In the next section, you will learn how your employer can help you to get coverage, if the employer is willing.

Prescription Plans

Whenever possible, make sure you have a prescription plan. Fertility drugs are expensive, particularly injectable FSH. Buying a prescription plan is well worth the price in most instances.

Ask If Your Employer Can Help

We may not always think of our employer as being able to advocate for us. But if you get your insurance through work, your employer is the customer, and the customer, in this instance, has a lot of clout. If you are willing to talk to Human Resources, you can go to the head of the department and ask if they will offer you an infertility rider. The information you give the HR department must be kept strictly confidential. You may have to pay for the rider, which may be more cost effective than paying out of pocket yourself.

Your medical practice can also initiate this. The doctor's office cannot and should not identify you to the company. They cannot provide your name, but the insurance counselor or head of the billing department can call Human Resources and tell them that they have a patient or, as is sometimes the case, a group of patients who work for their company. The billing head can then advocate for you by asking whether or not the company would consider adding an infertility rider. If you work for a large company, this may be a win-win situation for the employees and the company. The company is not paying any more money—because they don't pick up the costs—but they are offering a desired service to their employees, who very much want it and are willing to pay for it. Even smaller companies may be sympathetic. Each year your employer makes a decision about what will and will not be covered. If you are willing to talk to your employer—and not everyone is—you may be able to get the coverage you need.

There is power in numbers. Many women understand the pain of not being able to conceive easily, and many know someone who went through infertility. Gathering a group of people to go to HR and ask for infertility coverage can make a difference.

Make Sure Your Premiums Are Current

Many people are afraid that if they change plans, they will be seen as having a preexisting condition and be denied coverage. This should not happen if you do not let your insurance lapse. But a gap in coverage could cause problems, especially if you fail to pay your premiums on time. This is most likely to happen when you are receiving benefits through COBRA. Make sure that you keep your premiums current and don't let your coverage lapse when changing insurers.

Contact Your Insurer

Before you pick up the phone to call your insurer, get out a notebook. Write down the date you called, the name of the person to whom you spoke (try to get a last name if you can), the question you asked, and the answer. This will help you, if you later get a written denial. You are starting a paper trial trail of who said what when. If you can e-mail your questions, that's even better. Print out your e-mails and save them.

When you call the insurer, you are most likely going to reach someone in a pool of people trained to read your benefits to you. As suggested previously, this person may tell you that you are covered when you are not. For instance, if you say you are having an office visit, sonograms, and blood work, you may be erroneously told that you are covered for these procedures even when your insurance does not cover infertility services. You may get different opinions, because one person answering the phones may interpret your benefits differently than the next person in the pool. If the person working for the insurance company tells you that you are covered, don't take a verbal affirmative as the final response. Ask to be faxed a letter stating that you are covered. A letter of predetermination can help, but these letters often contain disclaimers stating that the authorization number does not necessarily guarantee that you are indeed covered. Still, a letter is another valuable document in your paper trail.

If you can't get a faxed letter from the person to whom you speak, ask to talk to the supervisor. Sometimes that person may not know the real answer to your question either, but may take enough of an interest to investigate the question for you. It's always good to have someone on your side. A little courtesy and knowledge about your care and treatment can go a long way. Knowing your diagnosis codes and the names of the procedures you are planning to have will help you communicate with the insurer.

Sometimes people are given a lifetime maximum benefit for infertility. Problems can arise when the insurer doesn't let the patient know when her benefit is running out. Many times doctor's offices won't know when benefits are set to expire, either. You may have to call or write your insurer for the answer. The same principles apply. Try to get an answer in writing.

DOES YOUR STATE MANDATE INFERTILITY CARE? OR: MOVE TO MASSACHUSETTS

In most states, insurers are not required to provide or to offer insurance for infertility treatment. At the time of this writing, only Arkansas, Hawaii, Illinois, Louisiana, Maryland, Massachusetts, Montana, New Jersey, New York, Ohio, Rhode Island, and West Virginia require insurers to provide coverage for infertility.

Mandates are not always what they appear to be. My own state of New York has a mandate that excludes the most important treatment for infertility—IVF. If you have no fallopian tubes, or blocked fallopian tubes, or you have a very low sperm count, and you live in New York, you really don't have mandated coverage. The New York state legislators who crafted this language came up with a law that appears to be what it is not, rather like the use of the term "peacekeepers" to describe rifles. The New York law is worded deceptively, because of very heavy lobbying by the Catholic interest group the New York State Catholic Conference. Some states have gotten around religious objections to IVF by inserting conscious clauses that allow religious institutions to avoid paying for something that is against their ethical directives. But in this instance, this conscious clause has been extended to everyone else.

But mandates can be good, such as those of Massachusetts and Illinois, which offer wide coverage. Mandates may or may not apply to HMOs, depending on the state. While some so-called mandates exclude IVF, some may cover IVF only after certain conditions are met. Some mandates may limit the number of cycles you can try or put a lifetime cap on benefits. In some states, the law mandating coverage only applies to employers of a certain size, such as twenty-five or even fifty or more.

As suggested, Massachusetts has the broadest language, requiring insurers to cover diagnosis and treatment of infertility. The generous coverage of infertility in this state has prompted some couples to move to Massachusetts to get the care they need. Because I practice in New York, I have personally known patients who have done just that.

Always find out what terms and conditions must be met before coverage for the service you need applies. Must you have failed with a certain number of IUIs to be eligible for coverage for IVF? Are there restrictions on age? What other conditions must be met before you will be covered? To find out what insurers must cover in your state, contact RESOLVE (see Resources), your state insurance commissioner (listed in the white pages of your local phone book or on the Web), or ask your IVF program for guidance.

DEALING WITH DENIALS

As most people can attest, there are some insurance companies that actively resist paying for any care for any condition. If you feel that you have been unfairly denied coverage, contact your insurer and ask for the address of the grievance department so that you can write a letter describing why you think your claim should be paid. Find out exactly how grievances are submitted and follow the procedure to the letter.

When writing, it's not enough to say that the claim should be paid because you pay a lot of money for insurance. You must show the insurer where it made a mistake. Legitimate grievances include having a medical emergency, since medical emergencies are covered under your plan, and knowing that the insurer paid for other claims for the same procedure under the same diagnosis.

If your problem doesn't neatly fit into either of these categories, just be sure to provide a concrete, logical reason why you think the claim should not be denied. Always send the letter "return receipt requested" so that the insurer cannot claim that it did not receive it, and be sure to file the grievance within the time period for filing grievances. If you're late, the insurer can ignore your request. Remember that insurers can make mistakes. You may be surprised how effective self-advocacy can be.

When You Are Still Having Trouble: The State Department of Insurance

When you believe that you have been denied benefits unfairly, or when you can't get a straight answer from your insurer about your benefits, your state insurance commission can be a major source of assistance. (The department may also be called the Department of Insurance or the State Insurance Fund.) If you have done everything you could to get an answer from your insurer, writing a letter to your state insurance commission can get action. In your letter, specify to whom you spoke in the insurance company and in your Human Resources department, if applicable. Specify the nature of the problem and the answers you got from the insurer. The state insurance commission can then send a letter of investigation. Documentation can help support your claim. You can find the address and phone number of your state insurance commission in the front section of your white pages or on the state commission's Web site, if there is one. While on the Web site, you may also find more valuable information about insurance laws in your state and the appropriate government regulatory agency for the type of health plan you have. The state may have an ombudsman service you can call for information.

KEEP TRACK OF YOUR DOCUMENTS

Knowing your medical history, exactly what was done when, by whom, and with what results, can help you communicate more effectively with your doctor, your insurer, and can help you really understand your health care. You will absolutely need these documents if you are disputing a claim or trying to sort out problems with the insurer.

You have a legal right to your medical records. A doctor's office or hospital cannot deny you access to your records, but they can charge for copies. A doctor who stands in the way of your access is behaving inappropriately. If this describes your doctor, you may want to think twice about continuing as a patient. To get a copy of your records, put your request in writing. Most likely, you will have to make a request from each doctor you have seen, but when you do this you will have a complete record of your medical history to keep for yourself.

MEDICAL LOANS AND SHARED RISK PROGRAMS

We know that medical expenses are the number-one cause of bankruptcy in the United States. Although the expenses that lead to bankruptcy are usually due to catastrophic illness, infertility patients often succumb to the temptation to use every resource at their disposal to get pregnant.

While this is understandable, you may want to remind yourself of the danger of spending beyond what you can really handle in the long run.

Unfortunately, some IVF programs offer incentives to patients who can't afford treatment. These medical loans or shared risk programs usually help the IVF program a lot more than they do the patient.

> *I've heard of couples taking out second mortgages on their home, spending their entire retirement savings, doing all sorts of fiscally irresponsible things, because they so desperately want to have a child. I am happy that my fertility benefit was a lifetime benefit. Once it was spent, it was done. It made me stop. But I can see how people get into a lot of trouble when they don't have a financial limit.* —LIZ

> *I wouldn't increase my mortgage. When you do that, you're stuck with that payment for the term of the loan. Try to be disciplined.* —MARY

Short-term Loans

Short-term loans are usually due in three to five months. It's worth asking yourself, if you can't pay for services now, how you will pay for them so soon?

Shared Risk Programs

Shared risk programs are among the newest gimmicks to attract young patients to IVF clinics. Qualified couples pay for a set number of IVF cycles and receive a partial or full refund if they don't get pregnant. If a woman gets pregnant early in the program, the clinic wins, taking the fee and thereby earning extra income. If a woman doesn't get pregnant and deliver a baby, the clinic loses money, with the patient getting as much as a 90 percent refund. Sound fair? Well, maybe. But there are often strict criteria for entering the program. A qualified person is someone with a good prognosis, such as young woman likely to have success. You may have to pay for a battery of tests that are not standard, such as immunological tests, and you may be charged more for these tests than for the procedure itself with no refund for these costs. Decisions that are normally your choice, such as how many embryos to put in your uterus, or even whether to use donor eggs, are made by the program to maximize the chance of conception. The clinic benefits, getting cash on the barrel, a young group of captive patients to boost its success rates, and if the patient gets pregnant early on, a much higher fee than the clinic would ordinarily receive, if the patient got pregnant on the first cycle. Although this type of arrangement may appeal to someone without insurance who is frightened that she won't get pregnant on the first or second cycle, the downside is if you do get pregnant on your first or second try, you are spending more money than you normally would, and you may be subjecting yourself to tests you may not need.

Equally troubling are the financial considerations the clinic must make to offer these programs. In order for a clinic to be financially viable, it must win more of these bets than it loses—just like a casino. Logically, more patients have to lose than win by paying more money for treatment than they should. Betting against someone when your respective knowledge and financial interests are unequal is de facto unethical. The American Medical Association has condemned these arrangements and discourages doctors from providing guarantees about medical care.

Less troubling is a model that is similar to but is not in fact a shared risk program. Advanced Reproductive Care, Inc. (ARC), offers packages to infertility patients for a certain number of IVF cycles with a percent refunded if the patient does not deliver a baby after treatment. The difference is that in the ARC program, a bank acts as the intermediary so that the clinic isn't serving as the bank. The people treating you are not reaching into their pockets and giving you money back if treatment doesn't work. As such, the program addresses, but perhaps does not entirely overcome, the ethical problem associated with shared risk programs.

———

Because of the urgent desire most people have for a baby, and the fifty-fifty chance of conceiving even with the most advanced techniques of assisted reproduction, having infertility care can be a little like gambling. You may, as many women and couples can attest, feel yourself being drawn into treatment far past your ability to pay for it. Debt is not easy. Think about what your limits are before you start treatment, even before your first consultation with your doctor. If you are partnered, discuss them as a couple. Set those limits so that you have a place to confer later, when and if you must consider quitting. It can be very painful to wind up without a child—and perhaps with limited or no funds for adoption, if you wanted to choose it—as well as financial hardship. For more information about finances and fertility, among other issues, you might want to look at Elizabeth Swire Falker's *The Infertility Survival Handbook: Everything You Never Thought You'd Need to Know,* published in 2004 by Riverhead Books.

AS WE LOOK TOWARD THE FUTURE OF IVF AND INFER-
tility treatment, it becomes evident that we are moving toward ever-
increasing control over reproduction. In the 1960s, we mastered fertility
through the development of contraception, and it appears that the next
horizon may very well be the mastery of infertility and the breaking of the
barrier of finite female reproductive capacity as we extend a woman's reproductive life past menopause.

FREEZING EGGS WILL REVOLUTIONIZE SOCIETY

By 2010, oocyte (egg) freezing should be an accomplished reality. A woman
who wants to preserve her eggs for future reproduction could have a pro-

cedure similar to egg retrieval for in vitro fertilization (IVF), harvesting, freezing, and banking her eggs. Although the procedure may be as expensive as one cycle of IVF, it could guarantee that a woman who delays childbearing will still be able to have her own biologically related children when she chooses. A woman who wants to have children with her own eggs, but who hasn't found the right mate by the time she is thirty-five, should probably freeze her eggs, if the technology exists. It might be even better to do this by age twenty-five or thirty. Even if technology for oocyte freezing does not come along as early as predicted, a woman who is absolutely sure that she doesn't want to use donor eggs or adopt a child can get donor sperm, create embryos with that sperm, and freeze those embryos. If she later meets the right person with whom to start a family and gets pregnant without assistance, she could donate the embryos to another couple, donate them to medical research, or have them destroyed.

When women can freeze their eggs with reliability and efficacy early in their adulthood for use later on, we will undoubtedly see dramatic social changes. Today, a woman faces a difficult choice between using her most fertile years to give birth and mother children or using that same youthful time to make headway in her career, which can equate with greater income and security. Right now women are penalized either way, sacrificing fertility when the focus is career or giving up advancements in career, having to start on the ground floor in the workplace when her children are more independent. When women are no longer forced to make this choice, we will certainly see people becoming parents much later in life. Women will not have to concentrate on finding a mate before their fertility declines, and many parents will be in a much better position to help their children with more income and savings for school, living in better homes, and possibly better school districts. And when parents no longer have to divide their energies between climbing the proverbial slippery pole to economic success, they will, as later-life parents, have more time to devote to their children's needs.

It may go without saying that when women are able to compete unfettered by the ticking biological clock, we will see a lot more women in positions of power. Hopefully, some of them will be the CEOs of health insurance companies. All of these changes fit nicely into the tremendous increase in life expectancy we have experienced since the beginning of the last century. Today, a woman who is seventy years old is more like a woman of fifty in the past. More couples are having children later in life, with both men and women putting off having children, or creating new families in new relationships in the second half of life.

In the future, the use of donor eggs may be reserved mostly for people who choose not to use their own eggs because of a genetic disorder. It's almost certain that oocyte freezing will make it possible for egg donors to be tested, have their eggs quarantined, and then be retested for health issues before the release of their eggs, just the way sperm donors are tested now.

WE WILL GET THE EMBRYO RIGHT AND GET THE RIGHT EMBRYO

Today, we look at embryos under a microscope to try to determine which will have the best chance of attaching to the uterine lining and developing into a fetus. But judging an embryo this way is a bit like walking down the street and looking at a person walking the other way. All you know is what that person looks like. But if you could extract that person's genes, draw his or her blood, and check metabolism, you would know a lot more. In the future there will be ways to find out if that embryo is viable and healthy by measuring markers in and around the embryo in the laboratory. When this happens, we will be able to select the embryo that has the very best chance of implanting and transfer only that one embryo, eliminating the chance of multiple pregnancy.

The patient with a good prognosis who today just has to do IVF often enough until it works will probably only have to do IVF once or twice, because she will have chosen the right embryos. Women who will never make viable embryos know this right away, saving themselves repeated unsuccessful IVF attempts, with all the emotional and financial loss that this entails. And for all we know, there may be a small population of women for whom the problem is not the embryo, but the uterus. We may only discover these women have uterine problems when we put in the right embryos but get the wrong result—failure. Even further down the line, there may be a way for young women who freeze their embryos to make sure they are freezing good embryos so that fifteen to twenty years later when they want to become parents, they can.

UTERINE RECEPTIVITY: DISCOVERING A RIGHT TIME TO IMPLANT?

Purportedly, there are markers that tell us when the uterus is most receptive to implantation. One of the most well known of these markers is something called integrin beta. The lack of this protein is associated with the absence of implantation. It seems to be missing in many women who have unexplained infertility and in women with endometriosis. Treatment—for example, removing endometriosis—is associated with greater likelihood of implantation. But this appears to be more important for women who are not being treated with IVF. Because the uterine lining is exposed to high levels of hormones during ovarian stimulation, IVF seems to overcome this type of implantation problem. Other markers for uterine receptivity have been described. These are at best of theoretical importance, but in my experience not of proven clinical significance.

The bottom line is that there are probably factors in the uterus that allow or prevent implantation. We don't know enough about them now, but in the future, we will.

BEYOND IVF: IVM (IN VITRO MATURATION) AND OVARIAN TISSUE BANKING

Oocytes (eggs) sit in the ovary in a very immature state. When you take injectable FSH, those eggs ripen and mature and can be used to create embryos. But imagine if you didn't have to take fertility drugs to get mature eggs for fertilization. What if we could grow oocytes to maturity with efficiency in the laboratory? This is the next step in the evolution of ART. Eggs put into media culture in vitro grow spontaneously, but the reproductive potential of those oocytes is still very low. Right now, researchers are working on ways to retrieve the immature eggs of women with polycystic ovarian syndrome without having to put women through ovarian stimulation. The aim is to grow those oocytes to maturity in the lab without damage to the eggs. If this technique, called *in vitro maturation* (IVM), is successful, and it is likely to be, women may not have to go through ovarian stimulation, repeated blood tests, and numerous sonograms to get pregnant with IVF.

Once we can grow oocytes in vitro without damage to their reproductive potential, reliable ovarian tissue freezing will be in the offing. Currently, scientists are freezing ovarian tissue to give women who go through early menopause as the result of chemotherapy a chance to have children with their own eggs when chemotherapy is over. Although it is being done without definable success today, in the future an ovary or piece of ovary could be removed through a relatively noninvasive surgery called laparoscopy. When replaced or grafted back under the skin, the ovary or part of the ovary will function as it did before, releasing hormones and preventing menopause. Just as the use of donor eggs helped women with genetic disorders in the past, eventually reaching the larger population, ovarian tissue freezing and banking could prolong reproductive life for women in the mainstream.

REPRODUCTION WITHOUT SPERM?

While it seems as if we have done everything we can to assist male fertility, there may be more advances ahead. ICSI allows men who have sperm found only at testicular biopsy to become fathers. But will there be a way to help men with absolutely no sperm cells at all at any stage of development? Could we take another type of cell from a man and prompt it to divide as a gamete does, halving its forty-six chromosomes to twenty-three? Could we then fuse that cell with an egg to produce offspring? Some researchers are looking at this possibility.

Very far off in the future, we may find an agent that turns sperm production on and off without affecting the testicle itself. Theoretically, this agent could be taken by injection or perhaps even be orally active in pill form.

It may be impossible, but it's not unthinkable, that we could one day convert eggs into cells that have the genetic potential of a sperm cell. Although this is highly theoretical, this may mean that we could create an embryo from two women's eggs. In their very early stages, eggs go through what's called parthenogenesis, where the cell divides on it own, sometimes up to a four-cell stage. To some degree, it's possible that conversion could take place at this very early stage. Were this ever to be a reality, it would have tremendous consequences for lesbian couples.

REPRODUCTION ON DEMAND AND WHAT IT MEANS FOR THE FUTURE

Today, couples can choose the gender of their offspring by using a technology developed to identify genetic disorders in the embryo, a technique called preimplantation genetic diagnosis (PGD). And although the use of PGD for sex selection is banned in the UK, it turns out that many infertility patients in the United States would consider using PGD to choose their child's gender, if it were offered without charge.[1]

As we gain more knowledge about the human genome, the possibilities of PGD will magnify, allowing us to identify more genetic disorders and traits than we can at present. But as we learn more, will this technology also permit us to select embryos for cosmetic reasons, such as height, hair color, eye color, or bone structure?

At the same time that we are improving our understanding of the human genome, we are learning how to select the right embryo at the right time for implantation. In the future, the chance of getting pregnant on the first try with IVF will increase, at least in theory, to about 90 percent or more in certain patients. Few people will need repeated cycles of IVF to get pregnant and fewer reproductive endocrinologists will be needed in the field. Doctors may concentrate more on optimizing patients' conditions for IVF, such as taking out fibroids or blocked fallopian tubes. Reproduction on demand could become a reality. When this happens, we will be forced to confront questions about the effect of the use of these technologies and their impact on society.

Most likely, people will always want to have children in the usual way, finding a partner, getting married or forming a union, having sex, getting pregnant, and giving birth. But when some members of the population, conceivably affluent people, are able to use IVF to give their children a kind of "edge," will we think of the use of these technologies as being based in inequality? It is possible that clinics will begin taking care of people who don't have infertility but who just want, for lack of a better word, eugenics? Will clinics compete not only on the basis of services offered, but also on the basis of the quality of the "product" they can help create? Will doctors feel that they have the right to deny parents choice in their child's characteristics, if the choice is possible and in demand?

If PGD can be expanded to detect more disorders than at the present, how will we begin to think of people with what we might term as disabilities? We can certainly say there are some disorders and diseases that are so burdensome and so limiting to the quality of life as to be undesirable, but some conditions affect quality of life only debatably. Is deafness, for instance, something to be avoided? Many in the hearing-impaired community would protest. Who are we to say that those with hearing impairments don't have a terrific quality of life or that their lives are worth less than other people's lives? One of the problems with trying to control the physical characteristics of human beings is that when we say something is good, we imply its opposite is bad, bringing us back to the question of how we handle difference in our society. And who is to say that what we prize aesthetically is healthy or useful? We like tall, willowy people in this culture, but such people are likely to suffer bone fractures that are more severe than those experienced by short, squat people. Is there a risk in deliberately choosing tallness for future generations?

When we can deliberately choose the type of children we want, how can we make sure that we will make the best choice? Will we destroy diversity or will we create more diversity as we exercise individual autonomy?

Almost ten years ago, Peter Kramer raised similar questions in his book *Listening to Prozac*. One might argue that if all people are more functional and happier on SSRI drugs, shouldn't everyone be on these drugs? If the most productive people in our culture are a bit hypomanic—somewhere between manic and normal—should we develop a pill to make us all hypomanic, or should we try to even everyone out?

We don't have to confront these issues in reproductive endocrinology today, but these realties are not far off. While legislating against medical procedures may not be the solution, open discussion of how we determine what we value may help us negotiate the muddy ethical waters of the future. Or perhaps the way to look at this is with a certain sense of libertarianism and scientific fundamentalism, allowing that if something is going to happen, we ought to let it happen and call it evolution.

BUT WILL THE COST OF TREATMENT STAY THE SAME?

No matter how some things change, some things stay the same. As assisted reproduction becomes less invasive, with less need for drugs and egg retrieval, one would imagine that the use of new technologies would make assisted reproduction more widespread, more user friendly, and perhaps less expensive. While the future will afford us more control over reproduction, the cost is unlikely to come down. There is historical precedent here. When angioplasty began to replace coronary bypass surgery, people expected to see the cost of treatment fall. It didn't. One of the reasons is that we simply replaced a procedure that was extremely expensive with a procedure that was only slightly less pricey. The upside is that as IVF technology becomes more efficient, success will virtually be guaranteed. Paying from $10,000 to $15,000 for an IVF cycle that is less invasive and that will almost certainly produce a baby is likely to be much more attractive than paying the same amount for a potentially rigorous process with fifty-fifty chance of having a child, which is the state of the art today.

Another reason why the cost of IVF won't be cheaper may have to do with the tenuous condition of health care in the United States. Inevitably, the current system of private insurance will collapse. It's too expensive, its focus is too far from patient care, and it leaves too many patients uncovered to be viable. If we do have a single payer system, the equivalent of Canada's National Health, infertility care is likely to be low on the list of covered services, unless women make a concerted political effort to highlight the need for services, much in the same way that women advocated for breast cancer research. On the other hand, advances in technology may so profoundly affect women's lives that women will be able to strike a compromise about the availability of care and the extension of coverage for care for many more people than at the present.

PROLONGING YOUR PRODUCTIVE LIFE *AND* YOUR REPRODUCTIVE LIFE

Society is always changing, and one of the major changes we witnessed during the course of the twentieth century is the increase in life span and the decrease in the risks associated with pregnancy and childbirth. Along with this change has come an improvement in the quality of life that extends through many more decades than ever before. When Social Security was first introduced, people were considered old at sixty-five and were expected to leave the workforce. Now people are active and very productive in the workplace far past that age. A woman who is seventy-five years old today is more like someone who was fifty-five years old in the past.

These changes have major implications for women who in their prime reproductive years have traditionally had to choose between starting a family and developing a career path early in adulthood when opportunities are highest. With the perfecting of oocyte freezing in the near future, women are on the cusp of being able to reliably choose motherhood *and* career, a development that will have a profound impact on society. Here is where these changes may afford us the possibility to leverage coverage for treatment. We know that natural reproduction, that is, conception without any medical intervention, is uncommon after forty-four. Could we use that age as a cutoff point for reimbursement for infertility treatment for both men and women in exchange for universal coverage for infertility, including IVF? Connecticut recently enacted an IVF mandate that is limited to women under forty. While affording more women the opportunity to compete in the workplace without forgoing motherhood, universal coverage will allow people to have IVF with single embryo transfers as many times as necessary to get pregnant—but with a single fetus. When we take away the need and incentive to put back multiple embryos, we reduce the risks of multiple pregnancy, including medical risks to the mother and the risk of having children with severe disabilities, saving enormous medical costs in the long-run.

I had been an empty nester for a while when I remarried. We made a decision to have children, and it seemed like a very natural process. Having had the opportunity to retire eight days before they were born was a whole new experience in parenting. Before, I was like everybody else, out there making a living, hustling. When I came home, I was exhausted. I may have helped my wife get the kids to bed, and I would hear what my children had accomplished during the day, but now I'm here to see it for myself. I'm here for everything. —MURRAY

My family was always supportive of my having children later in life. But when we meet people in the store or at school, they look at us twice. We always get, "Oh, you're out with the grandchildren." We were in a restaurant and the couple next to us said, "We just got rid of our grandchildren. How much longer do you have them?" and my husband looked at them and said, "The rest of our lives. They're ours. There's no one to give them back to." —DENISE

THE UNCERTAINTY OF PARENTHOOD

As a parent myself, I know, as we all inevitably learn, that being a parent is a very uncertain thing. This wasn't at all obvious to me until I had my children. We can't control who our children are, nor can we control what happens to them. Children can get sick or get into accidents, which sometimes change them dramatically. Although we don't always think this way when planning to have children, it behooves us to remember that it is not fair to punish children for not turning out as we hoped. This doesn't mean that we don't want to do everything that we can to give our children the best advantages. But at the risk of being flippant, just because a woman uses Viking sperm from a Scandinavian graduate student doesn't mean that her children will be above average height, of above average intelligence, or even that they will have athletic ability. As human beings, we tend not to reject our children, but I do worry that being able to choose the characteristics of our children will cause us to expect too much of those we love. We should never forget that parenting is an act of love and commitment and that it is our children who teach us how to be better human beings, not only the other way around.

Resources

General Support and Information

American Fertility Association
Toll free: 888-917-3777
http://www.theafa.org
E-mail: info@theafa.org

Centers for Disease Control and Prevention
Division of Reproductive Health
770-488-5200
http://www.cdc.gov/ART/index.htm
E-mail: ccdinfo@cdc.gov

International Council on Infertility Information
    Dissemination (INCIID)
703-379-9178
http://www.inciid.org
E-mail: inciidinfo@inciid.org

National Infertility Network Exchange (NINE)
516-794-5772
http://www.nine-infertility.org
E-mail: info@nine-infertility.org

RESOLVE: The National Infertility Association
Business office: 301-652-8585
Toll-free Helpline: 888-623-0744
http://www.resolve.org
E-mail: info@resolve.org

Single Mothers By Choice
212-988-0993
http://mattes.home.pipeline.com
E-mail: mattes@pipeline.com

Acupuncture and Traditional Chinese Medicine
National Certification Commission for Acupuncture and
    Oriental Medicine
11 Canal Center Plaza, Ste. 300
Alexandria, VA 22314
703-548-9004
http://www.nccaom.org
E-mail: info@nccaom.org

Adoption

Adoptive Families
646-366-0830
http://www.adoptivefamilies.com
E-mail: letters@adoptivefamilies.com

National Adoption Information Clearinghouse
703-352-3488 or 888-251-0075
http://naic.acf.hhs.gov
E-mail: naic@caliber.com

National Council For Adoption
703-299-6633
http://ncfa-usa.org
E-mail: ncfa@adoptioncouncil.org

Complementary and Alternative Medicine

NCCAM Clearinghouse
Toll free in U.S.: 888-644-6226
International: 301-519-3153; TTY: 1-866-464-3615
Live chat line: M–F 8:30 a.m. to 5:00 p.m. ET
http://www.nccam.nih.gov
E-mail: info@nccam.nih.gov

Drug Companies

Ferring Pharmaceuticals
Customer Service Line: 888-FERRING
http://www.ferringusa.com/

Organon USA
Customer Service: 800-241-8812
973-325-4500
http://www.organon-usa.com

Serono, Inc.
Toll free: 800-283-8088
http://www.serono.com

Genetic Testing

GeneTests
206-616-4033
http://www.genetests.org/
E-mail: genetests@genetests.org.

Legal Rights

National Center for Lesbian Rights (NCLR)
415-392-6257
http://www.nclrights.org
E-mail: info@nclrights.org

Medical Research Online

Medline Plus
http://medlineplus.gov

PubMed
National Library of Medicine
http://www.ncbi.nlm.nih.gov/entrez/query.fcgi
(Or type "PubMed" into your search engine window.)

Parents of Multiples

Mothers of Supertwins
631-859-1110
http://www.mostonline.org
E-mail: info@MOSTonline.org

Multiple Births Canada
705-429-0901
http://www.multiplebirthscanada.org
E-mail: office@multiplebirthscanada.org

The Triplet Connection
435-851-1105
http://www.tripletconnection.org
E-mail available through the Web site.

Professional Organizations
American Academy of Pediatrics
847-434-4000
http://www.aap.org/
E-mail addresses available on the Web site.

American College of Obstetricians and Gynecologists (ACOG)
202-638-5577
To order publications: 202-863-2518 or resources@acog.org
http://www.acog.org

American Médical Association
800-621-8335
http://www.ama-assn.org

American Society for Reproductive Medicine (ASRM)
205-978-5000
http://www.asrm.org
E-mail: asrm@asrm.org

Society for Assisted Reproductive Technology (SART)
205-978-5000 ext. 109
http://www.sart.org

Society for Maternal-Fetal Medicine
202-863-2476
http://www.smfm.org/
E-mail: smfm@smfm.org

Society for Reproductive Endocrinology & Infertility
http://www.socrei.org

Society of Reproductive Surgeons
205-978-5000 ext. 118
http://www.reprodsurgery.org
E-mail: asrm@asrm.org

Find a Urologist

Society for Male Reproduction and Urology (SMRU)
205-978-5000
http://www.smru.org
E-mail: asrm@asrm.org

Society for the Study of Male Reproduction
847-517-7225
http://www.ssmr.org
E-mail: info@ssmr.org

Third-Party Reproduction

American Association of Tissue Banks
703-827-9582
http://www.aatb.org
E-mail: aatb@aatb.org

Nightlight Christian Adoptions
714-278-1020
E-mail: info@nightlight.org (Indicate which adoption program you are
   interested in on the subject line of your e-mail.)

Surrogate Mothers Online
http://surromomsonline.com
E-mail: info@surromomsonline.com

TASC: The American Surrogacy Center, Inc.
http://www.surrogacy.com

Glossary

Adenomyosis: A condition where glands normally found in the uterine lining occur within the uterine wall.

Adhesions: Scar tissue that forms between surfaces in the body like cobwebs, strings, or ropes.

Amenorrhea: Absence or cessation of menstruation.

Anabolic steroids: Steroids that promote muscle growth.

Androgens: Male hormones that increase muscle mass, hair growth, and other male characteristics.

Aneuploidy: A condition in which one has more or less than the normal number of chromosomes, as in Down syndrome, which is a form of aneuploidy called trisomy.

Antiphospholipid antibody: A common blood clotting disorder associated with both early and late pregnancy loss.

Antisperm antibodies: A condition where the male or female immune system attacks sperm cells.

Antithyroid antibodies: An autoimmune condition, more common in women, where antibodies are directed against the thyroid gland.

ART: Assisted reproductive technology, for example IVF.

Artificial insemination: An older term for inseminations that were usually done vaginally, not through the cervix, as in intrauterine inseminations.

Asherman's syndrome: A condition in which the uterine walls are stuck together due to scarring, often caused by repeated or overly vigorous curetting or scraping of the uterus.

Aspermia: No sperm in the ejaculate.

Aspiration: A technique in which a needle or similar instrument is used to draw out fluid or tissue.

Assisted hatching: A microoperative technique performed on embryos to create a hole in the zona pellucida (shell or covering).

Autoimmune disorder: When one's own immune system attacks tissue from one's own body.

Azoospermia: No sperm in the ejaculate.

Basal body temperature: Your body's resting temperature. Basal body temperature charts are a way of determining your pattern of ovulation by charting your body's resting temperature each day.

Blastocyst: An embryo at day five or six of development.

Bromocriptine (Parlodel): A drug used to treat women who don't ovulate because of high levels of prolactin. Bromocriptine mimics the neurotransmitter dopamine, lowering prolactin levels.

Cerclage: A procedure in which a purse-string suture is put around the cervix to treat an incompetent cervix and potentially avoid pregnancy loss.j376

Cervical mucus: A fluid that plays a key role in escorting sperm from the vaginal canal through the cervix to the uterus, protecting sperm from the vagina's acidic environment.

Cervix: The neck or bottom of the uterus that opens into the uterus at the top of the vagina.

Chlamydia: A common sexually transmitted disease associated with tubal damage.

Chorionic villus sampling (CVS): A test for chromosomal abnormalities and genetic problems at ten to twelve weeks of pregnancy.

Chromosomes: Structures in the nucleus of a cell that contain genetic information.

Cilia (cilium): Tiny hairlike projections in cells that move the cell or move fluid or substances across the surface of the cell.

Clomiphene citrate (Clomid, Serophene): A fertility drug used to stimulate ovulation by fooling the pituitary into making more follicle-stimulating hormone (FSH).

Conception: An old-fashioned term meaning fertilization.

*Cone biopsy (*also called *conization):* A cervical biopsy in which a circular wedge-shaped piece of tissue is taken from the cervix for examination under a microscope.

Congenital bilateral absence of the vas deferens (CBAVD): A condition in which the vas deferens are absent. It is associated with cystic fibrosis and men who carry a mutation of a gene related to cystic fibrosis, called the CFTR gene.

Corpus luteum: The stage of the ovulated follicle at which it becomes a glandular structure that emits estrogen and progesterone during the second phase of your cycle. Literally, "yellow body."

Cryopreservation: Freezing of embryos or gametes such as sperm (or eggs).

Cryosurgery: A procedure to treat cervical dysplasia in which the abnormal tissue is frozen.

Cryptorchidism: Undescended testes.

Cytomegalovirus: A virus spread by human contact that can cause severe disease in people with compromised immune systems. CMV can be passed from a woman to her fetus or new child and is associated with severe birth defects.

Deoxyribonucleic acid (DNA): The material in the chromosomes in the nucleus of the cells responsible for transmitting genetic information.

Dexamethasone: A corticosteroid given in very low doses to treat women who don't ovulate because of elevated adrenal hormones.

Diethylstilbestrol (DES): A synthetic estrogen prescribed to prevent miscarriage until the beginning of the 1970s, when it was linked to high rates of vaginal cancer in daughters of women who took it. Subsequently it was linked to other reproductive disorders in sons and daughters, including fallopian tube abnormalities.

Dilatation and curettage (D&C): A procedure to open the cervix to gently scrape and remove the contents of the uterus.

Distal: The farthest end, such as the portion of the fallopian tube farthest from the uterus.

Dominant follicle: The lead follicle, or the follicle that is chosen to ovulate.

Donor sperm: Sperm provided by a usually anonymous male.

Down syndrome: A condition in which a person has an extra portion of the chromosome number 21 in their cells.

Ectopic pregnancy: A pregnancy that develops outside the uterus, often in the fallopian tube.

Egg retrieval (oocyte retrieval or egg harvesting): The procedure after ovarian stimulation in which your eggs are retrieved for fertilization. Under sterile conditions and under patient sedation, a needle is put through the vaginal wall to the ovary to draw up follicular fluid, which contains eggs, also called oocytes.

Ejaculatory duct obstruction: A rare condition in which the ejaculatory ducts are blocked.

Ejaculatory ducts: A tubular structure that conducts sperm and semen out of the body.

Electrocautery: A method of destroying tissue or sealing off tissue by using heat or electricity.

Embolization: A procedure done by an interventional radiologist in which a catheter is guided via X-ray through a small vessel in the body to open a blockage.

Embryo: A fertilized egg.

Embryologist: A lab technician who performs all aspects of IVF, including oocyte identification, fertilization, embryo culture, cryopreservation, and preparation of the embryo for transfer to the uterus.

Endometrial biopsy: A procedure in which a small sample of endometrial lining is removed to evaluate the endometrium for luteal phase defect or other abnormalities.

Endometrioma: A blood-filled cyst made up of endometrial (uterine) lining.

Endometriosis: A condition in which implants of endometrial tissue grow outside the uterus.

Endometrium: Uterine lining.

Erectile dysfunction: Impotence.

Estradiol: The major form of estrogen made by the ovaries. Estradiol promotes uterine growth and together with progesterone prepares the uterine lining for the implantation of an embryo.

Estrogen: Female hormone produced by the ovaries.

Factor V Leiden: A common gene mutation that may predispose a person to coagulation.

Fallopian tubes: The long tubes that extend from the uterus and open and fan near the ovaries to pick up the ovulated egg, which is then moved toward the uterus.

Fertilization: The fusing of the sperm with the egg.

Fetus: An implanted pregnancy beyond the embryonic stage.

Fibroid: A benign smooth muscle tumor in the uterus also known as leiomyoma or myoma.

Fimbria (pl. fimbriae): The fingerlike ends of the fallopian tube that pick up the egg newly ovulated from the ovary.

Fimbrioplasty: The removal of scar tissue from the fimbriated (or fingerlike) ends of fallopian tubes.

Follicle: Fluid-filled sacs in the ovary that contain the eggs that ripen and ovulate.

Follicle-stimulating hormone (FSH): The pituitary hormone that stimulates the ovary to develop follicles to produce estradiol and mature eggs.

Follicular phase: The phase in your cycle during which the follicle develops and ovulates.

Fundus: The top of the uterus.

Gamete: A germ cell.

Germ cell: An immature sperm cell.

Gonad: Testes or ovaries, the part of the body that produces sex cells, such as eggs or sperm.

Gonadotropin-releasing hormone (GnRH): The hormone secreted by the hypothalamus to stimulate FSH and LH, the hormones that activate sperm and testosterone production in men, and follicle development, ovulation, estradiol, and progesterone production in women.

Gonadotropin-releasing hormone agonist (Lupron, Synarel): An agent that initially causes ovarian stimulation before shutting down FSH and LH production within two weeks.

Gonadotropin-releasing hormone analogs: Drugs that are a modification of the hormone GnRH. They result in suppression of LH and FSH in both men and women. They are used to treat hormone-sensitive conditions such as endometriosis or prostate hypertrophy. They are also used to suppress a woman's LH surge to keep it from interfering with the timing of egg retrieval.

Gonadotropin-releasing hormone antagonist (Antagon, Cetrotide): An agent that quickly shuts down FSH and LH production.

Hamster egg test: An outdated fertility test in which the covering of a hamster's egg is removed to allow for penetration by a human sperm.

Homocysteine: An amino acid. High homocysteine levels have been shown to damage blood vessels.

Hormones: Chemical messengers that are carried through the bloodstream to affect other organs, including the ovaries or testicles.

Human chorionic gonadotropin (hCG) (Novarel, Pregnyl, Profasi): A drug given to emulate your LH surge before planning egg retrieval in an IVF protocol. In pregnancy, the placenta secretes hCG. It is the hormone commonly measured in a pregnancy test.

Hydrosalpinx: An advanced stage of blockage at the fimbriated end of the fallopian tube, resulting in tubal fluid accumulation and swelling.

Hyperthyroidism: Overproduction of thyroid hormone.

Hypospadia: A congenital condition in which the urethra does not reach the tip of the penis.

Hypothalamic amenorrhea: An intrinsic shutdown of FSH and LH usually due to metabolic or psychological stress. Examples of people who may be affected include high-endurance athletes, very thin women, and women with eating disorders.

Hypothalamus: An area at the base of your brain that controls the pituitary and many other body functions, such as appetite.

Hypothyroidism: Underproduction of thyroid hormone.

Hysterectomy: Surgical removal of the uterus.

Hysterosalpingogram (HSG): An X-ray of your uterus and fallopian tubes.

Hysteroscope: A thin telescopic instrument with a light that can be inserted through your vagina and cervix into your uterus to examine your uterine cavity and treat abnormalities.

Implantation: The attachment of the embryo to the uterine lining.

Impotence: Inability to have an erection.

Incompetent cervix: Cervical weakness.

Intracytoplasmic sperm injection (ICSI): A procedure that allows for the injection of a single sperm into an egg to promote fertilization.

Intramuscular injection: Needle injection into the muscle tissue.

Intrauterine device (IUD): A contraceptive device inserted into the uterus.

Intrauterine insemination: A procedure in which purified sperm is slowly infused into the uterus with the intent of achieving fertilization and pregnancy.

Intravenous immunoglobulin therapy (IVIG): Infusion of a blood product that contains antibodies pooled from screened donors' plasma. Usually used to treat people with diseases of immunosuppression, IVIG is a controversial treatment for recurrent pregnancy loss.

In vitro fertilization (IVF): The primary ART procedure in which a woman is usually given fertility drugs to produce more than one egg, which can then be retrieved from her ovary for fertilization with sperm in the laboratory. The fertilized eggs are then placed in her uterus for potential development.

Isthmus: The portion of the fallopian tube near the uterus.

Kallman's syndrome: A rare disorder in which a man's hypothalamus does not produce gonadotropin-releasing hormone (GnRH), the hormone that tells the pituitary to secrete FSH and LH to activate testosterone and sperm production.

Kartagener's syndrome: A defect in the cilia and microtubules that causes sperm to be immotile.

Karyotype: A picture of the chromosomes taken to detect abnormalities.

Klinefelter's syndrome: A condition in which a man inherits an extra X chromosome. Men with Klinefelter's syndrome may have isolated pockets of sperm within their testes.

Laparoscopy: A relatively noninvasive operation to visualize your entire reproductive system to detect the extent of problems, such as tubal damage, endometriosis, or scarring.

Laparotomy: Major surgery in which an incision is made into your abdomen used to treat many problems, including the removal of fibroids (myomectomy) and reversal of tubal ligation (tubal anastomosis).

LEEP (loop electrosurgical excision procedure): A method of treating cervical dysplasia in which a small electrically driven loop is used to remove abnormal cells on the surface of the cervix.

Leiomyoma: See *Fibroid.*

Letrozole: A drug that blocks estrogen synthesis, lowering the amount of estrogen in the body; used to help women with PCOS ovulate.

Leydig cells: Cells in the seminiferous tubules that produce testosterone.

Luteal phase: The phase of your cycle after ovulation, when the corpus luteum pumps out estradiol and progesterone, making your uterine lining secretory and preparing it for implantation of an embryo.

Luteal phase defect: A condition in which a woman either has inadequate progesterone production or her uterine lining does not respond sufficiently to progesterone.

Luteinizing hormone: A hormone secreted by the pituitary that stimulates the ovaries to produce estradiol and that triggers the release of an egg or eggs in ovulation.

Luveris: A manufactured form of luteinizing hormone (LH) that can be used to trigger ovulation.

Maternal fetal medicine specialist (MFM; also called perinatologist): A board-certified obstetrician-gynecologist with two to three additional years of education and clinical experience in the obstetrical medical, surgical, and genetic complications of pregnancy.

Meiosis: Division of reproductive cells that results in halving the number of chromosomes from 46 to 23.

Menopause: The period of a woman's life when her menstrual periods gradually stop completely and reproductive hormone production decreases, usually occurring in the late forties or early fifties. Menopause can also occur when the ovaries are removed or after some chemotherapy treatments that destroy ovarian function.

Menses: Menstruation or uterine bleeding.

Metformin: A drug used to help women with PCOS ovulate by enhancing the action of the insulin.

Microsurgical TESE: A procedure in which a small piece of tissue is taken from the testis to look for sperm that can be used in in vitro fertilization (IVF) with ICSI.

Miscarriage: Loss of a pregnancy before twenty weeks.

Miscarriage, multiple: Repeated pregnancy loss defined as three miscarriages in a row.

Mittelschmerz: Discomfort that some women feel at ovulation when the egg ruptures from the ovary.

Morphology, sperm: Refers to the shape of a sperm.

Mullerian ducts: In a female fetus, the tubes that eventually develop into part of the female reproductive system. The fallopian tubes and uterus develop from the Mullerian ducts.

Multifetal reduction: A procedure in which one or more fetuses are terminated in a pregnancy to attempt to provide better outcomes for the remaining fetuses in higher-order multiple pregnancies.

Myoma: See *Fibroid.*

Myomectomy: A surgical procedure to remove fibroids.

Nonobstructive azoospermia: A condition in which a man produces no sperm due to hormonal problems or problems with sperm production in the testicle.

Nucleus: A structure in a cell that contains DNA and RNA and governs cell reproduction, growth, and metabolism.

Obstructive azoospermia: A condition in which a man produces sperm normally, but a blockage prevents it from leaving the body.

Oligomenorrhea: Infrequent menstruation.

Oligospermia: Few sperm in the ejaculate.

Oocyte (egg): The female gamete.

Ova (eggs, oocytes): Ovum, plural.

Ovarian reserve: The number of follicles and the quality of the eggs that a woman has left in her ovaries. Day three FSH/estradiol tests measure ovarian reserve.

Ovaries: The female reproductive organs that produce ova, or eggs, and estrogen.

Ovulation induction (also called *ovarian stimulation):* The use of fertility drugs to stimulate the development and release of more than one oocyte (egg).

Ovum: Egg.

Pap smear: A test for cervical cancer in which cells are scraped from the cervix and examined under a microscope; also called a *Papanicolaou test.*

Percutaneous epididymal sperm aspiration (PESA): A procedure in which sperm is aspirated from the epididymis, potentially useful for men with obstructive azoospermia.

Perimenopause: The transition into menopause, usually between the ages of forty and fifty.

Perinatologist: An older term for Maternal Fetal Medicine subspecialist.

Peritubal adhesions: Scar tissue that can block fallopian tubes.

Pituitary gland: The "master gland" at the base of the brain at the hypothalamus that secretes a number of hormones, including FSH and LH.

Placenta: An organ that develops during pregnancy to connect the mother's system to the fetus and supply nutrients, oxygen, and other essentials to the fetus and remove wastes.

Polycystic ovarian syndrome (PCOS): A common complex disorder most typically causing lack of ovulation, accumulation of ovarian follicles, hormone imbalances, and which is often associated with insulin resistance and long-term health concerns.

Polyp: A mass (tumor) of glandular tissue in the uterine lining, or endometrium.

Postcoital test (PCT): A simple examination to test cervical mucus-sperm interaction after sexual intercourse.

Prednisone: A corticosteroid given in very low doses to treat anovulation due to elevated adrenal hormones.

Preeclampsia: Pregnancy-induced high blood pressure and other systemic disorders.

Pregnancy loss: Miscarriage; spontaneous abortion; missed abortion.

Preimplantation genetic diagnosis (PGD): A method by which embryos are tested for evidence of a genetic disorder by removing one or two cells (blastomeres or polar bodies).

Premature ovarian failure: Menopause prior to the age of forty.

Premenstrual syndrome (PMS): The time in the second half of a woman's cycle in which progesterone levels rise and in which certain symptoms, such as bloating, cramping, moodiness, food cravings, breast tenderness, and tingling, are present to the point of causing dysfunction.

Progesterone: An ovarian hormone that drives the uterine lining's development to support the early embryo.

Progestins: Synthetic progesterones, often used in birth control pills.

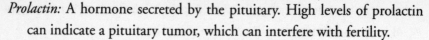

Prolactin: A hormone secreted by the pituitary. High levels of prolactin can indicate a pituitary tumor, which can interfere with fertility.

Prolactinoma: A typically benign pituitary tumor associated with elevated prolactin levels.

Prostaglandins: Hormone-like substances involved in a number of processes that cause the uterus to contract; for example, to shed its lining each month in menstruation.

Prostate gland: A gland that sits beneath the bladder and around the urethra in the male and supplies fluid to sperm on ejaculation.

Prostatitis: An inflammation of the prostate gland.

Recurrent miscarriage: Having three miscarriages in a row.

Reproductive endocrinologist (RE): An ob-gyn with an additional two to three years of approved fellowship training in reproductive endocrinology and infertility.

Retrograde ejaculation (RE): A common disorder in which semen doesn't exit the body on ejaculation but instead flows backward into the bladder.

Retrograde menstruation: A condition in which some of the menstrual flow moves backward through the fallopian tubes and which predisposes one to endometriosis.

Retroverted uterus: A uterus that is tipped toward the spine.

Salpingectomy: Removal of a fallopian tube.

Salpingitis isthmica nodosa (SIN): A severe abnormality of the fallopian tube at the isthmus, which is the portion of the tube near the uterus.

Salpingolysis: A surgical procedure to remove scar tissue from around fallopian tubes.

Salpingostomy: Opening up a blocked fallopian tube.

Scrotum: The exterior sac of skin that holds the testes.

Selective serotonin reuptake inhibitor (SSRI): A class of antidepressant drugs such as Prozac.

Semen analysis: The most important fertility test for men. It analyzes the sperm count and other components of semen.

Semen volume: Measurement of the amount of semen that is produced at ejaculation.

Seminal vesicles: Glands that sit behind the bladder, which contribute most of the fluid that will become semen.

Seminiferous tubules: Microscopic tubules tightly coiled inside the testis in which sperm are formed.

Septate uterus: A condition in which a septum, a wedge of tissue, divides the uterus. The septum does not get blood supply from outside the uterus and therefore a pregnancy that attaches in this area is unlikely to survive.

Sertoli-cell-only syndrome (SCO): A condition in which a man has no spermatocytes (germ cells).

Sertoli cells: Cells within the seminiferous tubules that support sperm development.

Sonogram: Ultrasound.

Speculum: A shoehorn-shaped instrument used to hold the vaginal walls apart.

Sperm: Male gamete or reproductive cell; spermatozoa.

Spermatocyte: Precursor cell to sperm.

Spermatogonium (pl. spermatogonia): Precursor cell to spermatocyte.

Sperm concentration: Sperm count.

Sperm morphology: The shape of the sperm.

Sperm motility: Movement of the sperm.

Sperm washing: A procedure to separate sperm from seminal fluid to isolate pure motile sperm for inseminations.

Spironolactone (Aldactone): A drug used to treat high blood pressure, but which also acts as an antiandrogen (male hormone) and which may help women who are hyperandrogenic to ovulate or to decrease hair growth (hirsuitism).

Tamoxifen (Nolvadex): An antiestrogen that can be used to help women ovulate. Also often used for breast cancer.

Tenaculum: A long-handled clamp used to steady the cervix in instrumentation procedures.

Testicular biopsy: A procedure in which a small piece of testicular tissue is taken to diagnose a number of male fertility problems, including azoospermia (no sperm).

Testicular sperm aspiration (TESA): A procedure in which sperm is drawn from the testis through a fine needle or other instrument.

Testicular sperm extraction (TESE): A surgical procedure in which a man's testis is opened under a microscope and small samples of testicular tissue are taken to look for sperm cells for use in IVF/ICSI.

Testis (pl. testes): Testicle.

Testosterone: The primary male sex hormone, an androgen.

Thyroid gland: An endocrine gland at the base of the neck that produces the hormone thyroxine, regulating growth and metabolism.

Thyroxine: A hormone produced by the thyroid that regulates growth and metabolism.

Tipped uterus: See *Retroverted uterus.*

Transvaginal ultrasound: An ultrasound test done with a vaginal probe to image the ovaries and uterus on a monitor.

Trisomy: A form of aneuploidy in which one has three chromosomes number 21 instead of two, such as with Down syndrome.

Tubal anastomosis (also called tubal reanastomosis): A procedure to reverse a tubal ligation by cutting out the damaged area of a tube and reconnecting the tube, usually involving a laparotomy (surgery through the abdomen).

Tubal catheterization: A procedure to unblock fallopian tubes, used with hysteroscope or hysterosalpingogram.

Tubal ligation: A procedure in which the tubes are cut or tied off to prevent conception.

Tubal pregnancy: A pregnancy that develops inside the fallopian tube, the most common form of ectopic pregnancy.

Turner's syndrome: A condition in females in which one of the two X chromosomes is missing. Also known as gonadal dysgenesis, or 45XO.

Ultrasound (also called sonogram): A painless procedure in which sound waves are used to create outlines of parts of the body visible on a monitor, such as a transvaginal ultrasound.

Undescended testicles: Cryptorchidism; testicles that do not descend during fetal development or infancy.

Urethra: The tube that connects the bladder to the outside of the body.

Urologist: A physician who specializes in treating problems of the urinary tract in men and women and male reproductive organs. Infertility urologists are fellowship-trained in male infertility.

Uterine septum: A wedge of tissue within the uterus.

Uterus: The major female reproductive organ in which a fertilized egg implants, is nourished, and develops into a fetus, growing until childbirth.

Vagina: In the female, the muscular tract leading from the cervix and uterus to the outside of the body.

Varicocele: A varicose vein in the scrotum.

Vas deferens: The long tubes that connect the epididymis to the ejaculatory ducts, carrying sperm from the testicles to the urethra.

Vasectomy: A male birth control method and simple surgery in which the vas deferens is cut, tied, clipped, or cauterized.

Vasectomy reversal: A procedure done to reconnect the vas deferens after a vasectomy.

Vasogram: An X-ray of the vas deferens.

Venography: An X-ray of a vein in which a contrast dye is injected into the vein to make it visible.

Zona pellucida: The protective covering of the egg (ovum).

Zygote: A fertilized egg, before cleavage.

1. Confronting Infertility

1. "Assisted Reproductive Technology Surveillance—United States, 2001," *MMWR* 53/SS01: 1–20 (April 30, 2004).
2. B. T. Ji, et al., "Paternal cigarette smoking and the risk of childhood cancer among offspring of nonsmoking mothers," *Journal of the National Cancer Institute,* 89, no. 3 (1997): 238–44.

2. Reproduction Quick and Easy

1. Baba K., et al., "Where does the embryo implant after embryo transfer in humans?" *Fertility & Sterility* 73, no. 1 (2000): 123–5.
2. A. J. Wilcox, et al., "Timing Sexual Intercourse in Relation to Ovulation: Effects on the probability of conception, survival of the preg-

nancy, and sex of the baby," *New England Journal of Medicine* 333, no. 23 (1995): 1517–21.

3. Get the Right Tests

1. P. J. Meis et al., "Prevention of recurrent preterm delivery by 17 alpha hydroxyprogesterone caproate," *New England Journal of Medicine* 348, no. 24 (2003): 2379–85.

2. A. Barash, et al., "Local injury to the endometrium doubles the incidence of successful pregnancies in patients undergoing in vitro fertilization," *Fertility & Sterility* 79, no. 6 (2003): 1317–22.

4. Get a Good Doctor

1. Society of Reproductive Endocrinology and Infertility (SREI), "Your physician is a member of the Society of Reproductive Endocrinology and Infertility (SREI) . . . What does that mean, and why should you care?" *Pamphlet,* no date. Available at www.socrei.org or by calling The American Society for Reproductive Medicine at 205-978-5000.

2. Practice Committee of the American Society for Reproductive Medicine and the Society for Assisted Reproductive Technology, "Revised minimum standards for practices offering assisted reproductive technologies," *Fertility & Sterility* 82, supp. 1 (2004): S4–S7. Reprinted with permission from the American Society for Reproductive Medicine.

5. Get the Right Treatment: For Women

1. A. Strandell, et al., "Hydrosalpinx and IVF outcome: Cumulative results after salpingectomy in a randomized controlled trial." *Human Reproduction* no. 11 (2001): 2403–10.

2. R. Hart, et al., "A prospective controlled study of the effect of intramural uterine fibroids on the outcome of assisted conception," *Human Reproduction,* no. 11 (2001): 2411–17.

6. Get the Right Treatment: For Men

1. Male Infertility Best Practice Policy Committee of the American Urological Association; Practice Committee of the American Society for Reproductive Medicine, "Report on evaluation of the azoospermic male," *Fertility & Sterility* 82, supp. 1 (2004): S132.

7. Fertility Drugs

1. M. A. Rossing, et al., "Ovarian tumors in a cohort of infertile women," *New England Journal of Medicine* 331, no. 12 (1994): 771–76.

8. Intrauterine Insemination (IUI)

1. L. Bujan, et al., "Insemination with isolated and virologically tested spermatozoa is a safe way for human immunodeficiency type 1 virus-serodiscordant couples with an infected male partner to have a child," *Fertility & Sterility* 82, no. 4 (2004): 857–62.

9. In Vitro Fertilization (IVF)

1. A. Thurin, et al., "Elective single-embryo transfer versus double-embryo transfer in in vitro fertilization," *New England Journal of Medicine* 351, no. 23 (2004): 2392–402.
2. M. Bonduelle, et al., "Prenatal testing in ICSI pregnancies: incidence of chromosomal anomalies in 1586 karyotypes and relation to sperm parameters," *Human Reproduction* 17, no. 10 (2002): 2600–14.

10. Recurrent Pregnancy Loss and Ectopic Pregnancy

1. The Practice Committee of the American Society for Reproductive Medicine, "Early Diagnosis and management of ectopic pregnancy," *Fertility & Sterility* 82, supp. 1 (2004): S147.

11. Multiple Pregnancy and Multifetal Reduction

1. ACOG Committee on Practice Bulletins—Obstetrics, the Society for Maternal Fetal Medicine and ACOG Joint Editorial Committee,

"ACOG Practice Bulletin: Clinical Management Guidelines for Obstetrician-Gynecologists," *Compendium of Selected Publications*, no. 56 (2004): 587.

12. Find Out About Alternatives

1. Susan L. Crockin, J. D., "Legally Speaking: Court Refuses to Recognize Genetic Mom Following Lesbian Partners' Breakup," *American Society for Reproductive Medicine News* 37, no. 3 (2003): 3.
2. Susan L. Crockin, J. D., "Legally Speaking: Dueling Insurance Companies Dispute Coverage for Gestational Carrier and Child," *American Society for Reproductive Medicine News* 37, no. 4 (2003): 4.

13. Acupuncture and Traditional Chinese Medicine for Infertility

1. W. E. Paulus, et al., "Influence of acupuncture on the pregnancy rate in patients who undergo assisted reproduction therapy," *Fertility & Sterility* 77, no. 4 (2002): 721–24.

14. Make Sure You Have Emotional Support

1. Alice D. Domar, Ph.D., *Conquering Infertility* (New York: Viking, 2002), 28.

Conclusion: The Future of Infertility Treatment: What's Next?

1. T. Jain, et al., "Preimplantation sex selection demand and preferences in an infertility population," *Fertility & Sterility* 83, no. 3 (2005): 649–58.

Index

sperm injection; Intrauterine inseminations

Azoospermia, 39
    nonobstructive, 141–44, 229–30
    obstructive, 144–49, 226–32
    pre-testicular, 141–43
    testes-originated, 143–44

Birth control pills, 39
    cervical mucus' relation to, 188
    menstrual cycle regulation with, 87, 167, 168, 204
Birth defects. *See* Genetics
Blastocysts, 210, 211, 317
    developmental stage of, 28
    disorders associated with, 218–19
    IVF transfer of, 75, 216–19
Blood clotting disorders (Thrombophilia), 34, 261
    miscarriage caused by, 256–58

Cancer, 65
    breast, 15
    clomiphene's relation to, 180
    fertility damage due to, 39
    injectable FSH and, 179–80
    IVF's relation to, 225
    ovarian, 180
    pregnancy risks during, 166
CBAVD. *See* Congenital bilateral absence of the vas deferens
Centers for Disease Control, 7, 72, 74, 366
Cervical mucus, 28
    disruptions to, 47, 187–88
    hostile, 46, 188
    interference of, 215
    testing of, 45–47, 55
Cervix, 28, 252–53
Cesarean section (C-section), 87, 275
Chemotherapy, 39, 139
Chorionic villus sampling (CVS), 255, 283
Chromosomal abnormalities, 9. *See also* Genetics
    age's relation to, 38, 222, 224, 238–39
    aneuploidy, 238–39, 248, 254
    ICSI's relation to, 224, 231
    IVF's relation to, 224
    karyotypes for, 34, 143, 238, 254, 260, 261
    miscarriage due to, 254–55, 262
    oligospermia's relation to, 150
Clomiphene Challenge Test, 54
Clomiphene citrate
    alternatives to, 161–62
    cervical mucus disruption by, 47, 187–88

cost of, 198
fertility treatment using, 43–44, 63, 65, 88, 90–91, 104, 149, 158–64, 171, 245
    infertility test using, 54
    IUI treatment with, 162–63
    PCOS treatment with, 90–91, 161
    side effects of, 160, 163–64, 171, 326
Coculture, 245
Congenital bilateral absence of the vas deferens (CBAVD), 144–45, 147–48, 228
Counseling. *See also* Support groups
    adoption, 318
    donor, 295, 307
    ectopic pregnancy, 270
    surrogacy, 314–15
    therapist, 339–40
Cramps, menstrual, 22
Cryopreservation
    developmental stage's relation to, 233, 317
    egg, 355–57
    embryo, 71, 72, 73, 75–77, 233–37, 317
    method of, 236
    ovarian tissue, 359
    problems with, 236
    sperm, 146, 148, 188, 194, 211
    success statistics for, 233–34
Cryotherapy, 187
Cryptorchidism, 55, 144
CVS. *See* Chorionic villus sampling
Cystic fibrosis, 147–48, 240

Day three FSH/estradiol test, 31, 54–55, 63
    overview of, 37–39
    PCOS testing with, 89–90
    post-miscarriage, 34, 262
D&C. *See* Dilatation & curettage
DES. *See* Diethylstilbestrol
Diabetes, 10, 15, 56–57, 262, 275
    PCOS's relation to, 86–87, 90, 92
    retrograde ejaculation's relation to, 152
Diethylstilbestrol (DES), 48, 97, 252, 265
Dilatation & curettage (D&C), 123–24, 252
    unviable pregnancies and, 258, 260–61
Diminished ovarian reserve, 93
Doctors. *See also* Fertility clinics
    changing of, 79–80
    embryology, 80–82, 210
    evaluation of, 78–80
    fertility clinics and, 70–78
    hucksterism by, 67
    laparoscopic, 100–103, 107–8, 130–35
    MFM, 275, 276–77, 282–83